W0227560

Metabolic Syndrome and Complications of Pregnancy

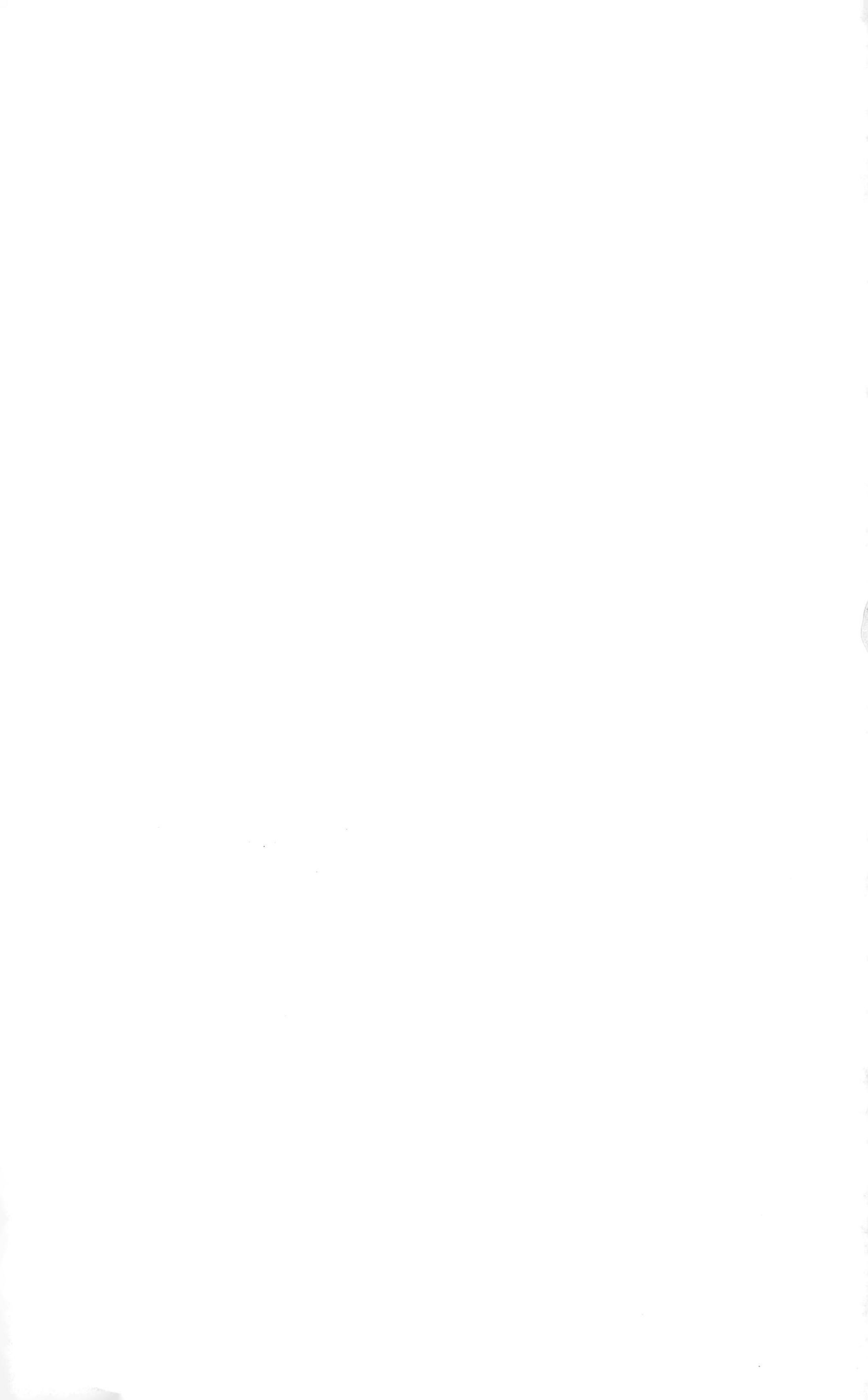

Enrico Ferrazzi • Barry Sears
Editors

Metabolic Syndrome and Complications of Pregnancy

The Potential Preventive Role of Nutrition

Foreword by Roberto Romero

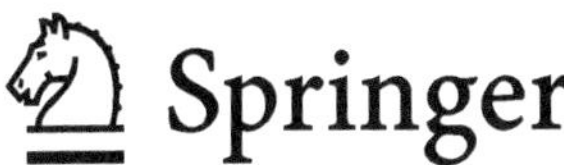

Editors
Enrico Ferrazzi
Woman, Mother and Neonate Department
University of Milan,
Buzzi Children's Hospital
Milan
Italy

Barry Sears
Inflammation Research Foundation
Marblehead, MA
USA

ISBN 978-3-319-16852-4 ISBN 978-3-319-16853-1 (eBook)
DOI 10.1007/978-3-319-16853-1

Library of Congress Control Number: 2015943063

Springer Cham Heidelberg New York Dordrecht London

Printed on acid-free paper

Springer International Publishing AG Switzerland is part of Springer Science+Business Media (www.springer.com)

Foreword

The concept of metabolic syndrome was articulated by Gerald Reaven in 1988 at the Banting Lecture of the American Diabetes Association annual meeting. Reaven proposed that insulin resistance led to hyperglycemia, hyperinsulinemia, hyperlipidemia, central obesity, and hypertension [1]. The term "syndrome X," a *physiologic construct*, was introduced to emphasize the role of insulin resistance in the clustering of the clinical manifestations. Ten years later, after the recognition that this cluster increased the risk for cardiovascular disease, the World Health Organization (WHO) proposed clinical criteria to identify such individuals, and the term *metabolic syndrome* was coined [2, 3]. Fast forward a few years and a large number of publications, scientific societies promoted harmonization of the diagnostic criteria for metabolic syndrome [4]. These include an elevated fasting glucose, elevated triglycerides, low high-density lipoprotein cholesterol (HDL-C), elevated waist circumference, and elevated blood pressure [4]. The diagnosis required 3 of the 5 to be present. The popularity of the subject is beyond dispute (at the time of this writing, there are over 54,000 publications recorded in PubMed). In 2010, Reaven reflected on the evolution of, utility, and insight provided by the term metabolic syndrome [5].

The evolutionary origin of insulin resistance can be attributed to viviparity. The fetus is an obligate parasite, requiring fuel (i.e., glucose and lipids) and nutrients for growth and survival. Relative insulin insensitivity is a transient and normal physiologic adaptation of pregnancy. The mechanisms responsible for the relative insulin resistance of pregnancy are largely attributed to the endocrine milieu, and particularly, placental lactogens. However, recent observations suggest that the gut microbiome of pregnant women may also play a role. The gut microbiota of pregnant women changes dramatically from the first to the third trimester, and when stool from pregnant women in third trimester is administered to germ-free mice, this results in adiposity and insulin resistance [6, 7]. Since microorganisms interact primarily with the host immune system, the observations support a role for a complex interaction among the maternal diet (which can alter the microbiota), the maternal immune system, and the placenta.

However, this process can go awry and have profound short- and long-term implications for mother and child. Gestational diabetes can be viewed as excessive carbohydrate intolerance during pregnancy, which can become maladaptive when there is fetal overgrowth (macrosomia). Metabolic syndrome is a risk factor for preterm delivery [8], preeclampsia [9], and unexplained fetal death [10]. However, the problem does not stop here. Longitudinal studies have shown that the offspring of diabetic mothers who are large for gestational age at birth are more likely to develop metabolic syndrome than those whose birthweight is appropriate for gestational age at birth and born to mothers without gestational diabetes [11, 12]. This also applies to fetuses of obese mothers [13].

What are the implications of this? Prevention in medicine can be primary, secondary, or tertiary. For diabetes, primary prevention could be exercise and weight control to avoid insulin resistance. Secondary prevention is the administration of insulin once carbohydrate intolerance is diagnosed, while tertiary prevention consists of treatment of end-organ damage (i.e., retinopathy). Yet, the most powerful preventive strategy is the one that begins in utero. The compelling role of environmental factors during fetal life in determining health and disease during childhood and in adult life and the opportunities to intervene through maternal nutrition and lifestyle during pregnancy and breastfeeding represent a new frontier in medicine [14].

The publication of *Metabolic Syndrome and Complications of Pregnancy* with an emphasis on the preventive role of nutrition is timely, important, and visionary. Professor Enrico Ferrazzi of the University of Milan, Italy, and Professor Barry Sears of the Inflammation Research Foundation in Massachusetts, USA, have brought together the leading experts in the field and provide a uniquely informed treatise that integrates the current understanding of the importance of diet, inflammation, metabolism, with an emphasis on pregnancy and its outcomes. This important contribution will enrich the reader, promote research and understanding of this fascinating field, and I believe will set the stage for a fundamental reappraisal of the role of diet and nutrition in pregnancy.

Roberto Romero, M.D., D.Med.Sci.
Chief, Perinatology Research Branch,
Program Head for Perinatal Research and Obstetrics,
Intramural Division, *Eunice Kennedy Shriver* NICHD,
NIH, Bethesda, MD and Detroit, MI, USA

Professor of Obstetrics and Gynecology, University of Michigan,
Ann Arbor, MI, USA

Professor of Epidemiology and Biostatistics,
Michigan State University, East Lansing, MI, USA

Professor of Molecular Obstetris and Genetics,
Center for Molecular Medicine, Wayne State University,
Detroit, MI, USA

References

1. Reaven GM. Banting lecture 1988. Role of insulin resistance in human disease. Diabetes. 1988 Dec;37(12):1595–607. Review.
2. Alberti KG, Zimmet PZ. Definition, diagnosis and classification of diabetes mellitus and its complications. Part 1: Diagnosis and classification of diabetes mellitus provisional report of a WHO consultation. Diabet Med. 1998;15:539–53.
3. Expert Panel on Detection, Evaluation, and Treatment of High Blood Cholesterol in Adults. Executive Summary of Third Report of the National Cholesterol Education Program (NCEP) Expert Panel on Detection, Evaluation, and Treatment of High Blood Cholesterol in Adults (Adult Treatment Panel III). JAMA. 2001;285:2486–97.
4. Alberti KG, Eckel RH, Grundy SM, et al. Harmonizing the metabolic syndrome: a Joint Interim Statement of the International Diabetes Federation Task Force on Epidemiology and Prevention; National heart, Lung, and Blood Institute; American Heart Association; World Heart Federation; International Atherosclerosis Society; and International Association for the Study of Obesity. Circulation. 2009;120:1640–5.
5. Reaven GM. The metabolic syndrome: time to get off the merry-go-round? J Intern Med. 2011;269:127–36.
6. Koren O, Goodrich JK, Cullender TC, et al. Host remodeling of the gut microbiome and metabolic changes during pregnancy. Cell. 2012;150:470–80.
7. Romero R, Korzeniewski SJ. Are infants born by elective cesarean delivery without labor at risk for developing immune disorders later in life? Am J Obstet Gynecol. 2013;208(4):243–6. doi: 10.1016/j.ajog.2012.12.026. Epub 2012 Dec 26.
8. Chatzi L, Plana E, Daraki V, Karakosta P, Alegkakis D, Tsatsanis C, Kafatos A, Koutis A, Kogevinas M. Metabolic syndrome in early pregnancy and risk of preterm birth. Am J Epidemiol. 2009;170:829–36.
9. Hooijschuur MC, Ghossein-Doha C, Al-Nasiry S, Spaanderman ME. Maternal metabolic syndrome, preeclampsia and small for gestational age infancy. Am J Obstet Gynecol. 2015. pii: S0002-9378(15)00521-9. doi: 10.1016/j.ajog.2015.05.045. [Epub ahead of print].
10. Yao R, Ananth CV, Park BY, Pereira L, Plante LA; Perinatal Research Consortium. Obesity and the risk of stillbirth: a population-based cohort study. Am J Obstet Gynecol. 2014;210:457.e1–9.
11. Boney CM, Verma A, Tucker R, Vohr BR. Metabolic syndrome in childhood: association with birth weight, maternal obesity, and gestational diabetes mellitus. Pediatrics. 2005;115:e290–6.
12. Moore TR. Fetal exposure to gestational diabetes contributes to subsequent adult metabolic syndrome. Am J Obstet Gynecol. 2010;202:643–9.
13. Catalano PM, Presley L, Minium J, Hauguel-de Mouzon S. Fetuses of obese mothers develop insulin resistance in utero. Diabetes Care. 2009;32:1076–80.
14. Gluckman P, Hanson M, Seng CY, Bardsley A. Nutrition & lifestyle for pregnancy & breastfeeding. Oxford: Oxford University Press; 2015.

Contents

Part I

Truncal Obesity, Inflammation, Metabolic Syndrome: An Insight

The Role of Diet in Inflammation and Metabolic Syndrome

1

Barry Sears

Contents

1.1 Introduction

The human body has developed an extraordinary number of systems to maintain stable blood glucose and to avoid broad swings in its level. These systems include hormones that are directly or indirectly generated by the diet as well as the ability to directly sense dietary nutrients to send appropriate neural signals to the brain

B. Sears, PhD
Inflammation Research Foundation, Marblehead, MA, USA
e-mail: bsears@drsears.com

E. Ferrazzi, B. Sears (eds.), *Metabolic Syndrome and Complications of Pregnancy: The Potential Preventive Role of Nutrition*,
DOI 10.1007/978-3-319-16853-1_1

(specifically the hypothalamus) to orchestrate fuel usage for either oxidation into energy or long-term storage. This metabolic flexibility is crucial for survival and reproduction. The central hormone in this metabolic communication system is insulin.

Insulin is the primary regulator of carbohydrate, fat, and protein metabolism [1–3]. It inhibits lipolysis of stored fat in the adipose tissue, it inhibits gluconeogenesis in the liver, it stimulates the translocation of the GLUT-4 protein to bring glucose into the muscle cells, it stimulates gene expression of proteins required for the optimal cellular function as well as cellular repair and growth, and it indicates the metabolic availability of various fuels to the brain. Therefore keeping insulin within balanced values or "appropriate zone" is critical for our survival.

In the past, access to adequate nutrients was a major concern. Today, we have a new concern: excess nutrient intake. However, even in this regard, insulin also plays a primary role in defending the body against the potential damage due the excess consumption of surplus nutrients using the adipose tissue, liver, and skeletal muscle as biological buffers against excess nutrient intake. This is important since all dietary nutrients are naturally inflammatory because their metabolism into other biological materials or conversion to energy can generate molecular responses that can activate increased inflammation [4]. This means that the intake of excess nutrients sets the foundation for the generation of excess inflammation. In the face of increased inflammation, the ability of insulin to orchestrate metabolism becomes compromised.

1.2 Inflammation

The body's inflammatory response needs to be maintained within a balanced zone. Too limited of an inflammatory response would make us easy targets for microbial invasion, and our physical injuries would never heal. Too strong of an inflammatory response or insufficient resolution of the inflammatory responses will generate chronic inflammatory damage to our organs.

All inflammatory responses ultimately start with the most primitive part of our immune system, the innate immune system that we share with plants. This is why many of the agents that turn on and turn off inflammatory responses can be found in our diet. Furthermore, these nutrients act through gene transcription factors to control the expression of our inflammatory genes. Thus the diet can either be proinflammatory or anti-inflammatory depending on its composition.

To add even further complexity is the fact that there are two separate biochemical phases that control inflammation [5]. The first is the initiation response that starts the inflammatory response. This is the cellular destruction phase normally associated with acute inflammation that represents the classical definition of inflammation in terms of heat, pain, swelling, and redness. However, inflammation is not like a burning log that eventually dies out. There is second active phase of inflammation known as the resolution phase that activates the expression of those genes necessary to bring the inflammatory system back to equilibrium. In an ideal world, both phases (initiation and resolution) of the inflammatory response are balanced. Unfortunately,

Table 1.1 Inflammatory potential of various nutrients

Proinflammatory	Anti-inflammatory
Omega-6 fatty acids	Omega-3 fatty acids
Saturated fatty acids	Polyphenols
Excess carbohydrates	

in the real world, there is often a mismatch of these two phases of the inflammatory response that can lead to chronic low-level inflammation that is beneath the perception of pain. This type of inflammation can be termed as cellular inflammation. As the levels of cellular inflammation rise, it can cause disruptions in signaling systems used by insulin that can lead to insulin resistance, metabolic syndrome, and eventually diabetes.

At the molecular level, this balance of the initiation and resolution responses can be focused on the gene transcription factor, nuclear factor-kappaB (NF-κB) that acts as the genetic master switch for inflammation. There are nutrients (directly or indirectly) that can either activate or inhibit NF-κB activity as shown in Table 1.1.

The body requires a balance of these proinflammatory and anti-inflammatory nutrients in the diet to maintain a balance in the initiation and resolution phases of the inflammatory process. However, an imbalance in either an excess of proinflammatory nutrients or deficiency of anti-inflammatory nutrients will increase the activity of NF-κB.

Once NF-κB is activated, it travels from the cytoplasm into the nucleus of the cell to cause the transcription of a wide variety of inflammatory proteins such as proinflammatory cytokines (IL-1β, IL-6, TNF-α, and others) as well as the increased production of the COX-2 enzyme which is needed for the production of proinflammatory eicosanoids such as prostaglandins. These inflammatory mediators expressed as a result of NF-κB activation act as paracrine hormones to activate nearby cells via their cytokine or prostaglandin receptors to amplify their inflammatory responses.

How these dietary factors impact both the initiation and resolution of inflammation at the molecular level is described in the next section.

1.3 Proinflammatory Nutrients

Foremost of the proinflammatory nutrients are omega-6 fatty acids as these are the building blocks required for the formation of hormones known as eicosanoids that are key players in the inflammatory process. Although there are hundreds of known eicosanoids, the primary eicosanoids important for the initiation phase of inflammation are prostaglandins and leukotrienes. In particular, the most common dietary omega-6 fatty acid, linoleic acid, must be first converted into arachidonic acid (AA) that is the building block for prostaglandins and leukotrienes. The synthesis of AA is tightly controlled by two distinct enzymes, delta-6 and delta-5 desaturase.

These two particular rate-limiting enzymes are controlled by the hormones insulin and glucagon that are generated by the balance of carbohydrates and protein in the diet [6]. It is the balance of these carbohydrates and protein at each meal that influences the secretion of insulin (an activator for both desaturase enzymes) and glucagon (an inhibitor of both desaturase enzymes). The dietary levels of long-chain omega-3 fatty acids (eicosapentaenoic acid (EPA) and docosahexaenoic acid (DHA)) are also important as they can be weak feedback inhibitors of the activity of both desaturase enzymes [6]. However, under conditions of insulin resistance, the levels of insulin in the blood will increase often causing an overproduction of AA because of the activation of both desaturase enzymes. This increases the potential for the generation of proinflammatory prostaglandins and leukotrienes derived from AA.

Linoleic acid is also very prone to oxidation thus increasing the formation of increased oxidative stress within the cell. Oxidative stress is another activator of NF-κB [7]. This is especially true if the diet is low in polyphenols that can function as powerful antioxidants to retard the oxidation of linoleic acid [8]. Finally, as the levels of omega-6 fatty acids increase in the diet, the endogenous production of anti-inflammatory omega-3 fatty acids (EPA and DHA) is decreased [9].

Saturated fatty acids are not as proinflammatory as omega-6 fatty acids, but they still have the potential to activate NF-κB. This is done by binding to toll-like receptors (TLR), especially TLR-4 [10]. Once TLR-4 is activated, through a series of signaling mechanisms, it can also increase the activation of NF-κB [11]. Saturated fatty acids also can increase the formation of lipid rafts in the cell membrane that amplifies the signals coming from TLR-2 and TLR-4 to further increase NF-κB activation [12].

The body (in particular the brain) needs a certain level of glucose for optimal function. Similar to linoleic acid, glucose is also prone to oxidation and can form advanced glycosylated end products (AGE), which are glycosylated proteins that can interact with their receptors (RAGE) on the cell surface that likewise activate NF-κB [13]. Excess intake of carbohydrates (especially those containing high levels of glucose such as grains and pasta) will increase the secretion of insulin by the pancreas to bring the elevated levels of blood glucose back within a normal operating range. However, with the development of insulin resistance, insulin levels remain continuously elevated increasing the likelihood of more dietary linoleic acid becoming transformed into AA.

1.4 Anti-inflammatory Nutrients

Just as there are proinflammatory nutrients that activate NF-κB, there is a wide range of nutrients that decrease its activity. Thus an anti-inflammatory nutrient is defined as one that ultimately inhibits activation of NF-κB.

The anti-inflammatory potential of EPA and DHA is manifold. As pointed out above, they are weak inhibitors of the delta-5 and delta-6 desaturase enzymes that will thus decrease the production of AA [6, 9]. Any decrease in AA will restrict the production of proinflammatory eicosanoids. They also compete with AA as substrates for the lipo-oxygenase (LOX) enzymes and cyclooxygenase (COX) enzymes required to make leukotrienes and prostaglandins. However, the bulky three-dimensional structure of DHA makes it a poor substrate for the COX enzymes. Since the COX-2 enzyme is one of those proteins that have increased expression by the activation of NF-κB, this suggests that EPA may be the more anti-inflammatory of the two omega-3 fatty acids to reduce the impact of diet-induced inflammation.

Omega-3 fatty acids also can be sensed by nutrient receptors such as GPR120 on the cell surface to signal the inactivation of NF-κB [14, 15].

Polyphenols also represent anti-inflammatory nutrients [16]. Although not as strong regulators of resolution as are the omega-3 fatty acids, they do act on different aspects of the initiation of inflammation and therefore are complimentary to omega-3 fatty acids.

The first of these polyphenol pathways is their action as antioxidants [16, 17]. Increased oxidation within the cell can increase NF-κB activation [7]. One of the primary sources of diet-induced inflammation is increased consumption of calories [4, 18]. Any excess calories that cannot be immediately converted into chemical energy are typically stored for future use. This conversion of excess calories into new molecules for long-term storage will generate excessive levels of free radicals that are the underlying cause of oxidative stress. As powerful antioxidants, polyphenols are key to preventing the excess buildup of free radicals. Furthermore, polyphenols can interact with other gene transcription factors, such as Nrf2, to cause the increased production of additional antioxidative enzymes such as superoxide dismutase and glutathione peroxidase that will further reduce oxidative stress [16, 17, 19].

At higher levels of dietary intake, polyphenols (as well as omega-3 fatty acids) can activate the anti-inflammatory gene transcription factor PPARγ which not only inactivates NF-κB but also increases the production of new healthy fat cells needed to prevent the lipotoxicity of stored fat from spreading into other tissues such as the liver and muscles that can increase insulin resistance in those organs [20, 21].

At still higher levels of dietary intake, polyphenols can activate the gene transcription factor SIRT-1 that causes the increased production of AMP kinase (AMPK) that acts as the controller of metabolism [22, 23]. With the activation of AMPK, catabolism and autophagy are activated to increase ATP levels and the anabolism is decreased [23].

1.5 Pro-resolution Nutrients

The definition of a pro-resolution nutrient is one that promotes the resolution of inflammation. This is a very different concept than simply the inhibition of inflammation. The initiation phase of inflammation will continue unless bought back to equilibrium by the resolution phase of inflammation. Increased levels of neutrophils at the injury site characterize the acute initiation of inflammation [5, 24]. On the other hand, increased levels of macrophages at the same site characterize the potential beginning of the resolution phase [5, 24]. However, without adequate levels of resolvins, these macrophages at the injury site are maintained in the activated M1 state and remain as potent generators of proinflammatory cytokines [25]. It is the resolvins that cause the reversion of the activated, proinflammatory macrophages in the M1 state to become anti-inflammatory M2 state macrophages (Fig. 1.1). Without this macrophage

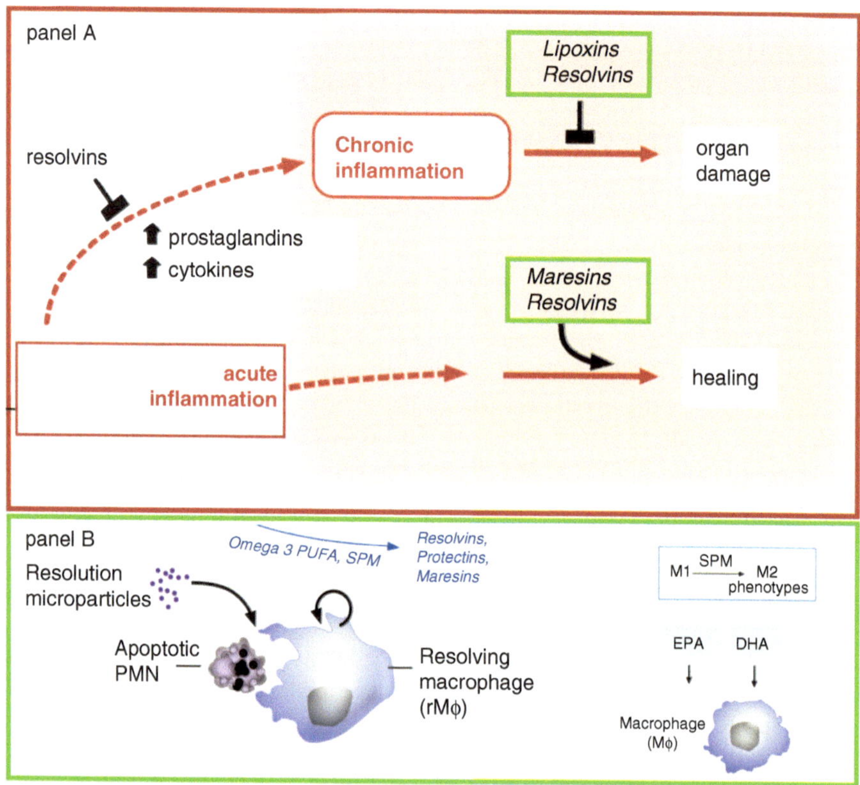

Fig. 1.1 PANEL (**A**) Specialized pro-resolving mediators (SPM) such as lipoxins, resolvins, protectins and maresins stimulate cellular events that counter-regulate pro-inflammatory mediators and regulate PMN, monocyte and macrophage response, leading to resolution. PANLE (**B**) Nutritional abundance of Omega-3, PUFA yields precursors of specialized pro-resolving mediators of inflammation, and eventually the M1 to M2 macrophage turnaround. Modified after Serhan [25]

transition mediated by resolvins, the inflammatory response continues at a lower but still proinflammatory level. This constitutes cellular inflammation.

The combination of adequate dietary intake of long-chain omega-3 fatty acids and polyphenols coupled with the dietary restriction of omega-6 and saturated fats as well as excess carbohydrates and calories represents the best therapeutic approach to maintain a balanced inflammatory response of initiation and resolution.

1.6 Adipose Tissue and Inflammation

The most effective site for storage of excess fat calories is the adipose tissue including those excess calories from carbohydrates that are converted to fat in the liver [26]. The fat cells of the adipose tissue are the only cells in the body that are designed to safely contain large amounts of fat. This is why the adipose tissue is extremely rich in stem cells that can be converted to new fat cells to contain large levels of

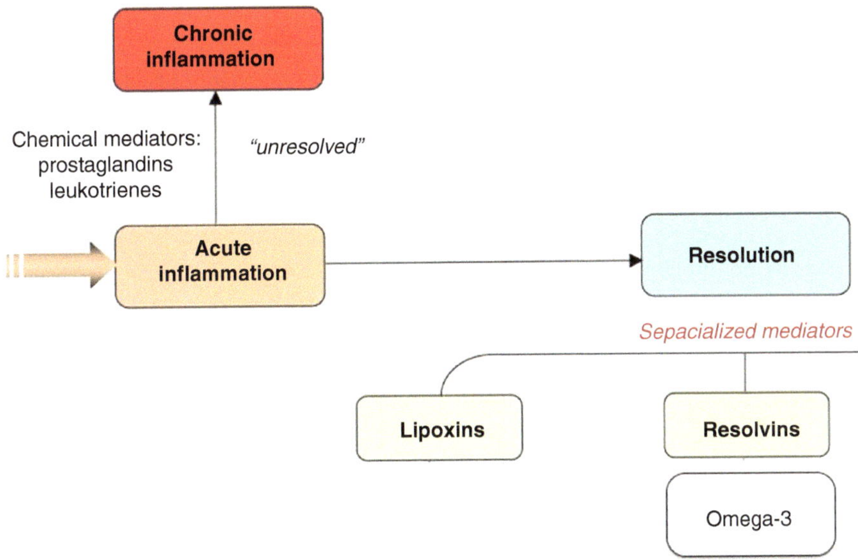

Fig. 1.2 Chronic inflammation can result from unresolved inflammatory responses. Arachidonic-acid-derived lipid mediators such as proinflammatory prostaglandins and leukotrienes can amplify this process. Bioactive products of omega-3 were originally isolated from mouse resolving exudates. The structure of these products was elucidated, and the biosynthesis of each new omega-3 family from EPA and DHA was recapitulated and analyzed in humans

excess energy as triglycerides [27]. As long as those fat cells are healthy, there are no adverse metabolic effects (except excess weight) for the person. This is why approximately one-third of obese individuals fall into the category of "metabolically healthy obese" [28]. They have excess body fat but no metabolic disturbances that characterize the manifestation of insulin resistance.

However, fat cells do not have an unlimited capacity to expand. Even though the adipose tissue is highly vascularized, the overexpansion of existing fat cells can create hypoxia that activates the HIF-1 gene [29, 30]. This results in the increased expression of both JNK and IKK, thereby creating inflammation within the fat cell [31]. This inflammation in turn creates insulin resistance within the fat cell.

In the adipose tissue, insulin is normally an anti-lipolytic hormone as it decreases the activity of the hormone-sensitive lipase (HSL) that is required to release stored fatty acids [32]. With the development of cellular inflammation and insulin resistance in the fat cell, higher levels of FFA can leave the fat cell to enter into the circulation to be taken up by other organs such as the liver and the skeletal muscles that are unable to safely store large amounts of fat. As described later, this leads to developing insulin resistance in these organs. With increased inflammation in the fat cells, there also is a migration of greater numbers of M1 macrophages into the adipose tissue with a corresponding release of inflammatory cytokines such as TNF-α and a family of proinflammatory cytokines that further increases insulin resistance and lipolysis [33] (Fig. 1.2). In the lean individual, only about 10 % of the adipose tissue mass is composed of macrophages, and those macrophages are primarily in the anti-inflammatory M2 state [34]. In the obese individual, up to 50 % of the mass of the adipose tissue may contain macrophages but now in the activated proinflammatory M1 state [34]. Theoretically, new healthy fat cells could be generated from stem cells within the adipose tissue. However, that process requires the activation of the gene transcription factor PPARγ [35]. The activity of this gene transcription factor is inhibited by inflammatory cytokines such as TNF-α [36]. On the other hand, the activity of PPARγ is increased in the presence of anti-inflammatory nutrients such as omega-3 fatty acids and polyphenols [37]. Without the ability to form new healthy fat cells, the continued expansion of the existing fat cells eventually leads to cell death and further adipose tissue inflammation caused by incoming neutrophils and macrophages to clean the cellular debris caused by the necrotic fat cells [38].

As stated earlier, insulin resistance can inhibit the action of hormone-sensitive lipase (HSL) leading to the elevation of insulin levels in the blood due to systemic insulin resistance in the muscle cells. Ironically, the increased hyperinsulinemia activates the lipoprotein lipase at the surface of the fat cell that hydrolyzes lipoprotein triglycerides to release free fatty acids [39] as well as increases the synthesis of fatty acid-binding proteins that bring the newly released FFA from the lipoproteins to the fat cells for deposition [40]. The increase in fatty acid flux into the fat cells also requires greater synthesis of the FFA into triglycerides, but this can lead to ER stress activating the JNK pathway thus further increasing insulin resistance in the fat cells [41]. This sets up a vicious cycle in which insulin resistance results in greater hunger (via insulin resistance in the hypothalamus) with increasing flux of FFA both into and out of the adipose tissue [42]. The cytokines being released by the proinflammatory M1 macrophages being attracted to the adipose tissue due to increasing cellular inflammation only increase this process by accelerating insulin resistance in the fat cells. This is why obese individuals with insulin resistance have greater levels of both the uptake and release of FFA into and from the adipose tissue. The increase in lipid influx causes an overload of the synthetic capacity to make triglycerides, and as a result, both DAG and ceramide levels begin to increase which only further increases insulin resistance in the fat cells [43].

The speed of the inflammatory changes in the adipose tissue is not as rapid as they are in the hypothalamus. Whereas inflammatory changes can be seen in the hypothalamus within 24 h after beginning an HFD, it often takes 12–14 weeks to see similar changes in inflammation in the adipose tissue [44].

If the fat cells cannot expand rapidly enough to store this increasing fatty acid flow, then the excess released fatty acids begin to accumulate in other tissues such as the liver and skeletal muscles, and this begins the process of lipotoxicity that further increases systemic insulin resistance [45]. It is with the development of lipotoxicity that the real metabolic consequences of insulin resistance begin.

We often think of obesity as the only cause of insulin resistance, yet the genesis of insulin resistance appears to start in the hypothalamus with a disruption in the normal balance of hunger and satiety signals. As hunger increases, so does calorie intake.

1.7 Hypothalamus

In many ways, early commands to develop insulin resistance in the body appear to start in the hypothalamus. The hypothalamus acts to match energy intake to energy expenditure to prevent excess accumulation of stored energy [46]. In particular, satiety signals from the gut are matched to adiposity (primarily leptin) and blood (primarily insulin) hormonal signals to control food intake [47]. Unfortunately, either excess calories or saturated fats (especially palmitic acid) can cause inflammation in the hypothalamus leading to resistance to the satiety signaling of both insulin and leptin [48, 49]. As a result, satiety is attenuated and hunger increases. Since the hypothalamus also contains GPR120 binding proteins, the presence of adequate levels of omega-3 fatty acids in this tissue can also decrease inflammation within the hypothalamus [50]. In fact, intracerebroventricular (icv) injections of omega-3 fatty acids into obese rats decrease insulin resistance [51]. Likewise similar icv injections of anti-TLR-4 and anti-TNF-α antibodies also decrease insulin resistance [52].

High-fat diet (HFD), especially those rich in saturated fats, is the standard method to cause diet-induced obesity. Increased inflammation appears in the hypothalamus within 24 h after beginning an HFD as indicated by increases in JNK and IKK proteins as well as increased expression of TLR-4 receptors and detection of ER stress [53]. IKK induces inflammation via activation of NF-κB that inhibits the normal hormonal signaling of leptin and insulin that is necessary to create satiety. Activation of JNK is often preceded by the increase in ER stress [54]. This sets up a vicious cycle of increased hunger that eventually leads to the accumulation of excess calories as stored fat in the adipose tissue. It should be noted that the inflammation in the hypothalamus precedes any weight gain in the adipose tissue [55]. This also explains why significant calorie restriction can reduce insulin resistance before any significant loss in excess body fat in the adipose tissue. These experimental observations suggest that the hypothalamus is the central control point for the development of insulin resistance.

Excess nutrient intake (especially saturated fat) can also indirectly cause inflammation in the hypothalamus by activation of the TLR-4 receptors in the microglia in the brain eventually causing inflammatory damage to neurons in the hypothalamus [49]. It has been shown that with an extended use of an HFD, there is a decrease in the number of neurons responsible for generating satiety signals in the hypothalamus [56].

HFD diets are also associated with increased production of palmitic acid-enriched ceramides in the hypothalamus which would provide still another link to the increased insulin and leptin resistance that gives rise to increased hunger as satiety depends on functioning insulin pathways in the hypothalamic neurons [57].

Besides the presence of the GPR120 receptors in the hypothalamus, which if activated by omega-3 fatty acids decreases inflammation, there are other fatty acid nutrient sensors in the hypothalamus that can be activated to increase inflammation. In particular, any increase in the free fatty acid (FFA) levels in the blood can be sensed by CD36/FATP-1 transporter at the surface of blood-brain-barrier (BBB). If those fatty acids are rich in palmitic acid (the primary product of de novo lipid production in the liver caused by excess dietary glucose), then the HPA axis is activated to release more cortisol that increases insulin resistance [58]. On the other hand, if the fatty acid being sensed is primarily oleic acid, there will be a reduction in NPY (a powerful appetite-inducing hormone) expression in the hypothalamus that promotes satiety [59].

Finally there is the interaction of the hypothalamus with the liver via signaling through the vagus nerve [53]. This may explain why any inhibition of TNF-α or TLR-4 signaling in hypothalamus also decreases glucose production in the liver [60, 61].

As you can begin to appreciate, the central regulation of appetite control by the hypothalamus is a very complex orchestration of the levels of inflammation and nutrient intake generated by the diet and the sensing of those levels by the hypothalamus.

1.8 Insulin Resistance

Although the definition of insulin resistance is deceptively simple (a condition in which cells are no longer responding appropriately to circulating insulin), the molecular causes of insulin resistance are diverse and extremely complex.

It is known that certain short-term dietary changes can rapidly reduce insulin resistance before any significant fat loss occurs. This would include strict calorie restriction that can reduce insulin resistance within a matter of days [62]. Likewise certain drugs such as corticosteroids can rapidly increase insulin resistance [63].

Furthermore, there are various metabolic adaptations to stressors that can induce insulin resistance. These stressors include pregnancy, hibernation, and sepsis [1]. The increase in insulin resistance in response to these stressors is a method of diverting stored nutrients to address the necessary metabolic adaptation. Likewise sleep deprivation is another effective way of increasing insulin resistance in the short-term [64].

However, the chronic insulin resistance appears to be directly or indirectly related to diet-induced inflammation. The mechanisms at the molecular level are complex and manifold, but they are based on the ability of increased cellular inflammation to interrupt insulin's action by disruption of the signaling mechanisms within the cell. The primary suspects appear to be the inflammatory cytokine tumor necrosis factor alpha (TNF-α) and other inflammatory protein kinases such as c-Jun N-terminal kinase (JNK) and the inhibitor of IκKβ kinase (IKK) [65].

TNF-α knockout models are resistant to the development of insulin resistance in animal strains prone to diet-induced obesity (DIO mice) or those that lack leptin (Ob/Ob mice) [31, 66]. Activation of JNK and IKK interrupts insulin-signaling pathways via separate mechanisms. Activation of IKK causes the dissociation of the inhibitory protein that prevents the translocation of NF-κB into the nucleus [67]. Once IKK releases that inhibitory protein from NF-κB, that gene transcription can now move to the nucleus to cause the expression of inflammatory proteins. The JNK pathway is stress activated and is associated with the presence of M1-activated macrophages [41].

The realization that inflammation was related to insulin resistance was more than century ago when it was observed that certain anti-inflammatory drugs (salicylates and aspirin) were effective in reducing the hyperglycemia observed in diabetes [68, 69]. It is now known that these drugs are inhibitors of IKK [70].

Additional molecular mechanisms of insulin resistance include the lipid overload hypothesis in which there is a buildup of diacylglycerides (DAG) or ceramides that inhibit the signaling of insulin as well as endoplasmic reticulum (ER) stress (induced by excess calories) or oxidative stress (induced by the generation of excess free radicals) [39–41, 71]. Making these diverse molecular mechanisms even more complex is that they are operative in some organs and not in others.

1.9 Individual Organ Responses to Diet-Induced Inflammation and Insulin Resistance

1.9.1 Liver

The liver can be viewed as the central manufacturing plant in the body. Raw materials (primarily carbohydrates and fats) are bought into the body to be processed by the liver and either stored (as liver glycogen) or repackaged as newly formed triglycerides (in the form of lipoproteins). The liver helps maintain stable glucose levels between meals by balancing glycogenesis (glycogen formation) and glycolysis of stored glycogen [72]. It should be pointed out that the glycogen stored in muscles can only be used internally as a source of energy and can't be released back into the circulation to help maintain stable blood glucose levels.

Unlike the adipose tissue that can safely store excess fat, the liver cannot. Therefore of the first adverse metabolic consequences of insulin resistance is the buildup of fatty deposits in the liver. This is known as nonalcoholic fatty liver disease or NAFLD. Currently 20–30 % of Americans have NAFLD and 90 % of obese type 2 diabetic patients have NAFLD [73]. Ominously, it is estimated that 50 % of all Americans will have NAFLD by 2030 [72].

Another difference between the liver and the adipose tissue is the lack of infiltrating macrophages. Whereas a significant increase is observed in the levels of macrophages in the adipose tissue upon inflammation, it is the internal macrophages (Kupffer cells) in the liver that become activated. These activated Kupffer cells can now release cytokines that will further activate NF-κB in the liver cells.

Like hypothalamic inflammation, NAFLD can be rapidly generated in animal models within 3 days of starting an HFD [74]. This may be due to the direct linkage of the hypothalamus to the liver via the vagus nerve [75]. Once NAFLD is established, the ability of insulin to suppress liver glucose production is diminished without changes in weight, fat mass, or the appearance of any indication of insulin resistance in the skeletal muscle [76].

Because of the rapid buildup of fatty acids in the liver, the ability to convert them to triglycerides is also overwhelmed and DAG formation in liver increases [77, 78]. This is why the levels of DAG in the liver are the best clinical marker that chronic insulin resistance has begun to develop in that organ. The primary source of the fatty acids coming to the liver is via the adipose tissue because as the adipose tissue develops insulin resistance, the increased flow of FFA from the fat cells into the blood and therefore into the liver increases [79]. De novo lipid synthesis of fats from glucose in the liver is a smaller contributor to this increased flux of FFA into the liver [80]. Furthermore, liver insulin resistance is related only to the fatty acid levels in the liver, not the levels of visceral fat [81]. This may explain why many normal-BMI individuals (especially Asians) can have high levels of insulin resistance in the liver [82].

Since the liver also controls cholesterol synthesis, insulin resistance in this organ is reflected in growing dysfunction in lipoprotein synthesis. In particular VLDL particles are increased and HDL levels are decreased [72]. This is easily measured by the TG/HDL ratio that is a good general clinical marker for liver insulin resistance [83].

1.9.2 Skeletal Muscle

Skeletal muscle represents the key site for glucose uptake. Thus reducing insulin resistance in this organ becomes a primary strategy for managing diabetes. Unlike the adipose tissue, where macrophage infiltration is a key indicator of inflammation, there is very little macrophage infiltration observed in the skeletal muscle in individuals with insulin resistance [84]. It appears that cytokines coming from other organs (adipose tissue and liver) may have the important impact on the development of insulin resistance in the muscle. However, enhanced signaling through the TLR-4 receptor by saturated fatty acids can reduce fatty acid oxidation of the lipids in the muscle [85]. In addition, palmitic acid is the preferred substrate for ceramide synthesis [86]. Whereas ceramide levels are not related to insulin resistance in the liver, they are strongly related to insulin resistance in the muscle [87]. This suggests that the molecular drivers of insulin resistance can be different from organ to organ.

1.9.3 Pancreas

Although the beta cells of the pancreas sense glucose levels in the blood and secrete insulin in response to those levels, the beta cells of this organ are not normally considered targets of insulin resistance. However, the beta cells are very prone to toxicity mediated by inflammatory agents. In particular, 12-HETE, derived from AA, is very toxic to the beta cells [88]. With the destruction of the beta cells by 12-HETE, the pancreas is no longer able to maintain compensatory levels of insulin secretion to reduce blood glucose levels, and the development of type 2 diabetes is rapid.

1.9.4 Gastrointestinal (GI) Tract

Like the pancreas, the GI tract is not considered a standard target organ for insulin resistance, but it is the first organ in the body for nutrient sensing of molecules that can ultimately affect insulin resistance. This begins in the oral region. Fatty acid receptors such as GPR120 and GPR40 and fatty binding proteins such as CD36 are present in the mouth and line the entire GI tract [89]. Essentially these receptors allow for the "tasting" of the fatty acid content of the diet. CD36 binds oleic acid and helps convert it into oleoylethanolamide (OEA) [90]. OEA activates PPARα gene transcription factor to increase satiety and also the expression of the enzyme required for fatty acid oxidation [91]. Thus the type of fat sensed in the mouth and gut provides satiety signals to the hypothalamus. The increased satiety lowers the overall caloric intake and reduces development of ER and oxidative stress thus indirectly reducing the development of insulin resistance.

Although the GI tract is a long and complicated organ, the enteroendocrine cells that produce hormones in the GI tract represent less than 1 % of its total cells. These specific cells sense and respond to specific nutrients by secreting more than 20 different hormones. The primary hormones secreted by these cells that relate to insulin resistance include CCK (from the proximal I cells) and GLP-1 and PYY (from the distal L cells).

CKK is the hormone secreted from the I cells in response to the fat content in a meal [92]. This is a short-acting hormone and works in association with serotonin to suppress hunger by directly interacting with the hypothalamus via the vagus nerve [77]. In animals being fed with an HFD, the satiety signals of CCK to the hypothalamus can become attenuated probably by increased inflammation in the hypothalamus [93]. CCK can also reduce glucose synthesis in the liver probably through its interaction with the hypothalamus [94], but only if its hormonal signal pathway is not being disrupted by inflammation within the hypothalamus.

PYY and GLP-1 are the hormones released by protein and glucose, respectively, when sensed by the L cells more distal in the GI tract. Both of these hormones are powerful inducers of satiety [78]. It has been shown that PYY responses are lower in obese individuals compared to lean individuals [95]. Animal models that have increased levels of PYY due to transgenic manipulation are resistant to diet-induced obesity [96]. It should be noted that PYY levels rapidly rise after gastric bypass surgery helping to explain the long-term weight loss success of this surgical intervention [97].

1.9.5 GI Microbiota

Finally, any mention of the GI tract would not be complete without discussing the microbial composition of the gut. It is known that the microbiota is different in lean and obese individuals [98]. The microbial composition also may be a source of low-grade intestinal inflammation especially via endotoxemia mediated by the lipopolysaccharide (LPS) component of gram-negative bacteria that interacts with the TLR-4 receptor. TNF-α is upregulated in the ileum of the GI tract by HFD before weight gain is observed in animal models [99]. It is also known that a single high-fat or high-carbohydrate meal can induce such endotoxemia during the increased permeability of the gut during digestion [100–102]. Any LPS fragments that enter the bloodstream are carried by chylomicrons to the lymph system where it can then

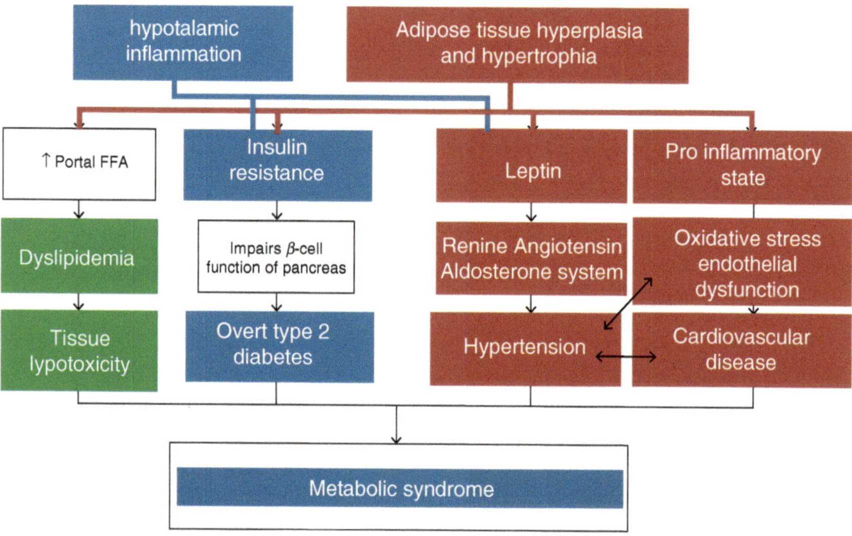

Fig. 1.3 Schematic representation of metabolic syndrome

interact with the TLR-4 receptors in the body to increase TNF-α levels that can generate insulin resistance in a wide variety of organs [103].

1.9.6 Cardiovascular System

The description of the impact of chronic inflammation of insulin resistance on the cardiovascular system would require a chapter by itself. Figure 1.3 summarizes for the purposes of this contribution the enormous impact that the proinflammatory state and the oxidative stress inflict to the endothelium and cardiovascular system as a whole. Oxidative stress, due to caloric overload and/or chronic low-grade inflammation induced by adipose tissue dysfunction, represents a vicious cycle favoring the progression of endothelial dysfunction, atherothrombosis, and cardiac overload and dysfunction. Increased food intake and insulin resistance have been shown also to rapidly enhance plasma leptin levels and subsequently tissue leptin resistance. Normal fluctuating levels of leptin do reduce appetite and enhance energy expenditure. Opposite to this, chronic elevated levels of leptin deregulate its original signals pathways, bringing into this scenario leptin resistance and the activation of the sympathetic nervous system to increase blood pressure and heart rate frequency. The higher heart rate in the hyperleptinemic individuals will impose a greater myocardial workload and eventually predispose the heart to pathophysiological changes that encroach on the other adverse conditions established by the "partners" of metabolic syndrome.

1.9.7 Metabolic Syndrome

All the above metabolic derangements concur to define both at a clinical level and a molecular level what we define as a metabolic syndrome (Fig. 1.3). Currently in the USA, there are 80 million individuals with metabolic syndrome and approximately 26 million with type 2 diabetes [104]. Metabolic syndrome is associated with increased mortality from both cardiovascular disease and non-cardiovascular causes [105].

The effects of constant hyperinsulinemia induced by insulin resistance will have adverse effects on pregnancy outcomes, especially in the long-term metabolic consequences such as obesity, diabetes, and heart disease for the offspring via fetal programming [106]. Therefore reduction of insulin resistance during pregnancy has major public health implications.

References

1. Odegaard JI, Chawla A. Pleiotropic actions of insulin resistance and inflammation in metabolic homeostasis. Science. 2013;339:172–7.
2. Zeyda M, Stulnig TM. Obesity, inflammation, and insulin resistance–a mini-review. Gerontology. 2009;55(4):379–86.
3. de Luca C, Olefsky JM. Inflammation and insulin resistance. FEBS Lett. 2008; 582(1):97–105.
4. Gregor MF, Hotamistigli GS. Inflammatory mechanisms in obesity. Ann Rev Immunol. 2011;29:415–45.
5. Spite M, Claria J, Serhan CN. Resolvins, specialized proresolving lipid mediators, and their potential roles in metabolic diseases. Cell Metab. 2014;19(1):21–36.
6. Brenner RR. Nutritional and hormonal factors influencing desaturation of essential fatty acids. Prog Lipid Res. 1981;20:41–7.
7. Kratsovnik E, Bromberg Y, Sperling O, Zoref-Shani E. Oxidative stress activates transcription factor NF-kB-mediated protective signaling in primary rat neuronal cultures. J Mol Neurosci. 2005;26(1):27–32.
8. Roche M, Dufour C, Loonis M, Reist M, Carrupt PA, Dangles O. Olive phenols efficiently inhibit the oxidation of serum albumin-bound linoleic acid and butyrylcholine esterase. Biochim Biophys Acta. 2009;1790(4):240–8.
9. Taha AY, Cheon Y, Faurot KF, Macintosh B, Majchrzak-Hong SF, Mann JD, et al. Dietary omega-6 fatty acid lowering increases bioavailability of omega-3 polyunsaturated fatty acids in human plasma lipid pools. Prostaglandins Leukot Essent Fatty Acids. 2014;90(5):151–7.
10. Kim JJ, Sears DD. TLR4 and insulin resistance. Gastroenterol Res Pract. 2010;2010:S1687–630X.
11. Saberi M, Woods NB, de Luca C, Schenk S, Lu JC, Bandyopadhyay G, et al. Hematopoietic cell-specific deletion of toll-like receptor 4 ameliorates hepatic and adipose tissue insulin resistance in high-fat-fed mice. Cell Metab. 2009;10(5):419–29.
12. Wong SW, Kwon MJ, Choi AM, Kim HP, Nakahira K, Hwang DH. Fatty acids modulate toll-like receptor 4 activation through regulation of receptor dimerization and recruitment into lipid rafts in a reactive oxygen species-dependent manner. J Biol Chem. 2009;284(40):27384–92.

13. Tobon-Velasco JC, Cuevas E, Torres-Ramos MA. Receptor for AGEs (RAGE) as mediator of NF-kB pathway activation in neuroinflammation and oxidative stress. CNS Neurol Disord Drug Targets. 2014;13(9):1615–26.
14. Oh DY, Talukdar S, Bae EJ, Imamura T, Morinaga H, Fan W, et al. GPR120 is an omega-3 fatty acid receptor mediating potent anti-inflammatory and insulin-sensitizing effects. Cell. 2010;142(5):687–98.
15. Oh DY, Olefsky JM. Omega 3 fatty acids and GPR120. Cell Metab. 2012;15(5):564–5.
16. Scapagnini G, Vasto S, Sonya V, Abraham NG, Nader AG, Caruso C, et al. Modulation of Nrf2/ARE pathway by food polyphenols: a nutritional neuroprotective strategy for cognitive and neurodegenerative disorders. Mol Neurobiol. 2011;44(2):192–201.
17. Rahman I, Biswas SK, Kirkham PA. Regulation of inflammation and redox signaling by dietary polyphenols. Biochem Pharmacol. 2006;72(11):1439–52.
18. Zhang X, Zhang G, Zhang H, Karin M, Bai H, Cai D. Hypothalamic IKKbeta/NF-kappaB and ER stress link overnutrition to energy imbalance and obesity. Cell. 2008;135(1):61–73.
19. Siriwardhana N, Kalupahana NS, Cekanova M, Le Mieux M, Greer B, Moustaid-Moussa N. Modulation of adipose tissue inflammation by bioactive food compounds. J Nutr Biochem. 2013;24(4):613–23.
20. Sears B, Ricordi C. Role of fatty acids and polyphenols in inflammatory gene transcription and their impact on obesity, metabolic syndrome and diabetes. Eur Rev Med Pharmacol Sci. 2012;16(9):1137–54.
21. Kim JY, van de Wall E, Laplante M, Azzara A, Trujillo ME, Hofmann SM, et al. Obesity-associated improvements in metabolic profile through expansion of adipose tissue. J Clin Invest. 2007;117(9):2621–37.
22. Chung S, Yao H, Caito S, Hwang JW, Arunachalam G, Rahman I. Regulation of SIRT1 in cellular functions: role of polyphenols. Arch Biochem Biophys. 2010;501(1):79–90.
23. Joven J, Rull A, Rodriguez-Gallego E, Camps J, Riera-Borrull M, Hernandez-Aguilera A, et al. Multifunctional targets of dietary polyphenols in disease: a case for the chemokine network and energy metabolism. Food Chem Toxicol. 2013;51:267–79.
24. Buckley CD, Gilroy DW, Serhan CN. Proresolving lipid mediators and mechanisms in the resolution of acute inflammation. Immunity. 2014;40(3):315–27.
25. Serhan CN. Pro-resolving lipid mediators are leads for resolution physiology. Nature. 2014;510:92–101.
26. Postic C, Girard J. Contribution of de novo fatty acid synthesis to hepatic steatosis and insulin resistance: lessons from genetically engineered mice. J Clin Invest. 2008;118(3):829–38.
27. Perrini S, Ficarella R, Picardi E, Cignarelli A, Barbaro M, Nigro P, et al. Differences in gene expression and cytokine release profiles highlight the heterogeneity of distinct subsets of adipose tissue-derived stem cells in the subcutaneous and visceral adipose tissue in humans. PLoS One. 2013;8(3):e57892.
28. Wildman RP, Muntner P, Reynolds K, McGinn AP, Rajpathak S, Wylie-Rosett J, et al. The obese without cardiometabolic risk factor clustering and the normal weight with cardiometabolic risk factor clustering: prevalence and correlates of 2 phenotypes among the US population (NHANES 1999-2004). Arch Intern Med. 2008;168(15):1617–24.
29. Lionetti L, Mollica MP, Lombardi A, Cavaliere G, Gifuni G, Barletta A. From chronic overnutrition to insulin resistance: the role of fat-storing capacity and inflammation. Nutr Metab Cardiovasc Dis. 2009;19(2):146–52.
30. He Q, Gao Z, Yin J, Zhang J, Yun Z, Ye J. Regulation of HIF-1(alpha) activity in adipose tissue by obesity-associated factors: adipogenesis, insulin, and hypoxia. Am J Physiol Endocrinol Metab. 2011;300(5):E877–85.
31. Hotamisligil GS. Inflammation and metabolic disorders. Nature. 2006;444(7121):860–7.
32. Jaworski K, Sarkadi-Nagy E, Duncan RE, Ahmadian M, Sul HS. Regulation of triglyceride metabolism. IV. Hormonal regulation of lipolysis in adipose tissue. Am J Physiol Gastrointest Liver Physiol. 2007;293(1):G1–4.
33. Hotamisligil GS, Murray DL, Choy LN, Spiegelman BM. Tumor necrosis factor alpha inhibits signaling from the insulin receptor. Proc Natl Acad Sci U S A. 1994;91(11):4854–8.

34. Weisberg SP, McCann D, Desai M, Rosenbaum M, Leibel RL, Ferrante AW. Obesity is associated with macrophage accumulation in adipose tissue. J Clin Invest. 2003;112(12): 1796–808.
35. Rosen ED, Sarraf P, Troy AE, Bradwin G, Moore K, Milstone DS, et al. PPAR gamma is required for the differentiation of adipose tissue in vivo and in vitro. Mol Cell. 1999;4(4):611–7.
36. Ye J. Regulation of PPARgamma function by TNF-alpha. Biochem Biophys Res Commun. 2008;374(3):405–8.
37. Scazzocchio B, Vari R, Filesi C, D'Archivio M, Santangelo C, Giovannini C, et al. Cyanidin-3-O-(sup)-glucoside and protocatechuic acid exert insulin-like effects by upregulating PPAR(sup) activity in human omental adipocytes. Diabetes. 2011;60(9):2234–44.
38. Cinti S, Mitchell G, Barbatelli G, Murano I, Ceresi E, Faloia E, et al. Adipocyte death defines macrophage localization and function in adipose tissue of obese mice and humans. J Lipid Res. 2005;46(11):2347–55.
39. Kraemer FB, Takeda D, Natu V, Sztalryd C. Insulin regulates lipoprotein lipase activity in rat adipose cells via wortmannin- and rapamycin-sensitive pathways. Metabolism. 1998; 47(5):555–9.
40. Chabowski A, Coort SL, Calles-Escandon J, Tandon NN, Glatz JF, Luiken JJ, et al. Insulin stimulates fatty acid transport by regulating expression of FAT/CD36 but not FABPpm. Am J Physiol Endocrinol Metab. 2004;287(4):E781–9.
41. Ozcan U, Cao Q, Yilmaz E, Lee AH, Iwakoshi NN, Ozdelen E, et al. Endoplasmic reticulum stress links obesity, insulin action, and type 2 diabetes. Science. 2004;306(5695):457–61.
42. Horowitz JF, Klein S. Whole body and abdominal lipolytic sensitivity to epinephrine is suppressed in upper body obese women. Am J Physiol Endocrinol Metab. 2000;278(6): E1144–52.
43. Summers SA. Ceramides in insulin resistance and lipotoxicity. Prog Lipid Res. 2006;45(1):42–72.
44. Lee BC, Lee J. Cellular and molecular players in adipose tissue inflammation in the development of obesity-induced insulin resistance. Biochim Biophys Acta. 2014;1842(3):446–62.
45. Unger RH. Weapons of lean body mass destruction: the role of ectopic lipids in the metabolic syndrome. Endocrinology. 2003;144(12):5159–65.
46. Thaler JP, Yi CX, Schur EA, Guyenet SJ, Hwang BH, Dietrich MO, et al. Obesity is associated with hypothalamic injury in rodents and humans. J Clin Invest. 2012;122(1):153–62.
47. Thaler JP, Schwartz MW. Inflammation and obesity pathogenesis: the hypothalamus heats up. Endocrinology. 2010;151(9):4109–15.
48. Yue JT, Lam TK. Lipid sensing and insulin resistance in the brain. Cell Metab. 2012; 15(5):646–55.
49. Milanski M, Degasperi G, Coope A, Morari J, Denis R, Cintra DE, et al. Saturated fatty acids produce an inflammatory response predominantly through the activation of TLR4 signaling in hypothalamus: implications for the pathogenesis of obesity. J Neurosci. 2009;29(2): 359–70.
50. Cintra DE, Ropelle ER, Moraes JC, Pauli JR, Morari J, Souza CT, et al. Unsaturated fatty acids revert diet-induced hypothalamic inflammation in obesity. PLoS One. 2012; 7(1):e30571.
51. Obici S, Feng Z, Morgan K, Stein D, Karkanias G, Rossetti L. Central administration of oleic acid inhibits glucose production and food intake. Diabetes. 2002;51(2):271–5.
52. Milanski M, Arruda AP, Coope A, Ignacio-Souza LM, Nunez CE, Roman EA, et al. Inhibition of hypothalamic inflammation reverses diet-induced insulin resistance in the liver. Diabetes. 2012;61(6):1455–62.
53. De Souza CT, Araujo EP, Bordin S, Ashimine R, Zollner RL, Boschero AC, et al. Consumption of a fat-rich diet activates a proinflammatory response and induces insulin resistance in the hypothalamus. Endocrinology. 2005;146(1):4192–9.
54. Tripathi YB, Pandey V. Obesity and endoplasmic reticulum (ER) stresses. Front Immunol. 2012;3:240.

55. Thaler JP, Guyenet SJ, Dorfman MD, Wisse BE, Schwartz MW. Hypothalamic inflammation: marker or mechanism of obesity pathogenesis? Diabetes. 2013;62(8):2629–34.
56. Moraes JC, Coope A, Morari J, Cintra DE, Roman EA, Pauli JR, et al. High-fat diet induces apoptosis of hypothalamic neurons. PLoS One. 2009;4(4):e5045.
57. Borg ML, Omran SF, Weir J, Meikle PJ, Watt MJ. Consumption of a high-fat diet, but not regular endurance exercise training, regulates hypothalamic lipid accumulation in mice. J Physiol. 2012;590(Pt 17):4377–89.
58. Auvinen HE, Romijn JA, Biermasz NR, Pijl H, Havekes LM, Smit JW, et al. The effects of high fat diet on the basal activity of the hypothalamus-pituitary-adrenal axis in mice. J Endocrinol. 2012;214(2):191–7.
59. Serrano A, Pavon FJ, Tovar S, Casanueva F, Senaris R, Dieguez C, et al. Oleoylethanolamide: effects on hypothalamic transmitters and gut peptides regulating food intake. Neuropharmacology. 2011;60(4):593–601.
60. Chaudhri OB, Field BC, Bloom SR. Gastrointestinal satiety signals. Int J Obes. 2008;32 Suppl 7:S28–31.
61. Morinigo R, Moize V, Musri M, Lacy AM, Navarro S, Marin JL, et al. Glucagon-like peptide-1, peptide YY, hunger, and satiety after gastric bypass surgery in morbidly obese subjects. J Clin Endocrinol Metab. 2006;91(5):1735–40.
62. Markovic TP, Jenkins AB, Campbell LV, Furler SM, Kraegen EW, Chisholm DJ. The determinants of glycemic responses to diet restriction and weight loss in obesity and NIDDM. Diabetes Care. 1998;21(5):687–94.
63. Pagano G, Cavallo-Perin P, Cassader M, Bruno A, Ozzello A, Masciola Dall'omo AM, et al. An in vivo and in vitro study of the mechanism of prednisone-induced insulin resistance in healthy subjects. J Clin Invest. 1983;72(5):1814–20.
64. Donga E, van Dijk M, van Dijk JG, Biermasz NR, Lammers GJ, van Kralingen KW, et al. A single night of partial sleep deprivation induces insulin resistance in multiple metabolic pathways in healthy subjects. J Clin Endocrinol Metab. 2010;95(6):2963–8.
65. Dali-Youcef N, Mecili M, Ricci R, Andres E. Metabolic inflammation: connecting obesity and insulin resistance. Ann Med. 2013;45(3):242–53.
66. Uysal KT, Wiesbrock SM, Marino MW, Hotamisligil GS. Protection from obesity-induced insulin resistance in mice lacking TNF-alpha function. Nature. 1997;389:610–4.
67. Cai D, Yuan M, Frantz DF, Melendez PA, Hansen L, Lee J, et al. Local and systemic insulin resistance resulting from hepatic activation of IKK-beta and NF-kappaB. Nat Med. 2005;11(2):183–90.
68. Ebstein W. Zur therapie des diabetes mellitus, insbesordere uber die anwendung des salicylsuaren natron bei demselben. Berliner Klinische Wochenschrift. 1876;13:337–40.
69. Hecht A, Goldner MF. Reappraisal of the hypoglycemic action of acetylsalicylate. Metabolism. 1959;8:418–28.
70. Hundal RS, Petersen KF, Mayerson AB, Randhawa PS, Inzucchi S, Shoelson SE, et al. Mechanism by which high-dose aspirin improves glucose metabolism in type 2 diabetes. J Clin Invest. 2002;109(10):1321–6.
71. Glass CK, Olefsky JM. Inflammation and lipid signaling in the etiology of insulin resistance. Cell Metabol. 2012;15(5):635–44.
72. Samuel VT, Shulman GI. Mechanisms for insulin resistance: common threads and missing links. Cell. 2012;148(5):852–71.
73. Tolman KG, Fonseca V, Dalpiaz A, Tan MH. Spectrum of liver disease in type 2 diabetes and management of patients with diabetes and liver disease. Diabetes Care. 2007;30(3):734–43.
74. Perry RJ, Samuel VT, Petersen KF, Shulman GI. The role of hepatic lipids in hepatic insulin resistance and type 2 diabetes. Nature. 2014;510(7503):84–91.
75. German J, Kim F, Schwartz GJ, Havel PJ, Rhodes CJ, Schwartz MW, et al. Hypothalamic leptin signaling regulates hepatic insulin sensitivity via a neurocircuit involving the vagus nerve. Endocrinology. 2009;150(10):4502–11.
76. Kraegen EW, Clark PW, Jenkins AB, Daley EA, Chisholm DJ, Storlien LH. Development of muscle insulin resistance after liver insulin resistance in high-fat-fed rats. Diabetes. 1991;40(11):1397–403.

77. Owyang C, Logsdon CD. New insights into neurohormonal regulation of pancreatic secretion. Gastroenterology. 2004;127(3):957–69.
78. D'Alessio D. Intestinal hormones and regulation of satiety: the case for CCK, GLP-1, PYY, and Apo A-IV. JPEN J Parenter Enteral Nutr. 2008;32(5):567–8.
79. De Fronzo RA. Dysfunctional fat cells, lipotoxicity and type 2 diabetes. Int J Clin Pract Suppl. 2004;143:9–21.
80. Diraison F, Yankah V, Letexier D, Dusserre E, Jones P, Beylot M. Differences in the regulation of adipose tissue and liver lipogenesis by carbohydrates in humans. J Lipid Res. 2003;44(4):846–53.
81. Fabbrini E, Magkos F, Mohammed BS, Pietka T, Abumrad NA, Patterson BW, et al. Intrahepatic fat, not visceral fat, is linked with metabolic complications of obesity. Proc Natl Acad Sci U S A. 2009;106(36):15430–5.
82. Azuma K, Kadowaki T, Cetinel C, Kadota A, El-Saed A, Kadowaki S, et al. Higher liver fat content among Japanese in Japan compared with non-Hispanic whites in the United States. Metabolism. 2009;58(8):1200–7.
83. McLaughlin T, Reaven G, Abbasi F, Lamendola C, Saad M, Waters D, et al. Is there a simple way to identify insulin-resistant individuals at increased risk of cardiovascular disease? Am J Cardiol. 2005;96(3):399–404.
84. Shoelson SE, Lee J, Goldfine AB. Inflammation and insulin resistance. J Clin Invest. 2006;116(7):1793–801.
85. Pang S, Tang H, Zhuo S, Zang YQ, Le Y. Regulation of fasting fuel metabolism by toll-like receptor 4. Diabetes. 2010;59(12):3041–8.
86. Straczkowski M, Kowalska I, Nikolajuk A, Dzienis-Straczkowska S, Kinalska I, Baranowski M, et al. Relationship between insulin sensitivity and sphingomyelin signaling pathway in human skeletal muscle. Diabetes. 2004;53(5):1215–21.
87. Adams JM, Pratipanawatr T, Berria R, Wang E, De Fronzo RA, Sullards MC, et al. Ceramide content is increased in skeletal muscle from obese insulin-resistant humans. Diabetes. 2004;53(1):25–31.
88. Wei D, Li J, Shen M, Jia W, Chen N, Chen T, Su D, et al. Cellular production of n-3 PUFAs and reduction of n-6-to-n-3 ratios in the pancreatic beta-cells and islets enhance insulin secretion and confer protection against cytokine-induced cell death. Diabetes. 2010;59(2):471–8.
89. Duca FA, Yue JT. Fatty acid sensing an the gut and the hypothalamus. Mol Cell Endocrinol. 2014;397:23–33.
90. Schwartz GJ, Fu J, Astarita G, Li X, Gaetani S, Campolongo P, et al. The lipid messenger OEA links dietary fat intake to satiety. Cell Metab. 2008;8(4):281–8.
91. Martinez de Ubago M, Garcia-Oya I, Perez-Perez A, Canfran-Duque A, Quintana-Portillo R, Rodriguez de Fonseca F, et al. Oleoylethanolamide, a natural ligand for PPAR-alpha, inhibits insulin receptor signalling in HTC rat hepatoma cells. Biochim Biophys Acta. 2009;1791(8):740–5.
92. Field BC, Chaudhri OB, Bloom SR. Bowels control brain: gut hormones and obesity. Nat Rev Endocrinol. 2010;6(8):444–53.
93. Arruda AP, Milanski M, Coope A, Torsoni AS, Ropelle E, Carvalho DP, et al. Low-grade hypothalamic inflammation leads to defective thermogenesis, insulin resistance, and impaired insulin secretion. Endocrinology. 2011;152(4):1314–26.
94. Cheung GW, Kokorovic A, Lam CK, Chari M, Lam TK. Intestinal cholecystokinin controls glucose production through a neuronal network. Cell Metab. 2009;10(2):99–109.
95. le Roux CW, Batterham RL, Aylwin SJ, Patterson M, Borg CM, Wynne KJ, et al. Attenuated peptide YY release in obese subjects is associated with reduced satiety. Endocrinology. 2006;147(1):3–8.
96. Boey D, Lin S, Enriquez RF, Lee NJ, Slack K, Couzens M, et al. PYY transgenic mice are protected against diet-induced and genetic obesity. Neuropeptides. 2008;42(1):19–30.
97. Ley RE, Turnbaugh PJ, Klein S, Gordon JI. Microbial ecology: human gut microbes associated with obesity. Nature. 2006;444:1022–3.
98. Shen J, Obin MS, Zhao L. The gut microbiota, obesity and insulin resistance. Mol Aspects Med. 2013;34(1):39–58.

99. Ding S, Chi MM, Scull BP, Rigby R, Schwerbrock NM, Magness S, et al. High-fat diet: bacterial interactions promote intestinal inflammation which precedes and correlates with obesity and insulin resistance in mouse. PLoS One. 2010;5(8):e12191.
100. Pendyala S, Walker JM, Holt PR. A high-fat diet is associated with endotoxemia that originates from the gut. Gastroenterology. 2012;142(5):1100–1101.e2.
101. Ghanim H, Abuaysheh S, Sia CL, Korzeniewski K, Chaudhuri A, Fernandez-Real JM, et al. Increase in plasma endotoxin concentrations and the expression of Toll-like receptors and suppressor of cytokine signaling-3 in mononuclear cells after a high-fat, high-carbohydrate meal: implications for insulin resistance. Diabetes Care. 2009;32(12):2281–7.
102. Laugerette F, Furet JP, Debard C, Daira P, Loizon E, Geloen A, et al. Oil composition of high-fat diet affects metabolic inflammation differently in connection with endotoxin receptors in mice. Am J Physiol Endocrinol Metab. 2012;302(3):E374–86.
103. Ghoshal S, Witta J, Zhong J, de Villiers W, Eckhardt E. Chylomicrons promote intestinal absorption of lipopolysaccharides. J Lipid Res. 2009;50(1):90–7.
104. Ford ES, Giles WH, Dietz WH. Prevalence of the metabolic syndrome among US adults: findings from the third National Health and Nutrition Examination Survey. JAMA. 2002;287(3):356–9.
105. Galassi A, Reynolds K, He J. Metabolic syndrome and risk of cardiovascular disease: a meta-analysis. Am J Med. 2006;119(10):812–9.
106. Yajnik CS. Fetal programming of diabetes: still so much to learn! Diabetes Care. 2010;33(5):1146–8.

Individual Food Clusters Excess and Low-Grade Inflammation in Pregnancy

2

Gabriele Piuri

Contents

2.1 Introduction

Pregnancy is a window of opportunity to prevent metabolic complications for the mother and for the unborn baby and its future development. A key role for an uneventful pregnancy is played by the immune system. Adverse effects of maternal immune adaptation to pregnancy may result from a variety of elements that interfere with the fabric of pregnancy: stress, infections, and nutritional habits stand among these. Higher maternal age at first pregnancy, obesity, and pregnancies conceived after assisted reproduction technology all pound on the natural adaptation to placental implantation and development and decidual immune trafficking.

In order to appreciate in full scale how nutrition in pregnancy can influence the process of immune tolerance, it might be useful to think from an evolutionary perspective. Nausea and vomiting in the first trimester and the cravings in the last

G. Piuri, MD, PhD
UNIMI – University of Milan, SMA LTd – Associated Medical Services, Milan, Italy
e-mail: gabriele.piuri@me.com

E. Ferrazzi, B. Sears (eds.), *Metabolic Syndrome and Complications of Pregnancy: The Potential Preventive Role of Nutrition*,
DOI 10.1007/978-3-319-16853-1_2

FIRST
TRIMESTER
= protection
• NAUSEA, VOMITING can protect pregnant women and their embryos from harmful substances in food.

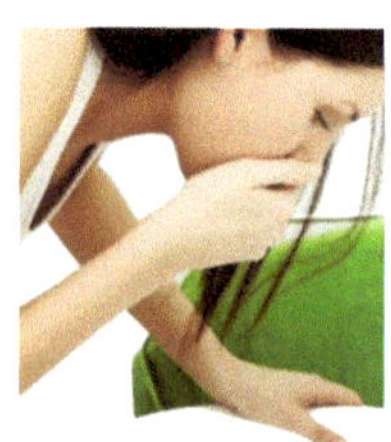

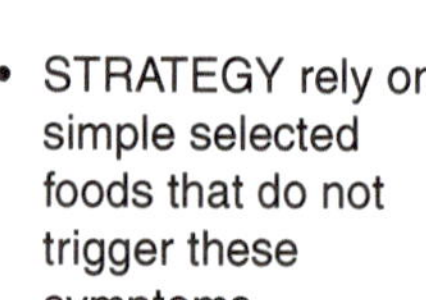

LAST
TRIMESTER
= knowledge
• CRAVINGS FOR FOODS can expose the fetus to an increased number of antigens to provide immune inprinting
• STRATEGY rely on a variety of foods within your "food culture".

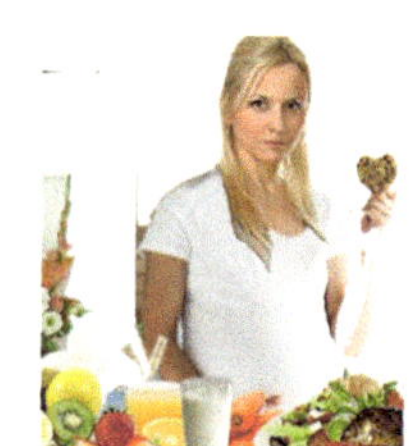

Fig. 2.1 A tentative holistic model of first trimester symptoms and third trimester eating habits

trimester of gestation might even represent the evolutionary necessity of restricting food variety during placentation and opposite to this to expose the fetus to an increasing number of antigens to educate the immune system to the alien world of food antigens (Fig. 2.1).

Food-specific immunoglobulin G (IgG) values may reflect exposure to specific antigens. The immune system does not recognize food antigens by a strong specificity, as is the case of IgE, but rather by an approach of similarity, reacting to food clusters that can reflect different eating habits of different populations. The excessive and recurrent intake of similar food clusters and the excessive production of corresponding antibodies could start a cause-effect reaction and an increase of inflammatory mediators. This mechanism, together with possible disease evolution, offers the very opportunity to avoid or to modulate the activation of inflammatory response.

2.2 Hormones and Cytokines Cross Talk

If in the past pregnancy was seen exclusively as a process to bring offspring to a stage of maturity sufficient for survival, similar to an incubation process, pregnancy is today interpreted as a complex process that determines the environment of the first stages of development and programs the genomic unfolding of fetal metabolism and its future health in adulthood.

The interaction between the mother and embryo begins with the implantation of blastocyst. The prerequisite of successful implantation depends on achieving

Table 2.1 Description of the positive or negative effects of cytokines in the process of implantation of the blastocyst [1, 4–7]

Cytokines	Effect on implantation of blastocyst	Description
IL-1	+	IL-1 stimulates endometrial IL-6 protein production, regulating the activity of this interleukin
IL-6	+	The crucial role of IL-6 during implantation is defined using IL-6-deficient mice, which show reduced implantation sites and reduced fertility. Leukemia inhibitory factor (LIF), a member of IL-6 family, is secreted from the uterus, and it is regarded as an important factor in both adhesive and invasive phases of implantation due to its anchoring effect on the trophoblast
IL-11	+	The lacking of the receptor of IL-11 brings female mice to infertility for a defective uterine response to implantation
TNF-alpha	–	TNF-alpha restricts the number of implantation sites, and TNF-alpha-induced inflammation has been shown to inhibit progesterone production in mouse ovaries, and TNF-alpha-receptor knockout mice have an increased fertility

appropriate embryo development to the blastocyst stage and at the same time the development of an endometrium that is receptive to the embryo. Implantation is a very intricate process, which is controlled by a number of complex molecules like hormones, cytokines, and growth factors and their cross talk. A network of these molecules plays a crucial role in preparing receptive endometrium and blastocyst [1]. Viviparity has many evolutionary advantages but brings in the problem of the semi-allogeneic fetus having to coexist with the mother for the duration of pregnancy. In species with hemochorial placentation, such as the human species, this problem is particularly evident as fetal trophoblast cells are extensively intermingled with maternal tissue and are directly exposed to maternal blood. Fascinating adaptations on both the fetal side and maternal side have allowed for this interaction to be redirected away from an immune rejection response, not only toward immune tolerance but, in fact, toward actively supporting reproductive success [2]. The implantation of the blastocyst is the result of a balance between inflammation and immune tolerance (Table 2.1). Inflammation-like responses are already induced by sperm and are necessary, or at least beneficial, for implantation [3]. Prominent roles for proinflammatory cytokines in implantation and decidualization have been attributed, for example, to IL-1, IL-6, and IL-11 [1, 4, 5], whereas TNF-alpha seems to have the opposite function in restricting the number of implantation sites. If progesterone is essential for pregnancy maintenance, Erlebacher et al. describe that TNF-alpha-induced inflammation has been shown to inhibit progesterone production in mouse ovaries [6] as well as TNF-alpha-receptor knockout mice have an increased fertility [7] (Fig. 2.2).

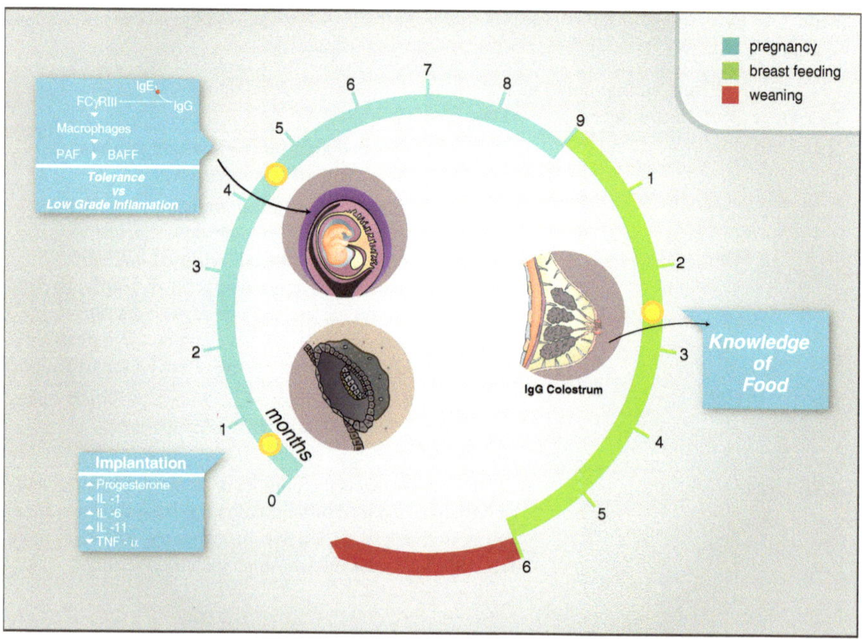

Fig. 2.2 Pregnancy expresses a balance between tolerance and inflammation with a intertalk between mother and offspring during pregnancy and breastfeeding until weaning. This process determines the environment of the first stages of development and programs the genomic unfolding of fetal metabolism and its future health in adulthood

2.3 A Balance Between Inflammation and Immune Tolerance

In a pregnancy that progresses normally, maternal adaptation to pregnancy occurs, resulting in the maintenance of fetal immune tolerance. The tolerance in pregnancy is the result of a complex network of changes that interest both the innate immune system with the rise of a new decidual natural killer population and adaptive immune system with the generation of CD4+ T reg and CD8+ T suppressor cells which together direct the production of cytokines and immunoglobulin with the aim of inducing tolerance in the maternal immune system. This successful adaptation is reflected by a well-developed immune system and a healthy child after birth [8, 9]. Adverse effects of maternal immune adaptation to pregnancy may result from or be aggravated by exogenous or endogenous threats [10]. Endogenous threats may include low amounts of maternal progesterone [11] and higher maternal age [12], whereas exogenous ones may include stress perception, infections [13] and possibly vitamin D deficiency [14], and last but not least nutritional habits. These threats may result in a failure to maintain fetal immune tolerance and may lead to pregnancy complications, such as infertility, fetal loss, preterm labor, hypertensive diseases of pregnancy, and poor fetal development. These complications may adversely affect children's health and compromise their immunity later in life.

2.4 An Evolutionary Perspective

For a better understanding of how the environment and in particular the diet of pregnant women can influence the process of immune tolerance, it is useful to look at these complex phenomena from an evolutionary perspective. Common symptoms such as nausea, vomiting, and cravings in pregnancy could also be interpreted from an evolutionary point of view. Sherman et al. find great support in the hypothesis that normal levels of nausea and vomiting in the first trimester of pregnancy (excluding hyperemesis) protect pregnant women and their embryos from harmful substances in food, particularly pathogenic microorganisms in meat products and toxins in strong-tasting plants [15]. Likewise the cravings in the last trimester of gestation might represent the evolutionary necessity of exposing the fetus to an increasing number of antigens raising immune contact with the outside world so as to provide immune imprinting.

As a matter of fact, recent studies have shown that food-specific immunoglobulin G (IgG) values may reflect exposure to a specific antigen [16, 17]. For the fetus, the immune knowledge of the outside world is achieved through the IgG produced by the mother. IgG antibodies cross the placental barrier, and colostrum and breast milk as well are rich in maternal IgG (Fig. 2.2).

IgG antibodies and in particular IgG4 are strictly connected to immune tolerance to food antigens. Protective antibodies have the capacity to modulate the response by preventing allergen binding to surface-bound IgE or inhibiting dendritic cell maturation [18]. IgG4 antibodies differ functionally from other IgG subclasses in their anti-inflammatory activity, which includes a poor ability to induce complement and cell activation because of low affinity for C1q and Fc receptors. In addition, these antibodies do not precipitate antigens owing to their ability to bind different antigens in different places [19].

IgG may be responsible for a process of attenuation of the immune response, but at the same time this class of immunoglobulins is also able to activate inflammatory processes. Studies with mouse models demonstrate two pathways of systemic anaphylaxis and activation of immune response: a classic pathway mediated by IgE, FcεRI, mast cells, histamine, and platelet-activating factor (PAF) and an alternative pathway mediated by total IgG, FcγRIII, macrophages, and PAF [20]. The importance of the alternative pathway in humans is discussed, but human IgG, IgG receptors, macrophages, mediators, and their receptors have appropriate properties to support this pathway if enough IgG and antigens are present [21].

According to this model, an excess of IgG may be responsible for the activation of an immune response even in pregnant women, altering the balance of immune tolerance to the fetus, which is a very delicate process. IgG antibodies express a previous immune contact with food. The production of IgG is linked to the "knowledge" of food and the delicate immune balance that allows alien food antigens to land on the gastrointestinal mucosa, the largest external surface of our body, two hundred times wider than our skin, to be accepted by the cross talk with the immune system and the microbiota. The excessive production of antibodies and the excessive and recurrent intake of food corresponding to these antibodies could overrun this balance and cause a reaction and an increase of inflammatory mediators (Fig. 2.2).

Western supermarket-to-fridge diet is prone to cause this unbalance: excess of refined carbohydrates, excess of long-chain saturated omega-6 fatty acids, excess of cholesterol, excess of proteins from red meat and dairy products, low insufficient consumptions of veggies and fruit, absence or poor consumption of freshly prepared food, absent or insufficient consumption of natural antioxidants and anti-inflammatory spices, iterative quasi-constant food items in the diet, and absence of seasonality in food consumption. All these factors conjure to determine excessive clusters of antibodies against food antigen clusters in parallel with unbalanced composition of the microbiota devoid of natural prebiotic (fibers) environment, whose role might even be overturned from an anti-inflammatory partner of dendritic cells of the intestinal mucosa into an aggressive bunch of proinflammatory bacteria.

2.5 BAFF and PAF, Two Cytokines at the Root of Maternal and Fetal Health

One of the main effectors of the inflammatory pathway supported by an excess of IgG is PAF (platelet-activating factor, also known as PAF-acether or AGEPC (acetyl-glyceryl-ether-phosphorylcholine)). PAF is a potent phospholipid activator and mediator of many immune functions, including platelet aggregation and degranulation, inflammation, and anaphylaxis. It is also active in vascular permeability, the oxidative processes, and chemotaxis.

In the chain of activation of the inflammatory response to IgG for food, it is essential to mention a second proinflammatory cytokine, called BAFF (B-cell-activating factor). BAFF and PAF have already been linked in nonatopic subjects to food reactions [22], and many studies suggest that BAFF could probably be one of the cornerstones of IgG pathway of immune reaction to food. A recent observational study by our group found a highly significant correlation between PAF and BAFF values in all three trimesters of pregnancy [23] in nonobese pregnant women with uneventful pregnancies. BAFF is a member of the TNF superfamily and an important regulator of peripheral B-cell survival and immunoglobulin class-switch recombination.

These properties of PAF and BAFF probably allow the use of any of these two molecules as a marker of inflammation in pregnancy and as a marker of the role of the IgG pathway in immune reaction. These findings are part of a larger research on immune system adaptation in pregnancy and their relation with the production of specific IgG for food, the enteric immune system, and the accelerated inflammation in pregnancy of women at risk of metabolic syndrome.

The excessive production of IgG associated with unbalanced nutrition may eventually generate an increase in low-grade inflammation through the activation of a pathway that involves IgG, PAF, and BAFF, probably. Future investigations should study the possible risks of immune response of the mother against the placenta. These changes in the levels of maternal inflammation may have an influence on the long-term health of the offspring. As mentioned previously, the increased levels of inflammatory cytokines like TNF-alpha reduce the maternal capacity to tolerate the trophoblast invasion and the production of progesterone and its effectiveness in the maintenance of pregnancy.

Table 2.2 Description of the five great food clusters in Italian population [24, 25]

Great food clusters	Description
Nickel	This group consists of foods with higher concentration of nickel salts such as tomatoes, kiwi, peanuts, almonds, buckwheat, and so on
Wheat	This great food cluster consists of wheat and related grains such as Kamut, barley, spelt and in general grains with gluten. Interestingly this group is part of the great food cluster of nickel
Milk	This cluster contains dairy products such as cow and goat milk as well as parmesan cheese, mozzarella cheese, and ricotta cheese
Yeasts	This group is about yeasts such as *Candida albicans* and *Saccharomyces cerevisiae* and contains also mushrooms. This group is probably connected with fermented foods
Natural salicylates	In this cluster, there are foods with higher concentration of natural salicylates such as honey, tea, courgette, orange, and so on

2.6 The Connection Between IgG for Food and Inflammation

A brief summary of a recent work conducted by our group could help sketch the connection between IgG and inflammatory responses [24, 25]. Specific IgG antibodies against 44 common food antigens were measured in sera of 11,488 Italian patients self-selected for gastrointestinal symptoms related to food reaction. Allergies, that is, IgE-mediated reactions, were not included.

In the study, we used an unsupervised hierarchical clustering algorithm to explore varying degrees of similarity among food antigens. The algorithm initially had 44 clusters (one for each food antigen) and then gradually grouped them together as a function of their similarities. The algorithm requires a notion of similarity between individual food antigens being clustered and between clusters. The algorithm stops when all food antigens belong to the same cluster.

We identified five great food clusters (Table 2.2). The first group consists of foods with higher concentration of nickel salts such as tomatoes, kiwi, peanuts, almonds, buckwheat, and so on. Within this group, it is possible to identify the second cluster that includes wheat and related grains such as Kamut, barley, spelt, etc. The third group contains dairy products starting from cow and goat milk as well as parmesan cheese, mozzarella cheese, and ricotta cheese. The fourth group gathers yeasts such as *Candida albicans* and *Saccharomyces cerevisiae* and contains also porcini mushrooms and champignon mushrooms. This cluster is probably connected with fermented foods. In the fifth group, less homogeneous contains foods with the higher concentration of natural salicylates: products such as honey, tea, courgette, orange, and so on.

The distribution of food in the different food groups most likely reflects different eating habits of the population. Presumably we can expect to identify different groups in different ethnic groups in accordance with the particular eating habits of each population.

In the Italian cuisine, which has wheat as a reference cereal, a high consumption of dairy products and fermented products (like bread and pizza), and higher concentrations of nickel- and salicylate-containing products, the great food groups are wheat, fermented products, nickel-containing foods, dairy products, and foods with higher content of natural salicylates. Instead, we can imagine that in the Japanese population the major food groups are rice, fish, soy, and also in this case fermented products.

As mentioned before, the levels of IgG against foods reflect exposure to foods, and the immune system recognizes foods by IgG not with a strong specificity, as is the case for IgE, but rather by an approach of similarity. This, on the one hand, determines a greater capacity to recognize foods and maintain tolerance and, on the other hand, determines the possibility of inducing inflammation not only with foods that are eaten more frequently but also with foods that the immune system recognizes as similar to those.

2.7 Food Personal Profile for a Balanced Nutrition During Pregnancy

These concepts and these findings altogether allow us to understand the importance of investigating antigen recognition pathways by the immune system and derive from this knowledge, albeit still incomplete, a proper nutritional approach for pregnant women [26]. IgG production represents the expression of the process – developed by millions of years of evolution started a long time before the definition of the current structure of our immune system – through which mammalians have learned to estimate the makeup of a specific food being introduced into the body for energy purposes, to understand if that food is suitable to get such an intimate contact with the organism as the alimentary one.

Nowadays, the evolution of science is leading toward a very important step into the understanding of events linked to nutrition and food-related inflammation. From the old concept of "food intolerances," no longer scientifically accepted, we are finally moving toward the understanding of the meaning of inflammatory food-related reactions, thanks to the ability of measuring and monitoring the levels of cytokines (inflammatory and signaling molecules) and of understanding the nutritional personal profile, upon which it is possible to define specific nutritional changes able to modulate inflammation.

Many studies already suggest that increasing food diversity in infancy reduces the risk of asthma and allergies in childhood [27]. In an interesting way, Nwaru et al. [28] noted that by 3 and 4 months of age, food diversity was not associated with any of the allergic end points. By 6 months of age, less food diversity was associated with increased risk of allergic rhinitis but not with the other end points. By 12 months of age, less food diversity was associated with increased risk of any asthma, atopic asthma, wheeze, and allergic rhinitis. This discrepancy in the results compared to the age of the child can be justified by the fact that probably in the first 3–4 months of life, the mother imprinting on the immune system of the unborn child is still determinant and it would be more useful to investigate maternal food variability. The increased variability in maternal food has never been considered either, and indeed in clinical practice for a long time, it is recommended to pregnant women to eliminate from their diet foods more allergenic with the result of further reduction of food variability. Although maternal avoidance of suspected allergenic foods during pregnancy and lactation has been perceived as a primary prevention strategy for the development of allergies in childhood, this strategy has not been effective thus far, and the recommendation on maternal dietary avoidance is now subject to change, and studies generally have not supported a protective effect of a maternal exclusion diet (including the exclusion of cow milk and eggs) during pregnancy on the development of atopic disease in infants [29]. Opposite to this, the increased variability of food in the maternal diet could contribute positively to the tolerance of the fetus. A repetitive diet is likely to lead to a higher production of IgG antibodies to food in response to major intake of foods belonging to the same great food group, and the subsequent continuous consumption of these foods is likely to activate the IgG-mediated pathway with the enhancement of inflammation and, consequently, reduction of the ability of immune tolerance of the mother.

2.8 Varying Diet for the Best Outcome

From a nutritional point of view, during pregnancy, it is important to promote as much as possible the variability of food, counseling pregnant women to vary as much as possible the foods on their table, for instance, a variety of cereals instead of a wheat-based diet and a variety of protein sources from fish, poultry, vegetables, and nuts instead of the red meat and cheese fast-food choice, and exploit the seasonality of fruit and vegetables around the 9 months of pregnancy. A broader contact antigenic food leads to the production of specific IgG for a large number of different foods without a large absolute prevalence for a specific food group. In this way it could be possible to avoid the activation of inflammatory response. If the consumption of a specific cluster of foods becomes excessive, the production of PAF and BAFF in response of IgG rises with the resulting increased level of inflammation. IgG is also reflected in the maintenance of food tolerance, and a wider and more varied contact with food is fundamental, especially in the third trimester, for a greater and better immune imprinting for the unborn child. In addition to this, the reduction of inflammation from food brings, on a clinical level, a reduction of disorders, major and minor, typical of the pregnancy from constipation to bloating, from the modulation of excessive weight gain to risk prevention of gestational diabetes and hypertensive diseases, conditions which are more and more recognized as a state of inflammation. In clinical practice, the determination of specific IgG to foods and the definition of a food personal profile, according to the logic of the great food clusters designed for each population, can be of great help in setting up a weekly rotation diet that does not point to the complete elimination of the food belonging to the food groups, but rather to a rebalancing of the immune contact with food with the aim of starting infant weaning from maternal feeding habits.

References

1. Singh M, Chaudhry P, Asselin E. Bridging endometrial receptivity and implantation: network of hormones, cytokines, and growth factors. J Endocrinol. 2011;210:5–14. doi:10.1530/JOE-10-0461.
2. Hemberger M. Immune balance at the foeto-maternal interface as the fulcrum of reproductive success. J Reprod Immunol. 2013;97:36–42. doi:10.1016/j.jri.2012.10.006.
3. McMaster MT, Newton RC, Dey SK, Andrews GK. Activation and distribution of inflammatory cells in the mouse uterus during the preimplantation period. J Immunol. 1992;148:1699–705.
4. Robb L, Li R, Hartley L, et al. Infertility in female mice lacking the receptor for interleukin 11 is due to a defective uterine response to implantation. Nat Med. 1998;4:303–8.
5. Stewart CL, Kaspar P, Brunet LJ, et al. Blastocyst implantation depends on maternal expression of leukaemia inhibitory factor. Nature. 1992;359:76–9. doi:10.1038/359076a0.
6. Erlebacher A, Zhang D, Parlow AF, Glimcher LH. Ovarian insufficiency and early pregnancy loss induced by activation of the innate immune system. J Clin Invest. 2004;114:39–48. doi:10.1172/JCI20645.
7. Cui L-L, Yang G, Pan J, Zhang C. Tumor necrosis factor α knockout increases fertility of mice. Theriogenology. 2011;75:867–76. doi:10.1016/j.theriogenology.2010.10.029.
8. Norwitz ER, Schust DJ, Fisher SJ. Implantation and the survival of early pregnancy. N Engl J Med. 2001;345:1400–8. doi:10.1056/NEJMra000763.
9. Solano ME, Jago C, Pincus MK, Arck PC. Highway to health; or how prenatal factors determine disease risks in the later life of the offspring. J Reprod Immunol. 2011;90:3–8. doi:10.1016/j.jri.2011.01.023.
10. Arck PC, Hecher K. Fetomaternal immune cross-talk and its consequences for maternal and offspring's health. Nat Med. 2013;19:548–56. doi:10.1038/nm.3160.
11. Hartwig IRV, Pincus MK, Diemert A, et al. Sex-specific effect of first-trimester maternal progesterone on birthweight. Hum Reprod. 2013;28:77–86. doi:10.1093/humrep/des367.
12. Arck PC, Rücke M, Rose M, et al. Early risk factors for miscarriage: a prospective cohort study in pregnant women. Reprod Biomed Online. 2008;17:101–13.
13. Bach J-F. The effect of infections on susceptibility to autoimmune and allergic diseases. N Engl J Med. 2002;347:911–20. doi:10.1056/NEJMra020100.
14. Brannon PM. Vitamin D and adverse pregnancy outcomes: beyond bone health and growth. Proc Nutr Soc. 2012;71:205–12. doi:10.1017/S0029665111003399.
15. Sherman PW, Flaxman SM. Nausea and vomiting of pregnancy in an evolutionary perspective. Am J Obstet Gynecol. 2002;186:S190–7. doi:10.1067/mob.2002.122593.
16. Ligaarden SC, Lydersen S, Farup PG. IgG and IgG4 antibodies in subjects with irritable bowel syndrome: a case control study in the general population. BMC Gastroenterol. 2012;12:166. doi:10.1186/1471-230X-12-166.
17. Speciani AF, Piuri G, Ferrazzi E. IgG levels to food correlate with nutritional exposure to food antigens but a methodological weakness of this research prevents the recognition of yeast-related foods as a possible cause of Irritable Bowel Syndrome (IBS). Comment to IgG and IgG4 antibodies in subjects with irritable bowel syndrome: a case control study in the general population. Published on 2014/02/20. BMC Gastroenterol. 2012;12:166. doi:10.1186/1471-230X-12-166. http://www.biomedcentral.com/1471-230X/12/166/comments
18. Wisniewski J, Agrawal R, Woodfolk JA. Mechanisms of tolerance induction in allergic disease: integrating current and emerging concepts. Clin Exp Allergy. 2013;43:164–76. doi:10.1111/cea.12016.
19. van der Neut Kolfschoten M, Schuurman J, Losen M, et al. Anti-inflammatory activity of human IgG4 antibodies by dynamic Fab arm exchange. Science. 2007;317:1554–7. doi:10.1126/science.1144603.
20. Finkelman FD. Anaphylaxis: lessons from mouse models. J Allergy Clin Immunol. 2007;120:506–15– quiz 516–7. doi: 10.1016/j.jaci.2007.07.033.
21. Khodoun MV, Strait R, Armstrong L, et al. Identification of markers that distinguish IgE- from IgG-mediated anaphylaxis. Proc Natl Acad Sci U S A. 2011;108:12413–8. doi:10.1073/pnas.1105695108.

22. Piuri G, Soriano J, Speciani MC, Speciani AF. B cell activating factor (BAFF) and platelet activating factor (PAF) could both be markers of non-IgE-mediated reactions. Clin Transl Allergy. 2013;3:O5. doi:10.1016/j.jaci.2007.07.033.
23. Piuri G, Bulfoni C, Mastricci AL, Speciani AF, Ferrazzi E. Two innovative inflammation biomarkers for the measurement of inflammation in pregnancy. Paper presented at the 24th European Congress of Perinatal Medicie (ECPM), Florence, 4–7 June 2014.
24. Speciani AF, Soriano J, Speciani MC, Piuri G. Five great food clusters of specific IgG for 44 common food antigens. A new approach to the epidemiology of food allergy. Clin Transl Allergy. 2013;3:P67. doi:10.1186/2045-7022-3-S3-P67.
25. Speciani AF, Piuri G, Soriano J, Ferrazzi E. A larger study of food-related IgG confirms the possible new epidemiological approach to non-IgE-mediated reactions and suggests five great food clusters. Paper presented at 3rd Food Allergy and Anaphylaxis Meeting (FAAM), Dublin, 9–11 Oct 2014.
26. Speciani AF. Measuring biomarkers for an innovative food personal profile. Lesson at 3rd international congress science in nutrition "anti-inflammation, quality of life and sport in nutrition." Milan 14–15 March 2014.
27. Roduit C, Frei R, Depner M, et al. Increased food diversity in the first year of life is inversely associated with allergic diseases. J Allergy Clin Immunol. 2014;133:1056–64. doi:10.1016/j.jaci.2013.12.1044.
28. Nwaru BI, Takkinen H-M, Kaila M, et al. Food diversity in infancy and the risk of childhood asthma and allergies. J Allergy Clin Immunol. 2014;133:1084–91. doi:10.1016/j.jaci.2013.12.1069.
29. Greer FR, Sicherer SH, Burks AW, Committee on Nutrition and Section on Allergy and Immunology. Effects of Early Nutritional Interventions on the Development of Atopic Disease in Infants and Children: The Role of Maternal Dietary Restriction, Breastfeeding, Timing of Introduction of Complementary Foods, and Hydrolyzed Formulas. Pediatrics. 2008;121:183–91. doi:10.1542/peds. 2007-3022.

3 The Effect of Diet and Probiotics on the Human Gut Microbiome

Lorenzo Morelli and Maria Luisa Callegari

Contents

3.1 Introduction

The term microbiome defines the overall amount of microbial genes harbored by the microbiota, the microbes inhabiting the human intestinal tract [1]. Probiotics, on the other hand, will be defined according to the FAO/WHO documents [2] as recently revised by an ISAPP consensus meeting [3]. Recent genomic studies are clearly suggesting that microbiota and microbiome are playing a role in a large number of physiological functions, far beyond the digestive ones. Just as examples it could be worthwhile to remind that the microbial community structure and its genomic composition strongly contribute to the relevant functions of the human host such as resistance to the infections, also influencing the immune system activity [4–6] which in turn modulates the composition of the gut microbiota (Fig. 3.1). Recent advances in neurosciences have also shown the relevant role of the so-called gut-brain axis, meaning that the bacterial load of the gut has a deep impact on the nervous system [7]. The role of gut bacteria and their genomic structure is then relevant for the human health and well-being; it seems worthwhile to elucidate which are the

L. Morelli (✉) • M.L. Callegari
Istituto Microbiologia, Facoltà di Scienze agrarie, alimentari e ambientali, Università Cattolica, Piacenza, Cremona, Italy
e-mail: lorenzo.morelli@unicatt.it

E. Ferrazzi, B. Sears (eds.), *Metabolic Syndrome and Complications of Pregnancy: The Potential Preventive Role of Nutrition*,
DOI 10.1007/978-3-319-16853-1_3

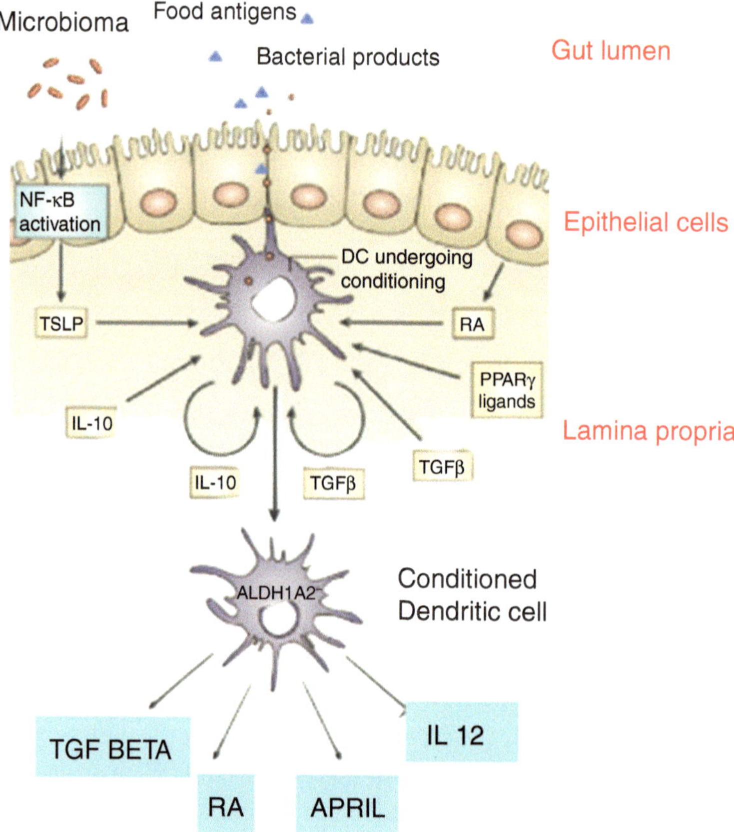

Fig. 3.1 Under eubiotic environment the intestinal endothelial cells secrete mucins and cytokines, which conditions dendritic cells to promote an antiinflammatory cellular and mediators to dampen effector responses

factors with a role in shaping the microbiota and microbiome composition. The composition of microbiota in terms of species is indeed influenced by several internal and external factors such as the initial intestinal colonization occurred at birth, the genetic background of the host, the antibiotic treatments, and, on top of that, diet (Fig. 3.2). As regards pregnancy the scenario is still under debate. A recent paper has demonstrated that gut microbiota is subjected to a dramatic remodeling over the course of pregnancy [8]. Authors reported that the first trimester is characterized by a gut microbiota composition very similar to those of healthy nonpregnant control group, whereas analysis of pregnant stool samples collected at the third trimester showed an enrichment in Proteobacteria and Actinobacteria, similar to the situation detected in inflammatory bowel disease and obesity. Furthermore, the number of health-related bacteria such as *Faecalibacterium*, a butyrate-producing bacterium with antiinflammatory effects, is less abundant in this trimester. However, these results are in contrast with those reported later by other studies [9, 10] in which little

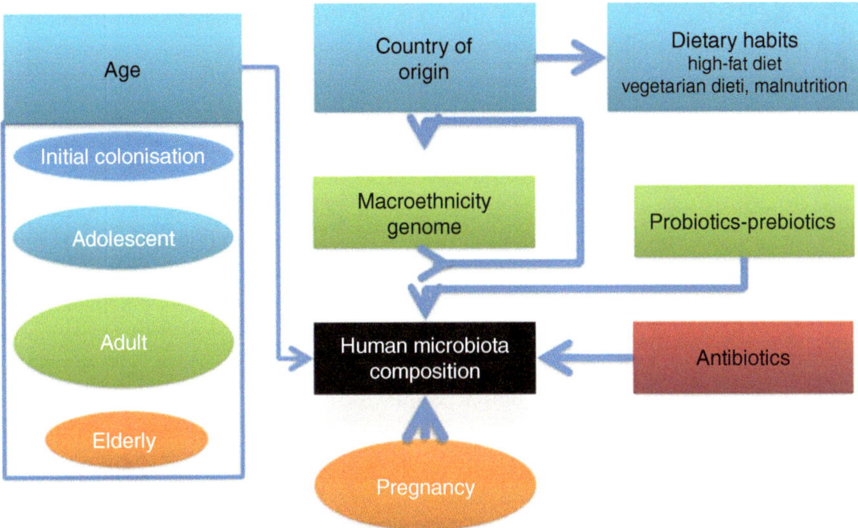

Fig. 3.2 Factors influencing the human microbiota composition

or no modifications of the fecal microbiota composition were reported during early and late pregnancy.

In the following sections, we will review some of the most recently published papers on the impact of diet on microbiota/microbiome structure, focusing on data obtained in humans.

3.2 Diet and Microbiota

The mutualistic relationship between the host and its microbiota leads to the production of beneficial microbial metabolites that contribute to the fitness of the host. The latter factor can influence the gut environment modifying the transit time, the pH, and, as regards the distal part, the richness in terms of carbohydrates, proteins, and fats related to food intake. These macronutrients are directly degraded by the host enzymes, while the degradation of plant structural polysaccharides, contained in the diet, is carried out by microbial enzymes encoded by specific microbial genes above all those of the colonic microbiota. Fermentation of these complex polysaccharides produces short-chain fatty acids such as butyrate, which represents one of the major energy sources for colonocytes, or propionate and acetate involved in gluconeogenesis and in lipogenesis respectively [11]. The dietary residues in the colon can represent a substrate for bacteria growth as well as the sloughed epithelial cells and mucin. The ability of bacteria to utilize different substrates may be crucial for the final microbiota composition, which is the final result of complex selection mechanisms of ingested bacteria.

Observational studies have shown that long-term diet influences the structure and activity of the trillions of microorganisms residing in the human gut, and it was also suggested that it could be possible to divide the human beings into three major groups according to their bacterial content.

Indeed, each of them is characterized by the dominance of *Bacteroides*, *Prevotella*, and *Ruminococcus*, respectively [12]. It is still unknown which environmental or genetic factors are involved in this clustering although it appears independent of nationality, sex, age, or other host properties. Wu et al. [13] described that dietary effects primarily distinguish the Prevotella enterotype (carbohydrate) from the Bacteroides enterotype (high protein and fat), and in this study a short diet intervention was insufficient for switching between the two groups. Moreover, it is important to underline that the enterotype hypothesis is a topic of debate. Some microbial groups exhibit high stability, but important quantitative fluctuation can be detected among bacteria that comprise the intestinal microbiota. These fluctuations move around an individual microbiota composition, and they can be due to variation of external environmental factors such as diet or drug treatments. When these species fluctuations do not exceed the limits that characterize a specific enterotype, but they remain at the borderline, no changes in enterotype can be detected.

This could be the reason of some contradictory reports. Indeed, recent data [14] described how even short-term intervention can modify gut microbiota composition: red meat based diets increase the prevalence of *Alistipes*, *Bilophila*, and *Bacteroides*, while decreasing the abundance of Firmicutes (plant polysaccharide metabolizers). The enterotype clusterization was not taken in consideration, and maybe this could justify the divergent results.

3.3 Microbiome, Macro Ethnicities, and Local Diets

A very interesting approach for evaluating the effect of diet on gut microbiota composition was adopted in a publication [15] in which the gut microbiota composition of children from a rural area in Africa (Burkina Faso) and Italian children were compared. The European subjects eat a typical Western diet (rich in proteins and fats), whereas the African children eat carbohydrate-rich diets with a very low supply of animal proteins. *Xylanibacter*, *Prevotella*, *Butyrivibrio*, and *Treponema* were distinctive of Burkina Faso children, whereas European children microbiota were characterized by the abundance of Firmicutes and Proteobacteria. The African children harbored microbiota in which it was possible to detect bacteria able to use xylan, xylose, and carboxymethylcellulose. It is possible to suppose that these polysaccharide-degrading bacteria are selected by the diet and are the responsible of short-chain fatty acids production using plant polysaccharides allowing the host to maximize the energy intake from the diet.

These results strongly indicate the important role of diet in shaping the microbial composition of the gut and revealed specific adaptations of gut microbiota communities to the lifestyles of the host. Confirmation of this founding is provided by a recent publication in which the gut microbiota composition of two different rural farming groups living in Tanzania (the Hadza population) was analyzed [16]. The gut microbiota of African voluntaries resulted in enriched *Prevotella*, *Treponema*, and unclassified Bacteroidetes. Interesting is the differences found comparing woman and men gut microbiota composition; indeed *Treponema* was more abundant in woman, whereas *Eubacterium* and *Blautia* were more represented in men. Women normally have a vegetarian diet, while men have the opportunity to eat meat and honey. Comparing the results of Hadza subjects with those obtained from the Italian control group, the total absence of *Bifidobacterium* was highlighted. Authors supposed that the postweaning in this population could explain this lack of bifidobacteria, while Western adult diet includes also meat, milk, and dairy products.

It is necessary to underline that Burkina Faso lifestyle differs from that of Tanzanian subjects overall in terms of diet; indeed around 70 % of Hadza diet is represented by plant foods (tubers, fruits, and vegetables) and the remaining 30 % by meat derived from hunting. Concerning Burkina Faso, children's diet [15] consists mainly of cereals, legumes, and vegetables; therefore, the content of carbohydrate, fiber, and vegetable protein is very high. Comparison between these populations and the European subjects showed that microbial composition reflects differences between herbivorous and carnivorous mammals, and for this reason it became relevant, for human's well-being, to try to modulate the composition of the bacterial population inhabiting the gastrointestinal tract. One of the key mechanisms to maintain gut health is the consumption of diet rich in nondigestible carbohydrates and poor in proteins and fats [17].

Alterations of the gut microbiota with the consequent dysregulation of interactions between host and microbial community have been described as implicated in a number of intestinal disorders and illnesses [18, 19].

3.4 Gut Microbiota and Probiotics

The rationale of probiotic use is to introduce microorganisms with specific and beneficial functions in order to obtain positive effects on the health of the host. Indeed the definition of probiotic is "live microorganisms which, when administered in adequate amounts, confer a health benefit to the host" [2].

The first condition to satisfy is to administer living probiotic cells. We know that sonicates, particles of dead probiotics, can stimulate the immune system, yet only viable bacteria cells may be able to reproduce and exercise a longer beneficial effect on the bacterial communities of the gastrointestinal tract. To achieve this goal, it is essential that probiotic bacteria pass beyond the gastric and ileal tract and reach in a viable form the large intestine. The second important aspect to be evaluated is the administration of an effective dose. This is a very unsettled frontier. Gut's pH, bile salt, and trilions resident microbiota outnumber low dose, short term supplementation of probiotics. All these factors play against the chances of an adequate impact on the microbial ecology of gut environment. Large doses, by hundred billions of viable cells for long periods of supplementation are required to provide beneficial effects.

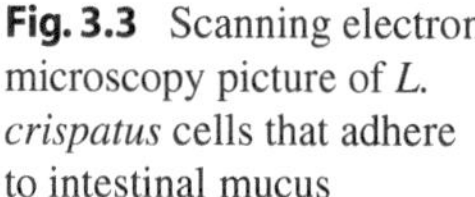

Fig. 3.3 Scanning electron microscopy picture of *L. crispatus* cells that adhere to intestinal mucus

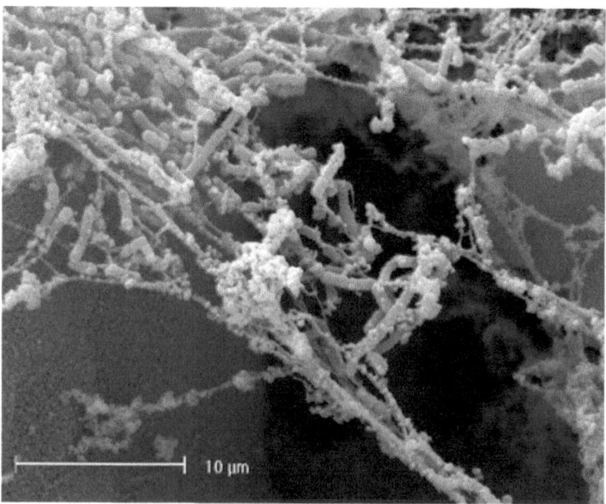

The definition of the effective dose is not easily defined depending on several factors, and it depends on the strain-specific feature, the chemical and physical characteristics of the vector food, and the host-related factors as well as the desired target effect [20].

The guidelines of the French Agency for Food Safety dedicated to probiotics and prebiotics [21] suggest that the number of viable cells in the gut present after consumption of product containing probiotic must be more than or equal to 10^6 CFU/ml in the small intestine and 10^8 CFU/g in the colon, even if the same agency acknowledges that "the scientific basis for these statements is relatively weak."

One of the more important concepts that need to be taken into consideration is that a probiotic must be a microorganism or a combination of microorganisms taxonomically well defined. The identification at species and strain level is very relevant for different reasons. The correct identification of a probiotic as a member of a recognized and well-known species corresponds to the evaluation of its safety. Indeed the bacterial species used as probiotic have a very long history of use in food, and this contributed to define them as safe for human consumption. On the other hand, the identification at strain level is relevant since the beneficial properties are strain specific that means the health benefit assigned to one strain is not necessarily applicable to another strain even belonging to the same species.

Adhesion to the intestinal mucosa is considered a prerequisite for bacterial colonization, and this event is important for the immune system modulation and for the antagonistic action of probiotic against pathogens. These adhesion properties can be mediated by secreted bacterial proteins that are able to interact directly with mucus (Figs. 3.3 and 3.4).

As already mentioned, probiotics have also important involvement concerning the immune response in enhancing signaling in host cells reducing the inflammatory response, delivering antiinflammatory molecules, and reducing the production of inflammatory substances [22–24]. Unfortunately, to demonstrate the positive effect of

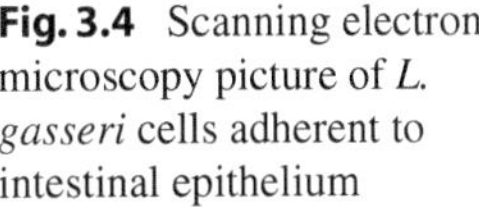

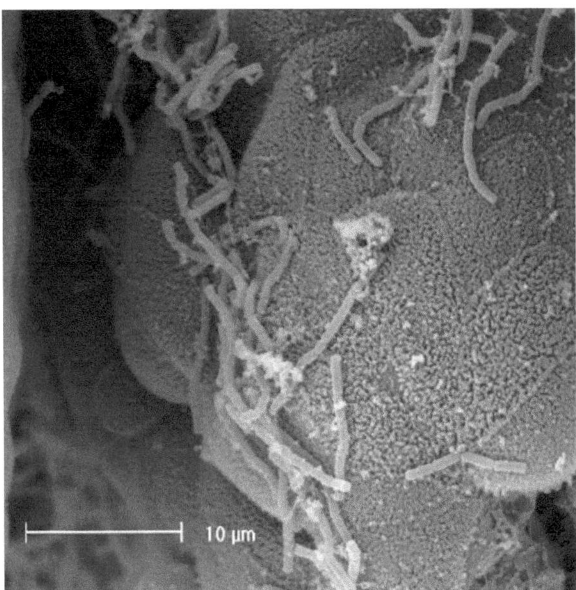

Fig. 3.4 Scanning electron microscopy picture of *L. gasseri* cells adherent to intestinal epithelium

probiotic bacteria intake in healthy adults is extremely difficult. One of the problems to face is the stability, in healthy adults, of the complex composition of the gut microbiota which unlikely can be altered by the introduction of a single bacterial strain and even a combination of more strains. For this reason the ecological use of probiotic should be held when specific conditions of altered microbiota occur as a consequence of inflammatory diseases or antibiotic treatments. In these conditions there are strong evidences concerning the benefit of probiotic administration [25–27].

However, it has been described that probiotic strains can replace other indigenous strains even if administered to healthy individuals with a stable microbiota. In these cases the introduction of probiotic strains did not alter the overall microbiota composition, but it was possible to obtain its beneficial modulation. This replacement effect was demonstrated in a study [28] in which a *L. paracasei* strain was administered to seven healthy subjects; after 15 days of administration no statistically significant difference in the total amount of lactobacilli was found, but the probiotic strain represented 66.6 % of the total facultative heterofermentative colonies isolated from fecal stools. The probiotic strain in these cases replaced the lactobacilli originally present in the fecal samples of the treated volunteers. Another aspect in which the administration of probiotic to healthy subjects could be very interesting is the impact of probiotics on intestinal transit. This is an increasingly important measure of well-being because of the high incidence of constipation particularly in the elderly women and overall in pregnant women. The probiotic administration can represent an efficacious and safe treatment well suited for these groups of individuals. The administration of probiotics for 4 weeks to 20 young pregnant women with functional constipation improved the defecation frequency [29] that significantly increased from 3.1 at baseline to 6.7 at the end of the trial. Also some secondary effects normally correlated with constipation such as stool consistency, sensation of incomplete evacuation, or abdominal pain were reduced, and no side effects were reported.

The common cold very common especially in winter is responsible for many absences at school and from job and causes important economic losses. In a recent meta-analysis [30] in which ten studies were taken in consideration, the effect of probiotics on the prevention of the common cold was evaluated. The total number of participant was 2,894 participants, including 1,588 in the probiotic group and 1,306 in the control group. The relative risk used to evaluate the efficacy of probiotic intake was of 0.92 for the control group whereas 0.87 for the group receiving probiotics. The authors report that probiotics have a marginal effect on the prevention of the common cold, but it is important to underline that probiotics do not correspond to a medication, and no side effects are related to their administration as it sometimes happens for drug treatments.

Probiotics might find another area of application in healthy individuals. Consistent data show that they can be used to treat babies suffering of infantile colics in the first months of life [31]. The cause of infantile colic still remains unclear, but this syndrome is observed with the same frequency in male and female babies (10–30 %), and is not associated with different feeding patterns. In 2007, it was described that *L. reuteri* ATCC 77530 was able to reduce infantile colic in the 95 % of the infants belonging to the supplemented group compared with only the 7 % reduction in the control group; unfortunately these interesting results were obtained in an unblinded study, where simethicone had been used as control intervention [31]. Six years later, the anti-colic properties of another *L. reuteri* strain, the DSM 17938, was evaluate in a double-blind study in exclusively and predominantly (>50 %) breastfed infants [32]. The primary outcome measures were the percentage of children achieving a reduction in the daily crying episodes (50 %) and the duration of crying at different sampling times. The administration of *L. reuteri* DSM 17938 gives beneficial effects to breastfed infants with infantile colic; indeed the crying time was significantly reduced as well as the duration of crying in this group compared with the control one. Even if some pediatricians consider insufficient the scientific evidence for recommending the use of probiotic to relieve colic, this application can represent a very interesting aspect of the use of probiotic in healthy subjects encouraged by these recent data that support the efficacy of the treatment [32].

Pregnancy induces dramatic immune and physiological changes finalized to accommodate fetus development. Many efforts are done to prevent maternal mortality and morbidity and enhance unborn health trying to prevent specific complications of pregnancy.

Supplementation with probiotics can be used as an alternative strategy to prevent intestinal dysbiosis, mucosal immunity, urogenital infections in pregnancy, and reduction of allergies in babies. Few clinical trials concerning probiotic supplementation in pregnancy are available, and they are focused on complication such as gestational diabetes mellitus, weight gain, preterm delivery, and preeclampsia (Table 3.1).

The maternal obesity and its subsequent health outcomes can impact public health, and prevention strategies are required. Overweight pregnant women provide an excess of energy to the fetus, which can in turn be overweight with risk of

Table 3.1 Primary and secondary outcomes of clinical trials concerning probiotic supplementation in pregnancy

Primary outcomes	Secondary outcomes	Strains	References
Lipid profile		*Lactobacillus rhamnosus* GG and *Bifidobacterium lactis*	[34]
Preeclampsia		*Lactobacillus rhamnosus* GG, *Bifidobacterium lactis* Bb12, and *Lactobacillus acidophilus* LA5	[35]
Gestational weight gain	*Gestational diabetes mellitus*	*Lactobacillus rhamnosus* GG and *Bifidobacterium lactis* Bb12	[33]
Gestational diabetes mellitus		*Lactobacillus rhamnosus* GG and *Bifidobacterium lactis* Bb12	[10]

complications at delivery. The overweight newborn has at risk of becoming overweight or obese adult. Strategies based on balanced diet and physical activity showed limited success, and for this reason alternative approaches are urgently needed. Overweight or obese women already have an altered gut microbiome, and these differences remain in pregnancy. Only few clinical trials of probiotic supplementation in pregnancy that focus on reported gestational weight gain and gestational diabetes mellitus are available.

A randomized trial on 256 Finnish pregnant women showed that a combination of diet and probiotic intervention with *L. rhamnosus* GG and *Bifidobacterium lactis* Bb12 reduced the risk of elevated concentrations of plasma glucose during and after pregnancy [10].

The only randomized placebo-controlled trial concerning probiotic efficacy in reducing the gestational weight gain consisted of 256 women who were enrolled in function of their prepregnancy body mass index.

Probiotic supplementation was not able to interfere with gestational weight gain or postpartum weight retention, but the postpartum waist circumference was decreased in the probiotic-treated group compared with the control group. Moreover a statistically significant reduction of gestational diabetes mellitus was noted in the probiotic-supplemented group compared with the control group [33].

Probiotics can represent a potential safe strategy for the prevention of pregnancy complications and adverse outcomes related to maternal metabolism. Randomized controlled trials are urgently required to provide more data for the role of probiotic in the prevention of metabolic disorders, such as overweight and obesity in pregnant women.

References

1. Ley RE, Lozupone CA, Hamady M, Knight R, Gordon JI. Worlds within worlds: evolution of the vertebrate gut microbiota. Nat Rev Microbiol. 2008;6:776–88.
2. FAO/WHO Expert Consultation. Health and nutritional properties of probiotics in food including powder milk with live lactic acid bacteria. Geneva: World Health Organization; 2001.

3. Hill C, Guarner F, Reid G, Gibson GR, Merenstein DJ, Pot B, Morelli L, Canani RB, Flint HJ, Salminen S, Calder PC, Sanders ME. Expert consensus document. The International Scientific Association for Probiotics and Prebiotics consensus statement on the scope and appropriate use of the term probiotic. Nat Rev Gastroenterol Hepatol. 2014;11:506–14.
4. Nicholson JK, Holmes E, Kinross J, Burcelin R, Gibson G, Jia W, Pettersson S. Host-gut microbiota metabolic interactions. Science. 2012;336(6086):1262–7.
5. Hooper LV, Littman DR, Macpherson AJ. Interactions between the microbiota and the immune system. Science. 2012;336(6086):1268–73.
6. Wardwell LH, Huttenhower C, Garrett WS. Current concepts of the intestinal microbiota and the pathogenesis of infection. Curr Infect Dis Rep. 2011;13(1):28–34.
7. Stilling RM, Bordenstein SR, Dinan TG, Cryan JF. Friends with social benefits: host-microbe interactions as a driver of brain evolution and development? Front Cell Infect Microbiol. 2014;4:147.
8. Koren O, Goodrich JK, Cullender TC, Spor A, Laitinen K, Bäckhed HK, Gonzalez A, Werner JJ, Angenent LT, Knight R, Bäckhed F, Isolauri E, Salminen S, Ley RE. Host remodeling of the gut microbiome and metabolic changes during pregnancy. Cell. 2012;150:470–80.
9. Jost T, Lacroix C, Braegger C, Chassard C. Stability of the maternal gut microbiota during late pregnancy and early lactation. Curr Microbiol. 2014;68:419–27.
10. Laitinen K, Poussa T, Isolauri E. Nutrition, allergy, mucosal immunology and intestinal microbiota group probiotics and dietary counselling contribute to glucose regulation during and after pregnancy: a randomised controlled trial. Br J Nutr. 2009;101:1679–87.
11. Modi SR, Collins JJ, Relman DA. Antibiotics and the gut microbiota. J Clin Invest. 2014; 124(10):4212–8.
12. Arumugam M, Raes J, Pelletier E, Le Paslier D, Yamada T, Mende DR, Fernandes GR, Tap J, Bruls T, Batto JM, Bertalan M, Borruel N, Casellas F, Fernandez L, Gautier L, Hansen T, Hattori M, Hayashi T, Kleerebezem M, Kurokawa K, Leclerc M, Levenez F, Manichanh C, Nielsen HB, Nielsen T, Pons N, Poulain J, Qin J, Sicheritz-Ponten T, Tims S, Torrents D, Ugarte E, Zoetendal EG, Wang J, Guarner F, Pedersen O, de Vos WM, Brunak S, Doré J, MetaHIT Consortium, Antolín M, Artiguenave F, Blottiere HM, Almeida M, Brechot C, Cara C, Chervaux C, Cultrone A, Delorme C, Denariaz G, Dervyn R, Foerstner KU, Friss C, van de Guchte M, Guedon E, Haimet F, Huber W, van Hylckama-Vlieg J, Jamet A, Juste C, Kaci G, Knol J, Lakhdari O, Layec S, Le Roux K, Maguin E, Mérieux A, Melo Minardi R, M'rini C, Muller J, Oozeer R, Parkhill J, Renault P, Rescigno M, Sanchez N, Sunagawa S, Torrejon A, Turner K, Vandemeulebrouck G, Varela E, Winogradsky Y, Zeller G, Weissenbach J, Ehrlich SD, Bork P. Enterotypes of the human gut microbiome. Nature. 2011;473(7346):174–80.
13. Wu GD, Chen J, Hoffmann C, Bittinger K, Chen YY, Keilbaugh SA, Bewtra M, Knights D, Walters WA, Knight R, Sinha R, Gilroy E, Gupta K, Baldassano R, Nessel L, Li H, Bushman FD, Lewis JD. Linking long-term dietary patterns with gut microbial enterotypes. Science. 2011;334(6052):105–8.
14. David LA, Maurice CF, Carmody RN, Gootenberg DB, Button JE, Wolfe BE, Ling AV, Devlin AS, Varma Y, Fischbach MA, Biddinger SB, Dutton RJ, Turnbaugh PJ. Diet rapidly and reproducibly alters the human gut microbiome. Nature. 2014;505:559–63.
15. De Filippo C, Cavalieri D, Di Paola M, Ramazzotti M, Poullet JB, Massart S, Collini S, Pieraccini G, Lionetti P. Impact of diet in shaping gut microbiota revealed by a comparative study in children from Europe and rural Africa. Proc Natl Acad Sci U S A. 2010;107: 14691–6.
16. Schnorr SL, Candela M, Rampelli S, Centanni M, Consolandi C, Basaglia G, Turroni S, Biagi E, Peano C, Severgnini M, Fiori J, Gotti R, De Bellis G, Luiselli D, Brigidi P, Mabulla A, Marlowe F, Henry AG, Crittenden AN. Gut microbiome of the Hadza hunter-gatherers. Nat Commun. 2014;5:3654.
17. Scott KP, Gratz SW, Sheridan PO, Flint HJ, Duncan SH. The influence of diet on the gut microbiota. Pharmacol Res. 2013;69:52–60.
18. DuPont AW, DuPont HL. The intestinal microbiota and chronic disorders of the gut. Nat Rev Gastroenterol Hepatol. 2011;8:523–31.

19. Clemente JC, Ursell LK, Parfrey LW, Knight R. The impact of the gut microbiota on human health: an integrative view. Cell. 2012;148:1258–70.
20. Aureli P, Capurso L, Castellazzi AM, Clerici M, Giovannini M, Morelli L, Poli A, Pregliasco F, Salvini F, Zuccotti GV. Probiotics and health: an evidence-based review. Pharmacol Res. 2011;63:366–76.
21. Agence Française de Sécurité Sanitaire des Aliments. Effets des probiotiques et prébiotiques sur la flore et l'immunité de l'homme adulte. http://www.isapp.net/docs/AFFSAprobioticprebioticfloraimmunity05.pdf. 2005.
22. Butel MJ. Probiotics, gut microbiota and health. Med Mal Infect. 2014;44(1):1–8.
23. Villena J, Kitazawa H. Modulation of Intestinal TLR4-Inflammatory Signaling Pathways by Probiotic Microorganisms: Lessons Learned from Lactobacillus jensenii TL2937. Front Immunol. 2014;4:512.
24. Dobson A, Cotter PD, Ross RP, Hill C. Bacteriocin production: a probiotic trait? Appl Environ Microbiol. 2012;78(1):1–6.
25. Sanders ME, Guarner F, Guerrant R, Holt PR, Quigley EM, Sartor RB, Sherman PM, Mayer EA. An update on the use and investigation of probiotics in health and disease. Gut. 2013;62:787–96.
26. Goldenberg JZ, Ma SS, Saxton JD, Martzen MR, Vandvik PO, Thorlund K, Guyatt GH, Johnston BC. Probiotics for the prevention of Clostridium difficile-associated diarrhea in adults and children. Cochrane Database Syst Rev. 2013;(5):CD006095.
27. McFarland LV. Systematic review and meta-analysis of *Saccharomyces boulardii* in adult patients. World J Gastroenterol. 2010;16(18):2202–22.
28. Morelli L, Garbagna N, Rizzello F, Zonenschain D, Grossi E. In vivo association to human colon of *Lactobacillus paracasei* B21060: map from biopsies. Dig Liver Dis. 2006;38:894–8.
29. de Milliano I, Tabbers MM, van der Post JA, Benninga MA. Is a multispecies probiotic mixture effective in constipation during pregnancy? 'A pilot study'. Nutr J. 2012;11:80.
30. Kang EJ, Kim SY, Hwang IH, Ji YJ. The effect of probiotics on prevention of common cold: a meta-analysis of randomized controlled trial studies. Korean J Fam Med. 2013;34:2–10.
31. Savino F, Pelle E, Palumeri E, Oggero R, Miniero R. Lactobacillus reuteri (American Type Culture Collection Strain 55730) versus simethicone in the treatment of infantile colic: a prospective randomized study. Pediatrics. 2007;119:e124–30.
32. Szajewska H, Gyrczuk E, Horvath A. Lactobacillus reuteri DSM 17938 for the management of infantile colic in breastfed infants: a randomized, double-blind, placebo-controlled trial. J Pediatr. 2013;162:257–62.
33. Ilmonen J, Isolauri E, Poussa T, Laitinen K. Impact of dietary counselling and probiotic intervention on maternal anthropometric measurements during and after pregnancy: a randomized placebo-controlled trial. Clin Nutr. 2011;30:156–64.
34. Hoppu U, Isolauri E, Koskinen P, Laitinen K. Maternal dietary counseling reduces total and LDL cholesterol postpartum. Nutr (Burbank Los Angel County Calif). 2014;30:159–64.
35. Brantsaeter AL, Myhre R, Haugen M, Myking S, Sengpiel V, Magnus P, et al. Intake of probiotic food and risk of preeclampsia in primiparous women: the Norwegian Mother and Child Cohort Study. Am J Epidemiol. 2011;174(7):807–15.

Part II

Inflammation and Physiology of Pregnancy

Pathology of the Placenta: A Continuum Spectrum of Inflammation from Physiology to Disease

4

Gaetano Pietro Bulfamante and Laura Avagliano

Contents

4.1 Introduction

Pregnancy is a biologic example of a successful semi-allogenic graft: at the feto-maternal interface, the semi-allogenic embryonic cells that adhere and "dig" into the decidua are protected from maternal immune rejection. The feto-maternal interface is localized between the maternal uterine mucosa and the trophoblastic cells [1].

G.P. Bulfamante, MD (✉) • L. Avagliano, MD, PhD
Department of Healt Sciences, San Paolo Hospital Medical School, University of Milan, Milan, Italy
e-mail: gaetano.bulfamante@unimi.it

E. Ferrazzi, B. Sears (eds.), *Metabolic Syndrome and Complications of Pregnancy: The Potential Preventive Role of Nutrition*,
DOI 10.1007/978-3-319-16853-1_4

Maternal decidua does not represent a passive tissue in which blastocyst implants and develops its placenta. Maternal tissues not only do not reject trophoblastic cells but play an active role to support the placental development and function: the endometrium undergoes a specialized tissue reaction called decidualization whereby cell morphology, cell activity, gene expression, and immune cell distribution contribute to support the blastocyst apposition, adhesion, and implantation within the decidua [2].

The placenta originates from the extraembryonic portion of the polar zone of the blastocyst that adheres to the uterus during the implantation process. From the adhesion process of the blastocyst to the uterine decidua, the trophoblastic tissue undergoes a series of differentiations to develop into its final aspect of villi composed of stromal tissue containing fetal vessels and surrounded by trophoblastic cells: cyto- and syncytiotrophoblast, the inner and outer villous trophoblastic layers, respectively [3]. Meanwhile, a specific type of villi, called anchoring villi, permits to anchor the placenta to the decidua, by means of cytotrophoblast cells, named trophoblastic anchoring columns. Some of these trophoblastic cells detach from the columns and migrate through the decidual stroma, reach the spiral arteries, penetrate the wall of the maternal vessels, and colonize the lumen of the spiral arteries. This ignites the complex and essential process of vascular remodeling of spiral arteries. Maternal inflammatory cells now start to work against their natural mission and tolerate and accept this invasion of these extravillous, semi-allogenic, trophoblastic cells.

A cross talk between trophoblast and decidua is a fundamental prerequisite to maintain maternal immune tolerance toward the semi-allogenic embryo and to allow trophoblast invasion, placental development, and pregnancy evolution. This cross talk includes the expression of immune cells, dynamically dependent on the pregnancy progression [4]:

- The first trimester of pregnancy is a phase of physiological inflammation [5]: leucocytes not only tolerate pregnancy but also they support gestation [6]. Immune cells in the first trimester are mainly natural killer (NK) cells (about 70 %) and macrophages (about 20 %), whereas the number of T cells is variable (about 10–20 %) and dendritic cells, B cells, and regulatory T cells are rare [7] (Fig. 4.1).
- The second trimester of pregnancy is a phase of predominant anti-inflammatory state. In this time frame, the mother and fetus are in symbiosis and the fetus undergoes rapid development and growth [5].
- The late third trimester of pregnancy is a phase characterized by a reconversion to a pro-inflammatory condition that characterizes human parturition of an altricial newborn [5].

4.2 Natural Killer Cells

In pregnancy, decidual natural killer cells have a characteristic and specific phenotype (CD56^{BRIGHT}, CD16^{-} , CD3^{-}). They change their structure as pregnancy progresses to adapt themselves to the role of pregnancy supporters.

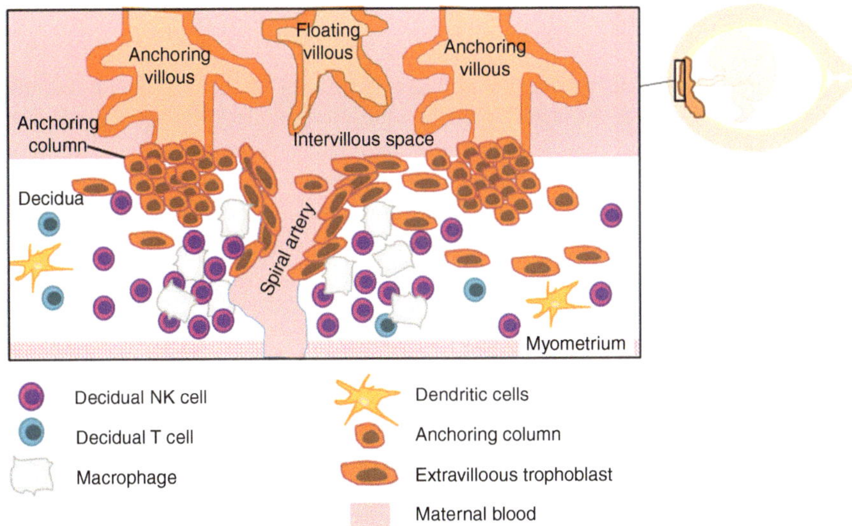

Fig. 4.1 Normal distribution of inflammatory cells at the feto-maternal interface. Decidual natural killer and macrophages accumulate near the maternal spiral artery during the remodeling process. The vessel undergoes dramatic anatomic modification, lacking the smooth muscular wall and the elastic fibers and transforming in a low-pressure, high-conductance vessel. Inflammatory cells play a role in the removal of dying cells and cellular debris, to facilitate trophoblast migration and invasion. Moreover, inflammatory cells contribute to maternal tolerance versus the semi-allograft conceptus. Extravillous trophoblasts invade into the decidua from the anchoring villi and progressively replace the endothelium of the vessel. This type of extravillous trophoblast takes the name of "endovascular trophoblast," and it is directly in contact with the maternal circulation. To avoid maternal reject reaction, extravillous trophoblast expresses a nonclassical major histocompatibility complex class I: it expresses a specific type of human leukocyte antigen (HLA), the HLA-G. HLA-G enters the maternal circulation and binds with the leukocyte immunoglobulin-like receptor on decidual natural killer cells, macrophages, and T lymphocytes, inactivating leukocytes and, in turn, inducing tolerance

During the first trimester, NK cells contain specific granules rich in angiogenic growth factor and vascular endothelial growth factor C. Moreover, during the first stage of pregnancy, decidual NK cells secrete matrix metalloproteinases MMP2 and MMP9. These enzymes break down the extracellular matrix. This process directly helps trophoblast migration and invasion. At this stage, NK cells play a decisive role for the proper placental development, promoting spiral artery remodeling. The number and the function of uterine NK cells are crucial for the physiological evolution of pregnancy. Their abnormalities have been associated with implantation failure [8], miscarriage [9], preeclampsia, and fetal growth restriction [10].

In the second trimester, decidual NK cells undergo a degranulation process. This will stop the production of angiogenic and vascular growth factors. Interferon-γ (INF- γ) secretion starts to oppose vascular development. During the third trimester, the uterine NK cells in the decidua are degranulated. In this stage, their production of INF-γ inhibits the trophoblastic invasiveness, protecting the uterus from a too deep trophoblastic migration [6].

4.3 Macrophages

At the feto-maternal interface, macrophages represent the second most abundant leukocyte population within the human decidua. Commonly, macrophages are classified in two different types: M1, the proinflammatory type, and M2, the immune-regulatory type [11]. The type of decidual macrophages appears to be predominantly M2 [12]. Their function is that of immune suppression, scavenging of apoptotic cells, clearing cellular debris, and promoting tissue remodeling.

4.3.1 Decidual Macrophages

Decidual macrophages are maternal cells and protect human pregnancy throughout gestation by inhibiting the immune response by decidual NK, T lymphocytes, and other circulatory macrophages [6]. Thanks to their additional production of matrix metalloproteinases 9 and vascular endothelial growth factor, decidual macrophages are believed to play a role in the spiral artery remodeling [12]. Despite this role in spiral artery modification, the association between abnormal number or function of decidual macrophages and preeclampsia is controversial [7].

4.3.2 Placental Macrophages

Placental macrophages, also called "Hofbauer cells," are $CD68^+$ fetal cells early detectable in pregnancy in the villous stroma. Since Hofbauer cells appear in the placental villi prior to the appearance of the fetal circulation, they may originate in the early stage of pregnancy from progenitor cells within the population of mesenchymal cells in the villous stroma; then, later in pregnancy, they may originate from penetration of embryonic bone marrow-derived monocytes into the villous stroma [3]. Generally, macrophages intervene in phagocytosis of apoptotic bodies and cellular debris as well as antigen presentation in response to inflammation and infectious insults; the specific role of placental macrophages has not been fully understood yet [13]. Their close contact with endothelial progenitor cells and primitive vessels suggests that Hofbauer cells intervene in early placental vascular genesis [14]. Moreover, the identification of proteins regulating branching morphogenesis localized to Hofbauer cells permits to hypothesize a role of placental macrophages in the development of the placental villous tree [15]. Alterations in the number and aspect of Hofbauer cells may be associated with complications of pregnancy such as fetal immune or nonimmune hydrops and fetal metabolic storage diseases such as GM1 gangliosidosis, glucuronidase deficiency, and type VII mucopolysaccharidosis [13]. Histological features of elevated concentration of Hofbauer cells have been related to adverse pregnancy outcome in association with villitis of unknown etiology or acute chorioamnionitis (see below) [13].

4.4 T Cells

T cells are poorly represented within the human decidua. Their role is not completely understood.

During the early stages of pregnancy, a successful implantation occurs in a finely regulated pro-inflammatory/anti-inflammatory microenvironment; T cells seem to play a crucial role in this balance. T-helper (Th) cells can be classified into Th1 cells, which are involved in cellular immunity, and Th2 cells, which are involved in humoral immunity [16]. In the past, maternal tolerance of the semi-allogenic graft was explained by an absolute predominance of the Th2-type immunity, which overrules Th1-type immunity, therefore protecting the fetus from maternal Th1-cell attack [17]. More recently, the role of Th1 has been reconsidered, showing that Th1 activity plays an important role in pregnancy, promoting Th2 response, regulating the placentation process, defending the maternal–fetal microenvironment against infections, and later cooperating in the initiation of delivery [18]; therefore, the concept of absolute Th2 predominance has been reconsidered and the hypothesis of "Th1–Th2 cooperation" has been introduced [18]. Moreover, it has been suggested that differences in the expression of the Th1 pro-inflammatory action and Th2 anti-inflammatory action depend on the phase of pregnancy: early and late pregnancy needs a Th1 milieu, whereas Th2 cells prevail in mid gestation (Table 4.1) [5]. Abnormal pregnancy outcome may occur in the presence of an aberrant Th1/Th2 profile: an excessive Th1 reaction may be associated with recurrent miscarriage, preterm delivery, and preeclampsia [18, 19], but even an increase of Th2 secretion at the feto-maternal interface could be associated with miscarriage and preeclampsia [18].

Histological features of placental elevated concentration of T cells have been associated with adverse pregnancy outcome as may occur in chronic deciduitis, chronic chorioamnionitis, and villitis of unknown etiology [7] (see below).

4.4.1 T Regulatory Cells

T regulatory cells (Treg) are a subset of T lymphocytes that act as strong suppressors of inflammatory immune response with a fundamental role in preventing destructive immune response and auto-inflammatory and autoimmune disease, warranting peripheral self-tolerance and immune homeostasis [20, 21]. Treg cells levels are high in maternal blood during the first and second trimesters of pregnancy and decline prior to delivery and postpartum [20]. Moreover, Treg cells physiologically accumulate in the maternal decidua. A deficiency in Treg cells number has been associated with recurrent miscarriage and preeclampsia [20]. Indeed, it is of interest to underline that there are two developmental pathways of Tregs: thymic (tTreg) and extrathymic or peripheral (pTreg). tTregs appear to suppress autoimmunity, whereas pTregs operate to downregulate responses to

Table 4.1 Inflammatory balance in pregnancy

Phase of pregnancy	Predominant immunological features	Physiological events	Comment
Early pregnancy	Th1	Blastocyst apposition to the uterus	In this phase, an inflammatory microenvironment needs for removing of apoptotic cells and cellular debris, for achieving an adequate repair of the uterine epithelium, and for the maternal tolerance versus the semi-allogenic embryo
		Decidual breaking for the blastocyst implantation	
		Trophoblast invasion of the decidua	
		Breaking into the spiral artery and disruption of the smooth muscular wall by the extravillous trophoblast, to warrant an adequate placental–fetal blood supply	
		Trophoblast replacement of the spiral arteries endothelium	
Mild pregnancy	Th2	Placental development	In this phase, an anti-inflammatory status predominates, but the mother maintains her ability to respond against infective–immunological insults
		Fetal growth	
		Fetal organ maturation	
Late pregnancy	Th1	Cervical ripening	In this phase, a recrudescence of an inflammatory status is necessary to promote parturition
		Myometrial contraction	
		Labor and delivery	
		Expulsion of the placenta	
		Uterine involution	

Modified from Mor [17]

antigens, such as those from ingested food, symbiotic bacteria, and allergens. Genomic analysis allowed to hypothesize that pTregs emerged in eutherian (placental) mammals to protect from maternal–fetal conflict. As a matter of fact, conserved noncoding sequence 1 (CNS1), which is required for pTreg development, has been detected present in all placental mammals, whereas it is absent in non-placental mammals such as the wallaby, opossum, and platypus, as it is expected to be absent in non-mammals such as zebra fish. pTregs specifically sort out paternal antigens in the trophoblastic cells and suppress effector T cells in an active process to induce tolerance [22]. Figure 4.2 shows the quasi-perfect correspondence between wild-type pregnant mice and knocked-out ones as regards embryonic reabsorption and number of females that presents reabsorbed embryos [23].

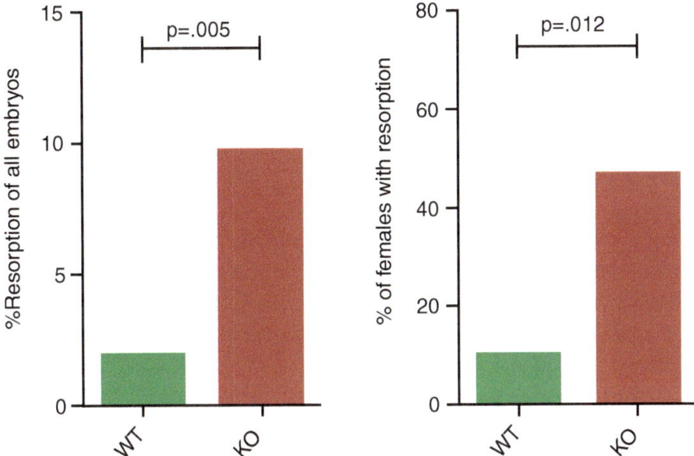

Fig. 4.2 Percent of resorbed embryos in CNS1-sufficient (wild type) and CNS1-deficient pregnancies in knockout mice

4.5 Dendritic Cells

Dendritic cells (DCs) are at the biological bridge between the innate and the adaptive immune system and their activation and modulation is critical for the outcome of the immune response. DCs localize in the peripheral tissue and act as sentinel of the immune response. After an inflammatory stimulus, DCs migrate via lymphatic vessels to the lymph node to present antigen to T cells [7]. According to their state (activated or not activated), DCs can secrete pro- or anti-inflammatory cytokines, thereby inducing immune responses or suppressing them, respectively.

In pregnancy, the number of DCs in the decidua is very low and the cells are phenotypically immature. The role of decidual DCs has not been fully elucidated; recently, it was suggested that DCs, as well NKs and macrophages, could act at the feto-maternal interface, intervening in the tissue remodeling and promoting maternal immune tolerance [7]. An increased number of phenotypically mature DCs have been associated with spontaneous miscarriage [24].

4.6 B Cells

B cells are a component of the humoral immunity of the acquired immune system. The main function of B cells is the production of antibodies (IgG, IgM, IgE, IgA), but B cells can also uptake, process, and present antigens and can produce several cytokines influencing immunity. The role of B cells during pregnancy has been poorly studied, but it was postulated that they may contribute toward pregnancy tolerance by regulating the production of the immune-modulatory cytokine IL-10 [25]. A physiological decrease of B cells was noted in the third trimester of normal pregnancy while preeclampsia has been associated with a persistence of a higher number of B cells. In women with autoimmune disease, it is possible that B cells compromise gestation, producing excessive autoantibodies [25].

4.7 Trophoblast as Regulator of Innate Immune Cell

Trophoblastic cells express pattern recognition receptors that act as "sensors" of the surrounding microenvironment [5]. These sensors allow the recognition of the presence of bacteria, viruses, damaged tissues, and dying cells by the trophoblast. Trophoblastic cells can secrete a specific set of cytokines influencing the immune cells within the decidua with the aim of instructing inflammatory cells to create an adequate microenvironment, to promote pregnancy evolution [5]. The success of the pregnancy depends on the trophoblastic ability to communicate with any immune cell type (monocytes/macrophages, pTreg and NK cells) and to coordinate their interrelated work [5, 26].

4.8 The Alteration of the Maternal–Fetal Equilibrium of the Inflammatory Cells

Alterations in type, number, aspect, or interrelationship of any component of the cells of the inflammatory milieu may be detrimental for pregnancy outcome. This might be the consequence of infections or of maternal immunological problems, either in clinical or in subclinical conditions.

Infection can reach the placenta and the fetus through the maternal blood circulation or by ascending into the uterus from the vagina or by descending into the uterus from the peritoneal cavity, by activation of the pathogenic phenotype of preexisting bacteria, or even by sudden immune reaction toward preexisting symbiotic bacteria.

4.8.1 Acute Chorioamnionitis

These processes could develop into acute chorioamnionitis. In these cases, most of infecting agents originate in the cervicovaginal tract and gain access to the uterine cavity breaching the normal cervical barrier. Maternal neutrophils infiltrate the chorionic plate and membranous chorioamnion (Fig. 4.3) [27]. Normally, neutrophils are a population of inflammatory cells that do not infiltrate placental compartments. When an infective insult occurs, neutrophils can invade placental structures; they can derive both from the intervillous space and the venules of decidua capsularis. In case of acute chorioamnionitis, a maternal and/or a fetal inflammatory response should be distinguished. The stage (progression of the disease) and the grade (intensity of the disease) of the inflammatory response are summarized in Table 4.2. Acute chorioamnionitis has been associated with adverse pregnancy and neonatal outcome, in relation to prematurity due to preterm delivery and/or preterm premature rupture of the membrane [29]. Fetal inflammatory response is the main factor that affected fetal–neonatal well-being; fetal inflammatory response involves

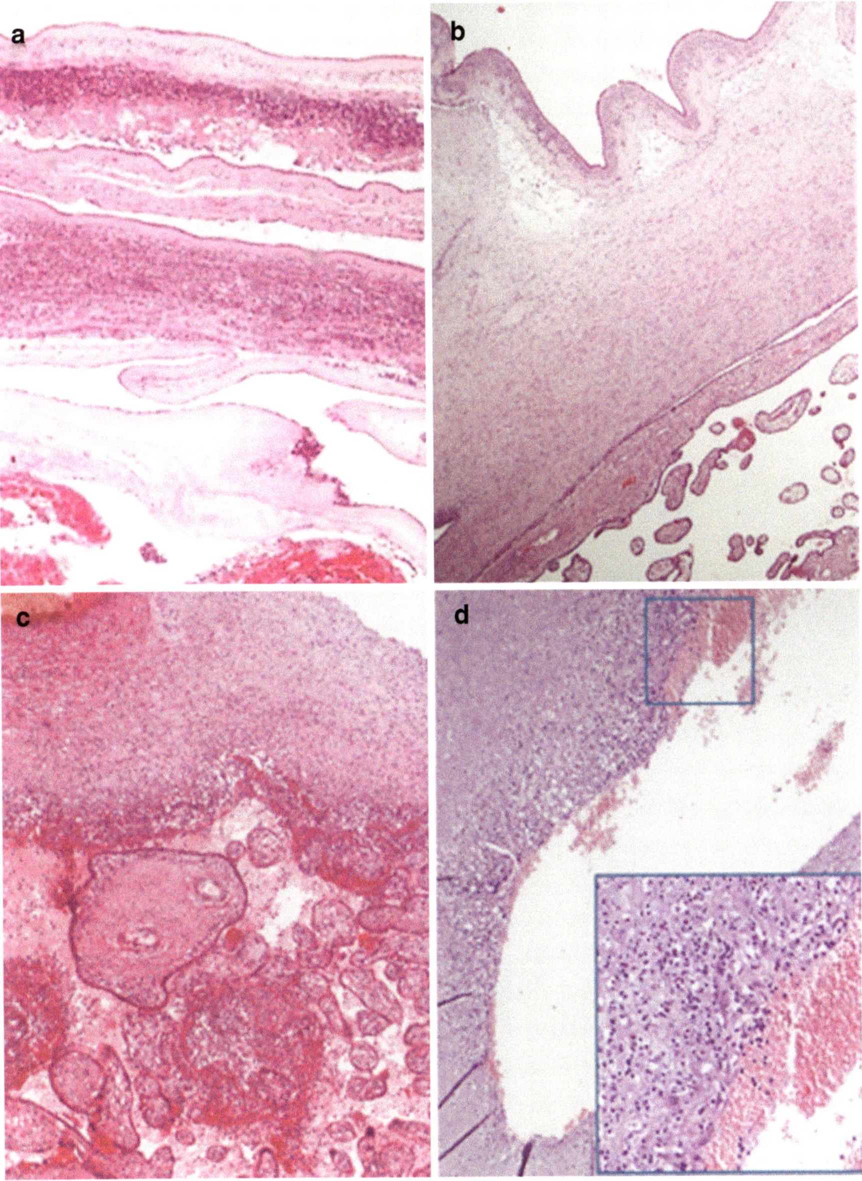

Fig. 4.3 Placental acute inflammatory lesions. Images show maternal and fetal inflammatory response in term placentas. *A* severe acute chorioamnionitis in the free membranes; note the patchy–diffuse accumulations of neutrophil in the subchorionic plate, involving also the chorion and amnion. *B* severe acute chorioamnionitis in the placental chorionic plate, involving both the amnion and chorion. *C* severe acute chorioamnionitis with acute intervillitis. Note the large accumulations of neutrophils (microabscesses) under the chorion and between placental villi. *D* fetal inflammatory response involving the umbilical vein. Note the accumulation of the inflammatory infiltration across the wall of the vessel

Table 4.2 Stages and grades of acute chorioamnionitis

	Maternal inflammatory response		Fetal inflammatory response	
	Definition	Description	Definition	Description
Stage 1	Acute subchorionitis/acute chorionitis	Patchy–diffuse accumulations of neutrophil in the subchorionic plate fibrin and/or membranous chorionic trophoblast layer	Chorionic vasculitis/umbilical phlebitis	Neutrophils in the wall of any chorionic vessel or in the umbilical vein
Stage 2	Acute chorioamnionitis	More than a few scattered neutrophils in the chorionic plate or membranous chorionic connective tissue and/or the amnion	Umbilical vasculitis	Neutrophils in one or two arteries and/or in umbilical vein
Stage 3	Necrotizing chorioamnionitis	Degenerating neutrophils (karyorrhexis), thickened eosinophilic amniotic basement membrane, and at least focal amniotic epithelial degeneration	Necrotizing funisitis or concentric umbilical perivasculitis	Neutrophils, cellular debris eosinophilic precipitate, and/or mineralization arranged in a concentric band around one or more umbilical vessels
Grade 1	Mild–moderate	Individual or small clusters of maternal neutrophils diffusely infiltrating amnion, chorionic plate, chorion leave, and/or subchorionic fibrin	Mild–moderate	Scattered neutrophilic infiltrate in the subendothelial or intramural portion of the vessel
Grade 2	Severe	Three or more chorionic microabscesses between the chorion and decidua in the membranes and/or under the chorionic plate or a continuous band of a confluent chorionic polymorphonuclear leukocyte	Severe	Vessels with near confluent neutrophils with attenuation and/or degradation of vascular smooth muscle cells

Modified from Redline et al. [28]

chorionic plate vessels and/or umbilical vein prior to the involving of umbilical arteries. The association between fetal inflammatory response and adverse neonatal condition and outcome takes place especially when umbilical arteries are involved. Neonatal sepsis could be a consequence of fetal inflammatory response but also neurological impairment may develop including cerebral palsy [30].

When fetal neutrophils are found in fetal capillaries and stroma of distal villi, with minimal intervillous component, the lesion is called *acute villitis* and it could represent an expression of intrauterine fetal sepsis due to a bacterial hematogenous infection such as *Escherichia coli* or group B streptococcus.

4.8.2 Chronic Chorioamnionitis

The differential diagnosis of acute chorioamnionitis includes chronic chorioamnionitis, a placental lesion characterized by an infiltration of maternally derived T lymphocytes $CD3^+$ in the chorioamniotic membranes [27]. Viral infection can be associated with chronic chorioamnionitis, but the actual cause of this lesion is still unknown. A frequent association between chronic chorioamnionitis and villitis of unknown etiology and the altered chemokine profile observed in the amniotic fluid of cases affected by chronic chorioamnionitis permit to hypothesize an immunological cause of this histological placental lesion, suggesting a reaction consistent in maternal anti-fetal rejection [31, 32]. Chronic chorioamnionitis has been associated with spontaneous preterm birth and intrauterine fetal growth restriction [27].

4.8.3 Chronic Villitis of Unknown Etiology

Chronic villitis of unknown etiology is a placental lesion characterized by the presence of villous mononuclear cell infiltrates composed of maternal $CD8^+$ T lymphocytes [33]. An increased number of placental Hofbauer cells may coexist and a histiocytic infiltrate within the intervillous space (chronic intervillositis) may accompany the chronic villitis. The origin of this lesion is still unknown but a maternal immune response against the fetus has been advocated, similar to host-versus-graft rejection [33]. Although a low grade of villitis of unknown etiology could affect placentas from normal pregnancies without clinical consequences, high-grade lesions could be associated with severe abnormal pregnancy outcome. Clinical associations are summarized in Table 4.3. Recurrent villitis in the subsequent pregnancies is associated with maternal obesity (a known condition of immune dysfunction) and multigravidity (in relation to the repeated exposure to the fetal antigens).

4.8.4 Chronic Villitis in Oocyte Donation

Pregnancies derived from donated oocyte also present a high prevalence of villitis of unknown etiology. Egg donation pregnancies represent an interesting challenge for the feto-maternal interface immunological aspect: the mother must tolerate a

Table 4.3 Chronic Villitis of unknown etiology

Grade	Histological features	Distribution	Association with other placental lesions	Possible clinical association
Low	Lesion affecting less than 10 villi per focus	Focal (only one slide involved) Multifocal (more than one slide involved)	No specific association	No specific association
High	More than 10 villi affected per focus	Patchy Diffuse (involving more than 5 % of all distal villi) Involving proximal stem villi Involving anchoring villi and the adjacent terminal villi (basal villitis)	Diffuse perivillous fibrin deposition Obliterative fetal vasculopathy Chronic deciduitis with plasma cells	IUGR, IUFD, PD NE, CP PL, SM

CP cerebral palsy, *NE* neonatal encephalopathy, *IUGR* intrauterine fetal growth restriction, *IUFD* intrauterine fetal death, *PD* preterm delivery, *PL* periventricular leukomalacia, *SM* spontaneous miscarriage

completely allogenic conceptus. The higher incidence of villitis of unknown etiology, as well as other placental histological lesions (chronic deciduitis, massive chronic intervillositis, increased infiltration of T-helper cells, and natural killer cells), in the basal plate of egg donation pregnancies seems to be related to a more pronounced immune-mediated response in this particular type of medical achieved pregnancies. The placental histological damages and the frequently abnormal clinical evolution of egg donor pregnancies may be the consequence of a reaction similar to graft-versus-host disease and/or organ rejection [34].

4.8.5 Chronic Deciduitis

Chronic deciduitis corresponds to a mixed lymphoplasmacytic infiltrate in the decidua, identifiable either in the free membrane or along the maternal surface, sometimes encroaching the anchoring villi. The presence of plasma cells in the endometrium is always considered an abnormal feature (Fig. 4.4). It may develop as a consequence of antigen-stimulating events related both to infection and noninfection insults [35]. A source of antigen is bacterial subacute endometritis that may cause recurrent acute chorioamnionitis and preterm delivery in the subsequent pregnancies [36]; otherwise, an alloimmune response may be at the base of chronic deciduitis. When there is not an acute inflammation, decidual plasma cells are associated with infertility, miscarriage, and chronic villitis [28].

In summary, an acute neutrophilic infiltrate of the placenta is generally related to infective insults, as occurs in acute chorioamnionitis; a chronic placental inflammatory infiltrate (including lymphocytes, histiocytes, plasma cells) generally represents

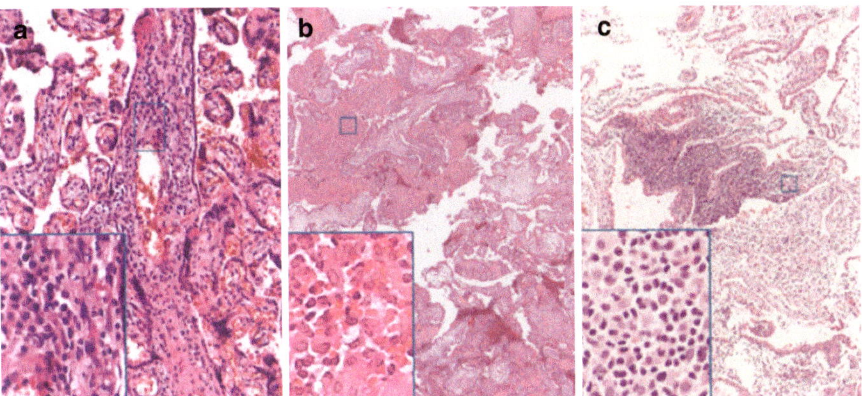

Fig. 4.4 Chronic placental inflammatory lesions. *A* chronic villitis of unknown etiology. Note the inflammatory infiltration within the placental villi. The *inset* permits to appreciate the characteristic predominant lymphocytic composition of the infiltrate. *B* chronic intervillositis. Note the aggregates of inflammatory cells in the intervillous space admixed with fibrin deposition. The *inset* permits to appreciate the characteristic predominant histiocytic composition of the infiltrate. *D* chronic deciduitis in first trimester spontaneous miscarriage. Note the massive plasma cells infiltration within the decidua (*inset*)

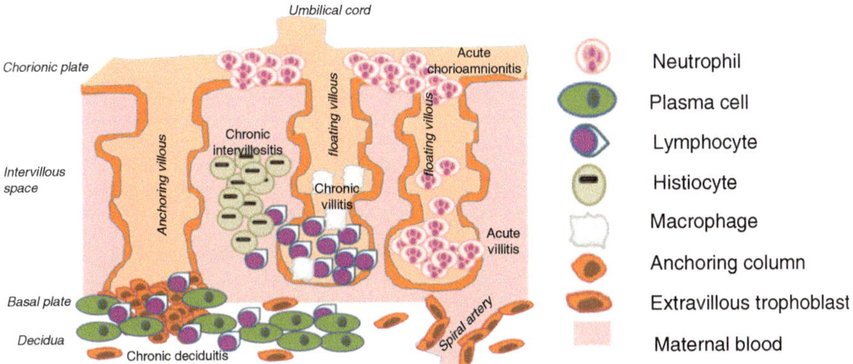

Fig. 4.5 Schematic example of the distribution of inflammatory cells during placental pathology. Many types of inflammatory cells may pathologically inhabit multiple compartments of the placenta, leading to damages of placental function and conducting to adverse pregnancy outcome. For a detailed description of any lesions, see the text

an inflammatory noninfective placental reaction, as occurs in chronic villitis, chronic chorioamnionitis, chronic intervillositis, and chronic deciduitis. These four last lesions often coexist as a tetrad, suggesting an alloimmune response. Maternal characteristics such as obesity and autoimmune disease (including systemic lupus erythematosus, antiphospholipid syndrome, type 1 diabetes mellitus, and thyroiditis) could constitute a predisposing factor for the development of these placental damaging lesions.

Schematic exemplification of the distribution of the inflammatory cell during the placental lesions is shown in Fig. 4.5

4.9 Inflammatory Lesions of the Decidua

Annetine Staff defines the decidua basalis "the decidual battleground" [37]. This is the place, the no man's land, where all these cells rush, live, cooperate, and fight in human reproduction. A more subtle immune-inflammatory lesion that dramatically impacts on placental function in late gestation is acute atherosis. This lesion affects 20–40 % of cases of late preeclampsia but is observed also as a minor lesion in a subset of "normal" pregnancies, suggesting a continuum of unbalanced interaction from subclinical to clinical to severe disease. This local process occurs without systemic vascular lesions. Histologically acute atherosis is characterized by CD68-positive subendothelial lipid-filled foam cells. These cells derive macrophages and possibly smooth muscle cells. This process is associated with an infiltration of inflammatory mononuclear cell like early stages of atherosclerosis in coronary artery disease. This lesion is seldom seen in the myometrial tract of spiral arteries and is not caused by hypertension. This process is immune-inflammatory in nature and not caused by dyslipidemia. It might be observed in pregnancies with fetal growth restriction and immune diseases. It is of interest to observe that this lesion might be found not only in abnormal spiral arteries as per early shallow trophoblastic invasion but also and mainly in normal spiral arteries. Atherosis ignites a vicious circle of under-perfusion, oxidative stress, inflammation, and atherosis. According to Staff and coworkers [38], the hyperlipidemia of normal pregnancy worsens in women with a pro-atherogenic lipid profile that develop preeclampsia.

These recent findings suggest a possible link between low-grade inflammation, dyslipidemia that characterize metabolic syndrome and excess, and/or severity of late gestation acute atherosis and late preeclampsia, associated with a normal fetal growth.

The full understanding of these pathological concepts should induce clinical counselors to underline the importance of prepregnancy lifestyle and nutrition for a successful pregnancy.

References

1. Red-Horse K, Zhou Y, Genbacev O, Prakobphol A, Foulk R, McMaster M, Fisher SJ. Trophoblast differentiation during embryo implantation and formation of the maternal-fetal interface. J Clin Invest. 2004;114(6):744–54.
2. Gellersen B, Brosens IA, Brosens JJ. Decidualization of the human endometrium: mechanisms, functions, and clinical perspectives. Semin Reprod Med. 2007;25(6):445–53.
3. Huppertz B. The anatomy of the normal placenta. J Clin Pathol. 2008;61(12):1296–302.
4. Oreshkova T, Dimitrov R, Mourdjeva M. A cross-talk of decidual stromal cells, trophoblast, and immune cells: a prerequisite for the success of pregnancy. Am J Reprod Immunol. 2012;68:366–73.
5. Mor G. Inflammation and pregnancy. The role of toll-like receptors I trophoblast-immune interaction. Ann N Y Acad Sci. 2008;1127:121–8.
6. Rapacz-Leonard A, Dąbrowska M, Janowski T. Major histocompatibility complex I mediates immunological tolerance of the trophoblast during pregnancy and may mediate rejection during parturition. Mediators Inflamm. 2014;2014:821530.

7. Erlebacher A. Immunology of the maternal-fetal interface. Ann Rev Immunol. 2013;31: 387–411.
8. Tuckerman E, Mariee N, Prakash A, Li TC, Laird S. Uterine natural killer cells in peri-implantation endometrium from women with repeated implantation failure after IVF. J Reprod Immunol. 2010;87:60–6.
9. Quenby S, Bates M, Doig T, Brewster J, Lewis-Jones DI, Johnson PM, Vince G. Pre-implantation endometrial leukocytes in women with recurrent miscarriage. Hum Reprod. 1999;14:2386–91.
10. Williams PJ, Bulmer JN, Searle RF, Innes BA, Robson SC. Altered decidual leucocyte populations in the placental bed in pre-eclampsia and foetal growth restriction: a comparison with late normal pregnancy. Reproduction. 2009;138:177–84.
11. Mantovani A, Sica A, Sozzani S, Allavena P, Vecchi A, Locati M. The chemokine system in diverse forms of macrophage activation and polarization. Trends Immunol. 2004;25:677–86.
12. Gustafsson C, Mjösberg J, Matussek A, Geffers R, Matthiesen L, Berg G, Sharma S, Buer J, Ernerudh J. Gene expression profiling of human decidual macrophages: evidence for immunosuppressive phenotype. PLoS One. 2008;3:e2078.
13. Tang Z, Abrahams VM, Mor G, Guller S. Placental Hofbauer cells and complications of pregnancy. Ann N Y Acad Sci. 2011;1221:103–8.
14. Seval Y, Korgun ET, Demir R. Hofbauer cells in early human placenta: possible implications in vasculogenesis and angiogenesis. Placenta. 2007;28:841–5.
15. Anteby EY, et al. Human placental Hofbauer cells express sprouty proteins: a possible modulating mechanism of villous branching. Placenta. 2005;26:476–83.
16. Saito S, Nakashima A, Shima T, Ito M. Th1/Th2/Th17 and regulatory T-cell paradigm in pregnancy. Am J Reprod Immunol. 2010;63:601–10.
17. Wegmann TG, Lin H, Guilbert L, Mosmann TR. Bidirectional cytokine interactions in the maternal-fetal relationship: is successful pregnancy a TH2 phenomenon? Immunol Today. 1993;14:353–6.
18. Wilczynski JR. Th1/Th2 cytokines balance – yin and yang of reproductive immunology. Eur J Obstet Gynecol Reprod Biol. 2005;122:136–43.
19. Sykes L, MacIntyre DA, Yap XJ, Teoh TG, Bennett PR. The Th1:th2 dichotomy of pregnancy and preterm labour. Mediators Inflamm. 2012;2012:967629. doi: 10.1155/2012/967629. Epub 2012 Jun 7. Review. PMID: 22719180
20. Guerin LR, Prins JR, Robertson SA. Regulatory T-cells and immune tolerance in pregnancy: a new target for infertility treatment? Hum Reprod Update. 2009;15:517–35.
21. La Rocca C, Carbone F, Longobardi S, Matarese G. The immunology of pregnancy: regulatory T cells control maternal immune tolerance toward the fetus. Immunol Lett. 2014;162:41–8.
22. Williams Z. Inducing tolerance to pregnancy. N Engl J Med. 2012;367:1159–61.
23. Samstein RM, Josefowicz SZ, Arvey A, Treuting PM, Rudensky AY. Extrathymic generation of regulatory T cells in placental mammals mitigates maternal-fetal conflict. Cell. 2012;150: 29–38.
24. Askelund K, Liddell HS, Zanderigo AM, Fernando NS, Khong TY, Stone PR, et al. CD83(+) dendritic cells in the decidua of women with recurrent miscarriage and normal pregnancy. Placenta. 2004;25:140–5.
25. Fettke F, Schumacher A, Costa SD, Zenclussen AC. B cells: the old new players in reproductive immunology. Front Immunol. 2014;5:285.
26. Fest S, Aldo PB, Abrahams VM, Visintin I, Alvero A, Chen R, Chavez SL, Romero R, Mor G. Trophoblast-macrophage interactions: a regulatory network for the protection of pregnancy. Am J Reprod Immunol. 2007;57:55–66.
27. Kraus FT, Redline R, Gersell DJ, Nelson DM, Dicke JM. Atlas of nontumor pathology: placental pathology. First series. Fascicle 3. Washington DC: American Registry of Pathology; 2004.
28. Redline RW, Faye-Petersen O, Heller D, Qureshi F, Savell V, Vogler C, Society for Pediatric Pathology, Perinatal Section, Amniotic Fluid Infection Nosology Committee. Amniotic infection syndrome: nosology and reproducibility of placental reaction patterns. Pediatr Dev Pathol. 2003;6(5):435–48.

29. Goldenberg RL, Andrews WW, Hauth JC. Choriodecidual infection and preterm birth. Nutr Rev. 2002;60:S19–25.
30. Shatrov JG, Birch SC, Lam LT, Quinlivan JA, McIntyre S, Mendz GL. Chorioamnionitis and cerebral palsy: a meta-analysis. Obstet Gynecol. 2010;116:387–92.
31. Oggé G, Romero R, Lee DC, Gotsch F, Than NG, Lee J, Chaiworapongsa T, Dong Z, Mittal P, Hassan SS, Kim CJ. Chronic chorioamnionitis displays distinct alterations of the amniotic fluid proteome. J Pathol. 2011;223:553–65.
32. Redline RW. Villitis of unknown etiology: noninfectious chronic villitis in the placenta. Hum Pathol. 2007;38:1439–46.
33. van der Hoorn ML, Lashley EE, Bianchi DW, Claas FH, Schonkeren CM, Scherjon SA. Clinical and immunologic aspects of egg donation pregnancies: a systematic review. Hum Reprod Update. 2010;16:704–12.
34. Katzman PJ. Chronic inflammatory lesions of the placenta. Semin Perinatol. 2015;39:20–6.
35. Goldenberg R, Hautth J, Andrews W. Intrauterine infection and preterm delivery. N Engl J Med. 2000;342:1500–7.
36. Staff AC, Redman CW. IFPA Award in Placentology Lecture: preeclampsia, the decidual battleground and future maternal cardiovascular disease. Placenta. 2014;35:S26–31. doi: 10.1016/j.placenta.2013.12.003. Epub 2013 Dec 18. PMID: 24411701
37. Staff AC, Dechend R, Pijnenborg R. Learning from the placenta: acute atherosis and vascular remodeling in preeclampsia-novel aspects for atherosclerosis and future cardiovascular health. Hypertension. 2010;56:1026e34.
38. Kim CJ, Romero R, Kusanovic JP, Yoo W, Dong Z, Topping V, Gotsch F, Yoon BH, Chi JG, Kim JS. The frequency, clinical significance, and pathological features of chronic chorioamnionitis: a lesion associated with spontaneous preterm birth. Mod Pathol. 2010;23:1000–11.

Obesity and Inflammation in Pregnancy 5

Raffaella Cancello

Contents

5.1 Introduction

The role of obesity and obesity-linked chronic inflammation in adverse pregnancy outcomes is an intense developing research area. Maternal-fetal obesity is a complex paradigm, characterized by factors related to overnutrition, adipose tissue morphologic and molecular modifications, and inflammatory processes, impacting negatively the development of the fetus and compromising the maternal health state. Further studies are urgently required to better characterize the biology of adipose tissue in obese pregnant women.

Nutritional intervention is actually the only therapeutic target to reduce maternal-fetal complications. Weight loss, specific dietary interventions, and physical activity should

R. Cancello
Molecular Biology Laboratory (Centro Ricerche e Biotecnologie),
Department of Medical Sciences and Rehabilitation,
Istituto Auxologico Italiano, IRCCS, Milan, Italy
e-mail: r.cancello@auxologico.it

E. Ferrazzi, B. Sears (eds.), *Metabolic Syndrome and Complications of Pregnancy: The Potential Preventive Role of Nutrition*,
DOI 10.1007/978-3-319-16853-1_5

be encouraged in obese women who intend to be pregnant, while in obese pregnant women healthy food choices and moderate exercise, rather than a weight-loss program institution, should be encouraged in order to prevent excessive gestational weight gain and possible controlling/reducing complication appearance.

5.2 Obesity and Chronic Low-Grade Inflammation

Obesity is a condition of fat mass excess in the body associated with serious health consequences [1–4]. Obese individuals are more prone to several medical conditions such as cardiovascular disease, type 2 diabetes, and some cancers [1–4]. The most commonly used anthropometric tool to classify obesity is body mass index (BMI), which is expressed as the ratio of total body weight over height squared (kg/m^2). Individuals with a BMI ≥30 kg/m^2 are classified as obese and with a BMI ranging between 25 and 29.9 kg/m^2 as overweight, and individuals with a BMI between 18.5 and 24.9 kg/m^2 are in acceptable range of weight (Table 5.1). This index, despite some limitations, is strongly correlated with body fat mass amount. The distribution of fat mass excess in the body is also important: visceral and perivisceral adipose tissues are more linked to increased metabolic and cardiovascular risks than other depots (such as the subcutaneous adipose tissue in the gluteo-femoral region). In practice, waist and hip circumferences and waist to hip ratio (WHR) should be coupled to BMI calculation to estimate the distribution of fat mass excess, evaluate the risks, and recommend the optimal weight gain during pregnancy. There is evidence for age and ethnicity-linked variations in waist circumference and WHR. In fact, compared to Europeans, Asian populations have greater visceral adipose tissue, and African populations have less visceral adipose tissue or body fat percentage at

Table 5.1 BMI and recommended body weight gain in pregnancy

BMI (kg/m^2)	Classification	Waist circumference ≥88 cm	Waist to hip ratio (WHR) ≥0.85	Recommended weight gain in pregnancy
Below 18.5	Underweight	–	–	28–40 pounds (from 13 to 18 kg)
18.5–24.9	Normalweight	–	–	25–35 pounds (from 11 to 16 kg)
25.0–29.9	Overweight	High risk[a]	Risk substantially increased[a]	15–25 pounds (from 7 to 11 kg)
30.0 and above	Obese	Very high risk[a]	Risk substantially increased[a]	11–20 pounds (from 6 to 9 kg)

[a]Disease risk for type 2 diabetes, hypertension, and cardiovascular diseases

any given waist circumference [5, 6]. Women's BMI, waist, and WHR cutoff are reported in Table 5.1.

There is still an open debate regarding the concept of obesity as pathology or a simple consequence of overfeeding and physical inactivity. Anyhow, the excess of fat mass in the body should be always considered pathologic when in concomitance with a disease state. Even in the absence of a disease state, fat mass excess is associated with an increased risk of cardiovascular disease [7–9].

In humans we should talk about "obesities" instead of "obesity," since the same excess of fat mass can be generated by different mechanisms: primary obesity is due to excessive food intake coupled with decreased energy expenditure due to physical inactivity, whereas secondary obesity refers to obesity secondary to endocrine, metabolic, or even genetic disorders. Genetic forms of obesity are rare, explaining at most 3–4 % of human obesities [10–12].

Obesity alters lipid metabolism and it is characterized by a rise in total triglycerides, reduced HDL cholesterol, and an increase of VLDL, although total cholesterol and LDL cholesterol are significantly modified. In obesity also glucose metabolism is altered and characterized by hyperinsulinemia (reaching levels approximately twofold higher than those found in nonobese women) [8]. Besides metabolic complications, it is now widely recognized that obesity is associated with a state of "chronic low-grade inflammation" [13–15]. Serum levels of many pro-inflammatory and anti-inflammatory mediators are chronically altered in obesity, negatively affecting organs such as the liver, skeletal muscle, pancreas, gut, and heart [13–15]. This low-grade inflammation is then viewed as the common pathophysiological mechanism underlying the appearance of chronic and obesity-related complications such as hypertension, type 2 diabetes, metabolic syndrome, cardiovascular disease, and several type of cancers [8, 15–18]. Obesity-linked inflammation is characterized by a modest, but chronic, increase in circulating levels of mediators such as tumor necrosis factor alpha (TNFα), interleukin 6 (IL-6), interleukin 1 beta (IL-1), monocyte chemoattractant protein 1 (MCP-1), and serum amyloid A protein (SAA) together with the increase of leptin and decrease in circulating adiponectin, a cytokine with well-known anti-inflammatory properties [8, 13, 19].

5.2.1 Leptin and Adiponectin

Leptin and adiponectin are also called "adipokines" since these two cytokines are almost exclusively secreted by white adipose cells [19–21]. Leptin and adiponectin have a crucial role in inflammation modulation. Leptin exerts proliferative and anti-apoptotic activities in a variety of cell types, including T lymphocytes, leukemia cells, and hematopoietic progenitors, and its levels are acutely increased by inflammatory stimuli, such as in endotoxemia, and by pro-inflammatory cytokines such as TNFα and IL-1 [22]. Adiponectin has anti-inflammatory, antiatherogenic, antioxidant, and antiapoptotic effects, inhibiting TNF-induced endothelial adhesion and macrophage transformation to foam cells and suppressing TNF expression by macrophages, as well as by adipocytes [19, 20]. Of note, even a modest weight loss (5–10 % of weight) is able to positively modulate these inflammatory circulating mediators [23].

5.3 The Molecular Role of White Adipose Tissue in Obesity

During the last decade, white adipose tissue has been recognized as more than simply a storage depot for triglycerides. White adipose tissue is an active endocrine organ secreting adipokines, inflammatory mediators, and many bioactive molecules [19]. Obesity dramatically alters the morphology, as well as the molecular physiology, of white adipose cells [24]. In obesity, adipose tissue is characterized by hypertrophy and hyperplasia of unilocular adipocytes, with a dramatic change in the relative abundance of stromal vascular fraction cells, composed by adipocyte precursors (*i.e.*, preadipocytes), hematopoietic progenitor cells, endothelial cells, and immune cells, 10 % of which are $CD14^+/CD31^+$ macrophages [25]. The accumulation of adipose tissue macrophages (ATMs) in visceral adipose tissue of obese individuals has been well described [13, 14]. The number of macrophages in white adipose tissue (WAT) is directly correlated with adiposity and adipocyte mean size, with a higher abundance in visceral than in subcutaneous compartment [14]. The accumulation of T lymphocytes in adipose tissues (ATLs) was also demonstrated, and in mice submitted to high-fat diet, this phenomenon precedes the accumulation of ATMs. Moreover, the increased expression of T-lymphocyte markers was concomitant with the initiation of insulin resistance characterized by a reduction in systemic glucose tolerance and insulin sensitivity [25]. Early ATL infiltration in adipose tissue might be considered as a "primary" event that orchestrates the adipose tissue inflammation. In the adipose tissue of obese subjects, all lymphocyte types were detected: NK (natural killer) and NKT (natural killer T) cells that belong to the innate immune system, B lymphocytes and $CD4^+/CD8^+$ lymphocytes that belong to the adaptive immune system, and T lymphocytes responsible for the innate and adaptive immunity [25].

5.3.1 Extracellular Matrix in the Adipose Tissue

In addition to the inflammatory components in the adipose tissue, it should be noted that also the extracellular matrix components are modified in obesity [26]. The extracellular matrix is extremely important for the structure and functions of almost any cell type. Furthermore, it is involved in numerous processes such as cell adhesion, proliferation, differentiation, migration, apoptosis, and gene expression. During obesity progression, the connective fiber content of the adipose tissue increases dramatically, due to an upregulation of several types of collagens. As the collagen content increases, the overall rigidity of adipose tissue also increases, likely contributing to an increase in its mechanical strength. In adipose tissue, "fibrosis" appears to be initiated in response to adipocyte hypertrophy, which occurs as the initial step toward fat expansion through enlargement of the lipid droplet size in adipocytes [26]. The cellular factors associated with adipocyte

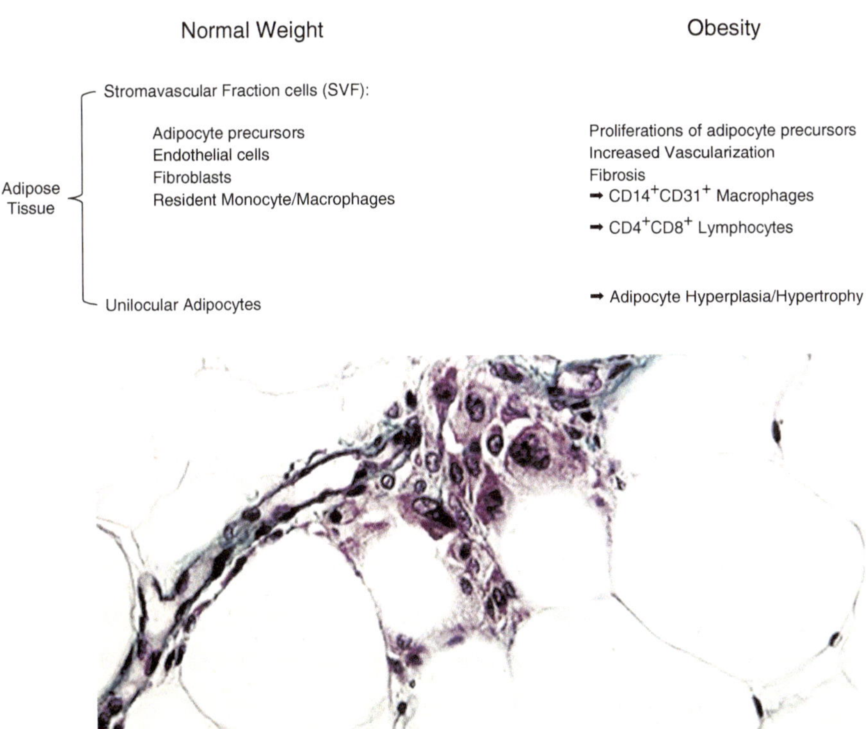

Fig. 5.1 List of cell types in adipose tissue of normal weight *vs*. obese subjects (*upper panel*). The *lower panel* shows the histology of human visceral adipose tissue from an obese donor. Fully mature hypertrophic adipocytes are clearly visible together with inflammatory infiltrations (macrophages and lymphocytes). Green fibers represent adipose tissue fibrosis (60×, Masson's Trichrom staining; R. Cancello, personal unpublished image)

expansion and collagen activation are currently unknown and a matter of intense investigations, but tissue hypoxia could be certainly involved. Fibrosis of the adipose tissue represents then another pro-inflammatory factor in dysregulation of adipocyte biology. The cellular components of adipose tissue in obesity are summarized in Fig. 5.1.

5.4 Obesity and Inflammation in Pregnancy

As a consequence of the rise in worldwide global obesity, the prevalence of obesity in reproductive-age women is currently 30 % and in the early pregnancy it is about 20 % [27–32]. Pregnancy is a physiological state characterized by changes in weight, maternal fat deposition, and fluid redistribution. An unambiguous assessment of the complications induced by obesity in pregnant women is made difficult by the frequent inability to distinguish the effects of obesity from those due to its complications [33, 34]. It is therefore interesting to focus our attention to the influence that excess of weight has on the mother. The literature shows that pregnancy in obese women is complicated by different medical conditions [33–41], such as:

- Higher incidence of adverse pregnancy outcome for the mother and newborn when compared to women with a BMI in a normal range
- Type 2 diabetes at the time of conception
- Hypertensive disease in pregnancy and preeclamptic toxemia
- Mechanical complication (i.e., pelvic pain and lower back pain)
- Reduced mobility during pregnancy (increased venous thromboembolism risk)
- Overall higher rate of labor induction with higher doses of oxytocin and prostaglandins
- Higher cesarean section rates
- Macrosomic babies with fat mass excess at birth
- Increased risk of postpartum depression

Pregnancy could be considered as a natural "pro-inflammatory" state, as demonstrated by the activation of maternal leukocytes and by mild elevations in circulating levels of both pro- and anti-inflammatory cytokines [39]. It has been suggested that at the local uterine/placental level, implantation (*i.e.*, early pregnancy phase) and delivery (*i.e.*, late pregnancy) may be considered as pro-inflammatory states while mid-pregnancy as an anti-inflammatory state [39]. However, few studies have examined longitudinal changes in circulating cytokines, during pregnancy progression and during postpartum transition.

Numerous studies have shown that maternal obesity is associated with an increased risk of gestational hypertension, but few studies have made a distinction between gestational hypertension and preeclampsia (PE) [35, 36, 41]. A maternal exaggerated inflammatory response to pregnancy, exacerbated by excessive body fatness, is associated with endothelial dysfunction, hypertension, proteinuria, and varying degrees of ischemic end-organ damage that characterizes PE [29–33]. The risk of developing gestational hypertension is directly correlated with maternal BMI [29–33]. However, the results are not entirely in agreement for high maternal BMI and increased risk for development of PE. Several studies show a strong association of maternal obesity with the PE (indicating a doubled risk for every increase of BMI of 5–7 kg/m^2), while others denote only a slight tendency in this direction [29–33]. The pathogenesis of vascular damage that underlies PE may also be explained as a manifestation of a state of insulin resistance.

A condition of hyperinsulinemia, typical of obesity, is able to alter the intracellular cationic pumps regulating vascular tone and blood pressure, to stimulate the sympathetic nervous system and to induce hypertrophy of smooth muscle cells [42–44]. An increased level of vasoactive peptides that is associated with hyperinsulinemia may then contribute to endothelial damage that is characteristic of PE. In confirming a strong correlation between obesity and the onset of PE, several authors have emphasized a common condition: the activation of the inflammatory system [42–44]. The finding of high serum concentrations of IL-6 and CRP in obese pregnant women is a key point in the condition of chronic inflammation typical of obesity, which correlates negatively with endothelial function and positively with the levels of fasting insulin, thus demonstrating a possible implication in the pathogenesis of gestational diabetes mellitus (GDM) [44, 45].

From these observations it emerges as the metabolic and inflammatory features of obese women may predispose to vascular damage then helping the mechanism through which the maternal adiposity is associated with the emergence of PE. Epidemiological studies demonstrated that women with pregnancies complicated by PE are more likely to develop coronary heart diseases later in life [29, 30]. However, TNF and IL-6 expression, well-known acute-phase reactant, are increased in obese pregnant women independently of PE, then suggesting the involvement of other sources to the circulation than the placenta itself. A role for maternal adipose tissue, particularly visceral fat, could then be suggested [8].

Abdominal obesity is frequently associated with a condition of hyperinsulinemia. High concentrations of insulin reduce the number of insulin receptors and, as a consequence, the effect of insulin itself. The maintenance of a euglycemia condition therefore requires a progressive increase in insulin secretion. Pregnancy, which is a condition of stress on carbohydrate metabolism, may affect this delicate balance. Multiple studies document an increased risk of GDM among obese pregnant women, in particular between those with morbid obesity (BMI > 35 kg/m^2) [42–46]. An incidence of 24.5 % for GDM in pregnant women with BMI greater than 40 kg/m^2 compared to 2.2 % in women with BMI between 20 and 24.9 kg/m^2 was reported [42–46]. Women who develop GDM are also more likely to develop diabetes in their lifetime [29]. Such considerations make it necessary to identify patients potentially at risk of developing GDM, in order to implement preventive measures. It is demonstrated that even a modest weight loss between two subsequent pregnancies modifies the risk of GDM development [42–46]. Obesity finally exposes pregnant women to a worsening of preexisting diabetes with an increased risk of fetal macrosomia, nervous system defects, cardiovascular diseases, and increased mortality risk, as well as an increased likelihood of developing obesity in childhood [29, 32–34].

5.5 Adipose Tissue in Pregnancy

The functional/morphologic changes of adipose tissue in pregnancy have been poorly studied in humans, but it is possible that the obesity-linked metabolic and inflammatory adipose tissue alterations represent an additional factor contributing to a pro-inflammatory state in pregnancy [35]. High subcutaneous abdominal adipose tissue thickness during pregnancy has been associated with elevated inflammatory marker levels [46]. It was described that abdominal thickness ≥15 mm (by ultrasounds techniques) is a strong predictor of high CRP and HbA1c circulating levels in pregnant women [47]. In addition, higher values of fat thickness during 24–28 weeks of gestation are associated with pregnancy-related complications that could be observed during later periods of gestation [47, 48]. Measurement of abdominal fat might then be helpful to identify groups at risk [47, 48].

The weight gain in pregnant women is due to the placenta, *fetus*, and increasing *uterus* and breast volumes, including increase of plasma mass and general body water retention. In pregnancy, the correct measurement of waist circumference or WHR, as well as calculation of BMI, might be difficult due to the progressive weight gain and fluid redistribution. Indeed, waist circumference measurement does not differentiate between visceral and subcutaneous depots and has not been validated for pregnant women. Changes in body-composition characteristics during pregnancy, such as hydration and frequently edema, may affect the validity of the interpretation of other instrumental measurements, such as body impedance analysis.

During pregnancy there is a progressive increase of fat deposits useful to protect the *fetus* from any nutritional deficiencies and to support lactation. The extent of these fat deposits is proportional to the increase of weight of the woman, and therefore, the greater the difference between the weight prepregnancy and that at the end of pregnancy, the greater the amount of adipose tissue remaining in the new mother [28]. Considering the methods and extent of weight loss in the *puerperium*, it is seen that the real cause of weight retention after pregnancy is to be found in increasing weight in pregnancy [28]. The demonstration of little influences of factors, such as maternal age, socioeconomic conditions, mode of delivery, smoking, type of work, and the use of oral contraceptives, underlines the importance of an adequate control of the pregnant weight, in order to avoid the onset of a condition of obesity from an overweight or worsen a pre-existing obesity [27–29].

5.5.1 Leptin and Adiponectin in Pregnancy

Focusing on adipokines, it is known that maternal leptin levels increase during the first and second trimesters, peaking in the late second or in the early third trimester. Leptin levels remain high throughout all the gestation period and drastically decline after delivery. Together with low-grade systemic inflammatory state, the high leptin levels of pre-gravid obese women are believed to be the primer for placental inflammation during pregnancies. The placenta itself is a source of leptin and significantly contributes to the increased circulating levels observed in pregnancy. High leptin concentrations during pregnancy are emerging as potential predictor of PE development in obese women [49–53].

Adiponectin plays an important role in maternal, placental, and fetal physiology. During gestation, there is an early increase in serum adiponectin levels followed by a decline in the second half of gestation. Interestingly, changes in serum adiponectin levels are correlated with maternal insulin sensitivity, and low adiponectin levels are associated with severe PE, GDM, and increased risk of delivering "large for gestational age" (macrosomic) infants. In normal weight pregnant women, serum adiponectin is inversely correlated with birth weight even though the molecular mechanisms underlying this relation are still unknown. Interestingly, with the exception of adiponectin, the placenta has a similar secretory profile as white adipose tissue [54–58].

Several studies demonstrated that the number of $CD68^{+}/CD14^{+}$ macrophages was increased two- to threefold in the placenta of obese, compared with lean, pregnant women [59]. Of interest, the source of the CD14+ macrophages in the placenta was confirmed to be of maternal and not fetal origin [60]. Based on these studies, maternal obesity seems to be the main cause of the inflammation involving maternal white adipose tissues, plasma, as well as placenta [33]. There is now agreement on the fact that many chronic diseases, including obesity, can negatively affect the *fetal programming*, *i.e.*, the epigenetic adaptation of cells and tissues to an early nutritional stress (with trans-generational heritable effects) [33, 40].

The biological mechanisms mediating these connections are not completely known at present, but are likely related to programming of insulin and leptin resistance *in utero*. Despite evidence of maternal obesity complications, inflammation, and negative effects in offspring, there is a little knowledge on the effectiveness of nutrients with anti-inflammatory properties during pregnancy in obese women.

References

1. Gallus S, Lugo A, Murisic B, Bosetti C, Boffetta P, La Vecchia C. Overweight and obesity in 16 European countries. Eur J Nutr. 2014. doi:10.1007/s00394-014-0746-4 [Epub a head of print]
2. Janssen I, Katzmarzyk PT, Ross R. Body mass index, waist circumference, and health risk: evidence in support of current National Institutes of Health guidelines. Arch Intern Med. 2002;162(18):2074–9.
3. Kelly T, Yang W, Chen CS, Reynolds K, He J. Global burden of obesity in 2005 and projections to 2030. Int J Obes (Lond). 2008;32(9):1431–7.
4. Webber L, Divajeva D, Marsh T, McPherson K, Brown M, Galea G, Breda J. The future burden of obesity-related diseases in the 53 WHO European-Region countries and the impact of effective interventions: a modelling study. BMJ Open. 2014;4(7). doi:10.1136/bmjopen-2014-004787 [Epub a head of print]
5. WHO, Global Database on Body Mass Index, World Health Organization. 2011. Available at: www.who.int/topics/obesity/en/
6. WHO. Waist circumference and waist–hip ratio: report of a WHO expert consultation. 2008; WHO Document Production Services, Geneva, Switzerland;p.1–39.
7. Onat A, Avci GS, Barlan MM, Uyarel H, Uzunlar B, Sansoy V. Measures of abdominal obesity assessed for visceral adiposity and relation to coronary risk. Int J Obes Relat Metab Disord. 2004;28(8):1018–25.
8. Bastien M, Poirier P, Lemieux I, Després JP. Overview of epidemiology and contribution of obesity to cardiovascular disease. Prog Cardiovasc Dis. 2014;56(4):369–81.
9. Burgio E, Lopomo A, Migliore L. Obesity and diabetes: from genetics to epigenetics. Mol Biol Rep. 2015;42(4):799–818. doi:10.1007/s11033-014-3751-z.
10. Loos RJ. Genetic determinants of common obesity and their value in prediction. Best Pract Res Clin Endocrinol Metab. 2012;26(2):211–26.
11. Loos RJ, Bouchard C. Obesity – is it a genetic disorder? J Intern Med. 2003;254(5):401–25.
12. Slomko H, Heo HJ, Einstein FH. Minireview: epigenetics of obesity and diabetes in humans. Endocrinology. 2012;153(3):1025–30.
13. Cancello R, Clément K. Is obesity an inflammatory illness? Role of low-grade inflammation and macrophage infiltration in human white adipose tissue. BJOG. 2006;113(10):1141–7.
14. Cancello R, Tordjman J, et al. Increased infiltration of macrophages in omental adipose tissue is associated with marked hepatic lesions in morbid human obesity. Diabetes. 2006;55(6):1554–61.
15. Gregor MF, Hotamisligil GS. Inflammatory mechanisms in obesity. Annu Rev Immunol. 2011;29:415–45. doi:10.1146/annurev-immunol-031210-101322.

16. Heilbronn LK, Campbell LV, et al. Adipose tissue macrophages, low grade inflammation and insulin resistance in human obesity. Curr Pharm Des. 2008;14(12):1225–30.
17. Hotamisligil GS. Inflammation and metabolic disorders. Nature. 2006;444(7121):860–7.
18. Hotamisligil GS. Endoplasmic reticulum stress and the inflammatory basis of metabolic disease. Cell. 2010;140(6):900–17.
19. Cancello R, Tounian A, et al. Adiposity signals, genetic and body weight regulation in humans. Diabetes Metab. 2004;30(3):215–27.
20. Ouchi N, Parker JL, et al. Adipokines in inflammation and metabolic disease. Nat Rev Immunol. 2011;11(2):85–97.
21. Tritos NA, Mantzoros CS. Leptin: its role in obesity and beyond. Diabetologia. 1997;14(12): 1371–9.
22. Fantuzzi G, Faggioni R, et al. Leptin in the regulation of immunity, inflammation and hematopoiesis. J Leukoc. 2000;68:437–46.
23. Cancello R, Henegar C, et al. Reduction of macrophage infiltration and chemoattractant gene expression changes in white adipose tissue of morbidly obese subjects after surgery-induced weight loss. Diabetes. 2005;54(8):2277–86.
24. Jo J, Gavrilova O, et al. Hypertrophy and/or hyperplasia: dynamics of adipose tissue growth. PLoS Comput Biol. 2009;5:e1000324.
25. Bouloumié A, Casteilla L, et al. Adipose tissue lymphocytes and macrophages in obesity and insulin resistance: makers or markers, and which comes first? Arterioscler Thromb Vasc Biol. 2008;28(7):1211–3.
26. Hammar EB, Irminger JC, Rickenbach K, Parnaud G, Ribaux P, Bosco D, et al. Activation of NF-kappaB by extracellular matrix is involved in spreading and glucose-stimulated insulin secretion of pancreatic beta cells. J Biol Chem. 2005;26(34):30630–7.
27. Aviram A, Hod M. Maternal obesity: implications for pregnancy outcome and long-term risks-a link to maternal nutrition. Int J Gynaecol Obstet. 2011;115(1):S6–10.
28. Norman JE, Reynolds RM. The consequences of obesity and excess weight gain in pregnancy. Proc Nutr Soc. 2011;70(4):514.
29. Papachatzi E, Dimitriou G. Pre-pregnancy obesity: maternal, neonatal and childhood outcomes. J Neonatal Perinatal Med. 2013;6(3):203–16.
30. Sattar N, Greer IA. Pregnancy complications and maternal cardiovascular risk: opportunities for intervention and screening? BMJ. 2002;325(7356):157–60.
31. Taylor PD, Samuelsson AM. Maternal obesity and the developmental programming of hypertension: a role for leptin. Acta Physiol. 2010;3:508–23.
32. Tenenbaum-Gavish K, Hod M. Impact of maternal obesity on fetal health. Fetal Diagn Ther. 2013;34(1):1–7.
33. Aune D, Saugstad OD. Maternal body mass index and the risk of fetal death, stillbirth, and infant death: a systematic review and meta-analysis. JAMA. 2014;311(15):1536–46.
34. Frias AE, Grove KL. Obesity: a transgenerational problem linked to nutrition during pregnancy. Semin Reprod Med. 2012;30(6):472–8.
35. Bashiri A, Heo HJ. Pregnancy complicated by obesity induces global transcript expression alterations in visceral and subcutaneous fat. Mol Genet Genomics. 2014;289:695–705.
36. Denison FC, Roberts KA. Obesity, pregnancy, inflammation, and vascular function. Reproduction. 2010;140(3):373–85.
37. Lindqvist P, Dahlback B. Thrombotic risk during pregnancy: a population study. Obstet Gynecol. 1999;94(4):595–9.
38. Molyneaux E, Poston L. Obesity and mental disorders during pregnancy and postpartum: a systematic review and meta-analysis. Obstet Gynecol. 2014;123(4):857–67.
39. Roberts KA, Riley SC. Placental structure and inflammation in pregnancies associated with obesity. Placenta. 2011;32(3):247–54.
40. Westermeier F, Sáez PJ. Programming of fetal insulin resistance in pregnancies with maternal obesity by ER stress and inflammation. Biomed Res Int. 2014;2014:917672. doi:10.1155/2014/917672. [Epub 2014 Jun 30].

41. Xu J, Zhao YH. Maternal circulating concentrations of tumor necrosis factor-alpha, leptin, and adiponectin in gestational diabetes mellitus: a systematic review and meta-analysis. Scientific World J. 2014;2014:926932. doi:10.1155/2014/926932 [Epub 2014 Aug 19].
42. Jeyabalan A. Epidemiology of preeclampsia: impact of obesity. Nutr Rev. 2013;71 Suppl 1:S18–25.
43. Jones CJ, Hartmann M. Ultrastructural localization of insulin receptors in human placenta. Am J Reprod Immunol. 1993;30(2-3):136–45.
44. Desoye G, Hartmann M. Location of insulin receptors in the placenta and its progenitor tissues. Microsc Res Tech. 1997;38(1–2):36–75.
45. Kirwan JP, Hauguel-de Mouzon S. TNF-alpha is a predictor of insulin resistance in human pregnancy. Diabetes. 2002;51(7):2207–13.
46. Radaelli T, Varastehpour A. Gestational diabetes induces placental genes for chronic stress and inflammatory pathways. Diabetes. 2003;52(12):2951–8.
47. Köşüş N, Köşüş A. Relation between abdominal subcutaneous fat tissue thickness and inflammatory markers during pregnancy. Arch Med Sci. 2014;10(4):739–45.
48. Straughen JK, Trudeau S. Changes in adipose tissue distribution during pregnancy in overweight and obese compared with normal weight women. Nutr Diabetes. 2013;3:e84. doi:10.1038/nutd.2013.25.
49. Tessier DR, Ferraro ZM. Role of leptin in pregnancy: consequences of maternal obesity. Placenta. 2013;34(3):205–11.
50. Hauguel-de Mouzon S. The known and unknown of leptin in pregnancy. Am J Obstet Gynecol. 2006;194(6):1537–45.
51. Masuzaki H, Ogawa Y. Non-adipose tissue production of leptin: leptin as a novel placenta-derived hormone in humans. Nat Med. 1997;3(9):1029–113.
52. Highman T, Friedman J. Longitudinal changes in maternal leptin serum concentrations, body composition and resting metabolic rate in pregnancy. Am J Obstet Gynecol. 1998;178(5): 1010–5.
53. Poston L. Leptin and preeclampsia. Semin Reprod Med. 2002;20(2):131–8.
54. Aye IL, Powell TL. Adiponectin-the missing link between maternal adiposity, placental transport and fetal growth? Placenta. 2013;34(Suppl):S40–5.
55. Briana DD, Malamitsi-Puchner A. Adipocytokines in normal and complicated pregnancies. Reprod Sci. 2009;16(10):921–37.
56. Mazaki-Tovi S, Kanety H. Maternal serum adiponectin levels during human pregnancy. J Perinatol. 2007;27(2):77–81.
57. Corbetta S, Bulfamante G. Adiponectin expression in human fetal tissues during mid- and late gestation. J Clin Endocrinol Metab. 2005;90(4):2397–402.
58. Haghiac M, Basu S. Patterns of adiponectin expression in term pregnancy: impact of obesity. J Clin Endocrinol Metab. 2014;99(9):3427–34.
59. Challier JC. Obesity in pregnancy stimulates macrophage accumulation and inflammation in the placenta. Placenta. 2008;29(3):274–81. doi:10.1016/j.placenta.2007.12.010.
60. Basu S, Leahy P. Molecular phenotype of monocytes at the maternal-fetal interface. Am J Obstet Gynecol. 2011;205(3):265.e1–8. doi:http://dx.doi.org/10.1016/j.ajog.2011.06.037.

The Role of Placental Inflammasomes in Linking the Adverse Effects of Maternal Obesity on Fetal Development

6

Irving L.M.H. Aye, Susanne Lager, and Theresa L. Powell

Contents

6.1 Introduction

In the United States, over two-thirds of women of reproductive age have a high body mass index (BMI >25 kg/m^2), and more than one-third are obese (BMI >30 kg/m^2) [1]. Maternal obesity represents significant health risks for both mother and child. Pregnant mothers who are obese have an increased risk of developing hypertension, preeclampsia, and gestational diabetes. Infants born to

I.L.M.H. Aye, PhD
Division of Basic Reproductive Sciences, Department of Obstetrics and Gynecology, University of Colorado School of Medicine, Denver, CO, USA

S. Lager, PhD
Department of Obstetrics and Gynaecology, University of Cambridge, Cambridge, UK

T.L. Powell, PhD (✉)
Division of Basic Reproductive Sciences, Department of Obstetrics and Gynecology, University of Colorado School of Medicine, Denver, CO, USA

Section of Neonatology, Department of Pediatrics, University of Colorado School of Medicine, Denver, CO, USA
e-mail: theresa.powell@ucdenver.edu

E. Ferrazzi, B. Sears (eds.), *Metabolic Syndrome and Complications of Pregnancy: The Potential Preventive Role of Nutrition*,
DOI 10.1007/978-3-319-16853-1_6

obese and gestational diabetic mothers are likely to have greater adiposity, elevated levels of proinflammatory cytokines, and insulin resistance [2]. Children of obese mothers are susceptible to childhood obesity and to develop cardiovascular disease, type 2 diabetes, and obesity as adults [3]. Animal models and clinical studies suggest that the intrauterine environment plays a critical role in mediating the adverse effects of maternal obesity on the offspring and therefore offers a unique window of opportunity for intervention. However, few strategies are currently available for the prevention of obesity or metabolic dysfunction in children of obese mothers. Recent studies demonstrate that children born to women who had undergone bariatric surgery and weight loss had a lower prevalence of obesity compared to their siblings born before surgical weight loss [4]. Although bariatric surgery is limited to morbidly obese patients, this finding establishes the importance of the maternal metabolic environment on the in utero transmission of obesity to the next generation.

In the past decade, the search for potentially unifying mechanisms underlying the pathogenesis of obesity-associated diseases has revealed a surprisingly close relationship between signaling pathways regulating cellular immune response and metabolic homeostasis. This has given rise to the concept of "metaflammation" (metabolically induced inflammation) which refers to a distinct set of inflammatory responses principally triggered by nutrients and metabolites [5]. In contrast to the acute innate immune response induced by microbial stimuli, metaflammation is characterized by multisystemic chronic low-grade inflammation leading to insulin resistance in several tissues including the adipose, liver, and muscle [6]. While pregnancy itself represents a physiologic inflammatory state, women entering pregnancy with preexisting obesity exhibit enhanced systemic inflammation associated with peripheral insulin resistance [7], which may lead to the development of gestational diabetes. In recent years, placental inflammation has emerged as a common observation in these pregnancy disorders [8–12], although the mechanisms regulating placental inflammatory processes in maternal obesity have been a matter for debate [8, 10, 11].

The human placenta is the direct interface between maternal and fetal circulations. The placenta performs many indispensable tasks including hormone production, nutrient transfer, and gas exchange. Optimal placental function is thus paramount to support the growth and development of a healthy infant. Maternal diet and disease can influence placental development and function, leading to changes in the supply of nutrients, hormones, and oxygen to the fetus. The placenta therefore plays a central role in determining the impact of maternal obesity on fetal development and the long-term health of the infant. Clinical studies now indicate that maternal obesity is associated with changes in placental function [13–17]. In particular, placental circulation [17, 18], nutrient transporters [13, 19, 20], and metabolic function [14, 15] have been reported to be influenced by maternal adiposity. Whether these changes are associated with or caused by placental inflammatory processes is currently unclear.

6.2 Inflammatory Mechanisms Involved in Metabolic Disorders

All tissues possess inflammatory mechanisms which mediate a highly coordinated homeostatic response to harmful stimuli. The short-term adaptive inflammatory response is a crucial component of tissue repair involving the integration of multiple signals in distinct cells and tissues. However, if left unresolved, long-term inflammation may result in permanent organ damage. The chronic nature of obesity produces low-grade inflammation that disrupts metabolic homeostasis over time. An adverse in utero environment may place individuals at risk of lifelong metaflammation predisposing the infant to the development of metabolic syndrome in later life.

Insulin resistance is a hallmark of the metabolic syndrome, occurring as a result of decreased insulin sensitivity in the adipose, liver, and muscle. To maintain homeostasis, insulin secretion from pancreatic β-cells is increased. Over time, β-cells may fail to meet the increasing demand for insulin, resulting in hyperglycemia and diabetes. A link between inflammation and insulin resistance was first established by the demonstration that TNFα knockout mice were protected against obesity-induced insulin resistance [21]. Compared to wild-type obese mice, TNFα-null obese mice exhibited increased insulin signaling in adipose and muscle tissues, improved glucose metabolism, and reduced circulating levels of free fatty acids. Indeed, TNFα levels during pregnancy predicted maternal insulin resistance even in euglycemic women [22], and a proinflammatory maternal *milieu* is associated with a number of pregnancy disorders.

Inflammation is initiated by cytokines and pathogen-associated molecular patterns (PAMPs), such as carbohydrates, lipoproteins, and lipopolysaccharide components of bacterial and fungal cell walls, that stimulate plasma membrane-bound cytokine receptors or toll-like receptors (TLR) to initiate an inflammatory signaling cascade. These signaling pathways in turn activate transcription factors which drive the expression of genes which collectively assist in the recruitment and activation of immune cells and removal of pathogens and accelerate tissue repair. In recent years, TLR4 has emerged as a sensor for both microbial products and nutrients. The archetypal TLR4 agonist is lipopolysaccharide (LPS), a component of Gram-negative bacteria cell wall. Interestingly, saturated fatty acids (SFAs) acylated in the lipid A moiety of LPS were sufficient to invoke TLR4-mediated biological effects [23], implicating a role for circulating fatty acids in the inflammatory response. The effect of fatty acids on TLR4 activity depends on chain length and saturation [24]. Saturated fatty acids such as palmitic (C16:0) and stearic (C18:0) acid promote TLR4-mediated inflammatory response, whereas the omega-3 polyunsaturated fatty acid (n-3 PUFA) docosahexaenoic acid (C22:6) attenuates TLR4 signaling. Additionally, TLR4 is activated by other endogenous molecules especially in response to stress. Otherwise known as danger-associated molecular patterns (DAMPs), these endogenous TLR4 agonists include heat shock proteins, oxidized lipids and sterols, and breakdown products of the extracellular matrix [25–27].

TLR4 activates two major signaling pathways, the mitogen-associated protein kinase (MAPK) pathways (p38 MAPK and c-Jun N-terminal kinases (JNK)) and

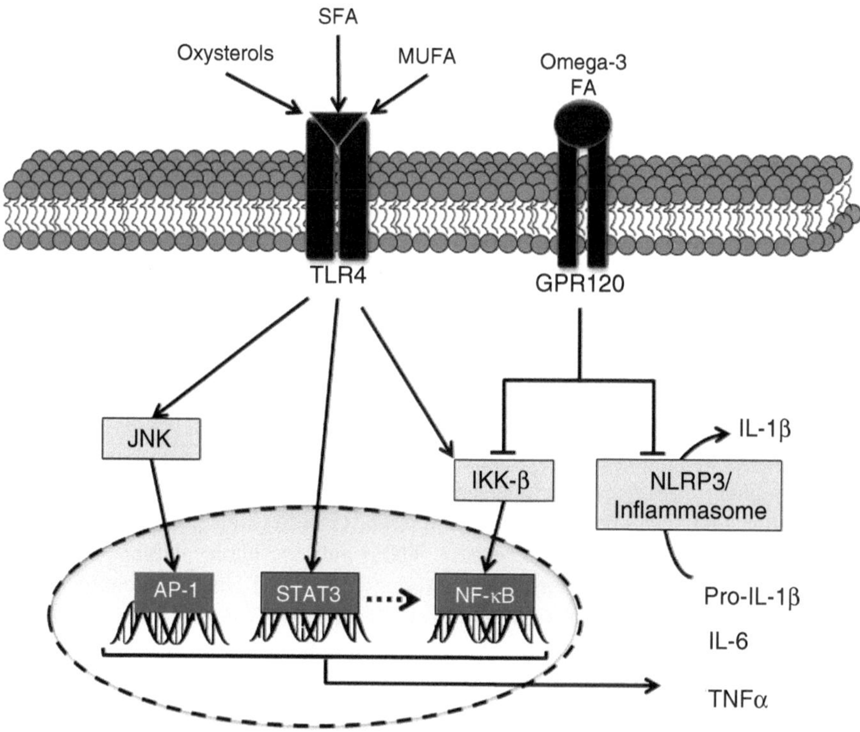

Fig. 6.1 Regulation of placental inflammatory response by dietary fatty acids. Saturated and monounsaturated fatty acids activate TLR4 leading to downstream inflammatory pathways JNK and NF-κB. JNK activates AP-1 transcription factors, while NF-κB subunits directly translocate to the nucleus and bind promoter regions of proinflammatory cytokines. Omega-3 fatty acids bind to the GPR120 plasma membrane receptor to inhibit inflammatory pathways. The intracellular NLRP3 inflammasome, which is responsible for IL-1β maturation, is also activated by dietary fatty acids and inhibited by omega-3 fatty acids. *AP-1* activating protein-1, *GPR120* G protein-coupled receptor 120, *IKK-β* inhibitor of nuclear factor kappa B kinase, *JNK* c-jun-N-terminal kinase, *MUFA* monounsaturated fatty acid, *NF-κB* nuclear factor kappa B, *NLRP3/Inflammasome* nod-like receptor 3 inflammasome, *SFA* saturated fatty acid

nuclear factor kappa B (NF-κB). Activation of JNK results in nuclear translocation where it regulates the activity of activating protein-1 (AP-1), a heterodimeric protein composed of multiple transcription factors belonging to c-Fos, c-Jun, ATF, and JDP families that regulate a vast array of genes. Conversely, NF-κB activation results in nuclear translocation of one of its five subunits which directly controls gene transcription. Moreover, reports of AP-1 regulation of NF-κB and vice versa suggest significant crosstalk between these signaling pathways [28, 29]. Collectively, activation of these signaling pathways results in increased transcription of cytokines, such as IL-6, IL-1β, and TNFα, which inhibit insulin signaling in many tissues. Research in the last decade provides significant evidence for the involvement of these pathways in the initiation, propagation, and development of metabolic diseases [30, 31]. Figure 6.1 illustrates an overview of the major inflammatory mechanisms implicated in metabolic disorders.

6.3 Placental Inflammation in Maternal Obesity

While there have been numerous animal models of maternal obesity in pregnancy demonstrating placental inflammation [18, 32–34], we have limited our discussion to human studies. Several studies show increased expression of proinflammatory cytokines IL-6, IL-1β, and TNFα in placental tissues of obese mothers [8, 10–12]. The mechanism(s) of placental inflammation in maternal obesity, however, has been a source of contention. Analogous to adipose tissues, increased accumulation of maternal macrophages in placentas of obese mothers has been reported by some investigators [9, 10], while others were unable to show any differences [11]. Similarly, Saben et al. have implicated placental JNK and NF-κB with maternal obesity [12, 35], while we could not find any changes in these pathways, but discovered increased STAT3 and p38 MAPK activity in placentas of obese mothers [8]. One possible explanation for these differences may be related to subject selection, since maternal obesity is also associated with several comorbidities including hypertension and gestational diabetes, conditions potentially more likely to invoke a greater multisystemic inflammatory response than obesity per se.

While activation of placental inflammatory processes in maternal obesity has been described [8, 12, 35, 36], the physiological significance of placental inflammation has not been addressed in adequate detail. Inflammation of the fetal membranes (chorioamnionitis) is a major risk factor for preterm birth, which may result in premature rupture of the membranes (PROM). Recent epidemiological studies demonstrate increased risk of preterm deliveries in obese mothers [37, 38]. However, it is currently unclear if placental inflammation associated with maternal obesity increases the risk of PROM. Systemic or placental inflammation may also result in endothelial dysfunction. Pre-gravid obesity increases maternal levels of markers of endothelial dysfunction [39] and is associated with impaired vascular function in placental arteries [17]. Consequently, this may impact upon fetal heart development, because uteroplacental circulation has been linked with fetal vascular function [40].

Previous work from our lab demonstrated that proinflammatory cytokines influence placental nutrient transport functions [41, 42]. Using concentrations similar to circulating cytokine concentrations in obese women, IL-6 and TNFα were shown to stimulate amino acid transport activity [41], while higher concentrations were required to stimulate fatty acid uptake into primary trophoblasts [42]. STAT3 activity was required for IL-6 (and leptin)-stimulated amino acid uptake [41, 43], while our preliminary data suggests a role for p38 MAPK in regulating the TNFα response (Aye et al, 2015 unpublished observations). In addition to cytokines, insulin and leptin (hormones elevated in maternal obesity) also significantly increase placental amino acid transport [44, 45]. Interestingly, IL-1β which is also upregulated in the placentas of obese mothers [8, 10, 11] was shown to inhibit insulin-dependent [46] and insulin-independent [47, 48] amino acid transport in placental primary trophoblasts and trophoblast cell lines. These findings suggest complex interactions between proinflammatory cytokines and maternal hormones in the regulation of placental nutrient transfer to the fetus.

6.4 The Emerging Role of Placental Inflammasomes in Pregnancy Disorders

Inflammasomes are multi-protein complexes composed of a cytoplasmic receptor, an apoptosis-associated speck-like protein (ASC) containing a caspase activation and recruitment domain (CARD) adaptor, and pro-caspase-1, which associate upon cellular exposure to microbial or endogenous danger signals. Upon activation, the inflammasome complex formation results in caspase-1 maturation leading to proteolytic cleavage of pro-IL-1β into mature IL-1β (Fig. 6.2). This is then followed by either secretion of IL-1β into the circulation which may lead to systemic inflammatory effects or more locally induced pyroptosis. Currently, six members of the nod-like receptor (NLR) family are known to function as "pathogen" or "danger" sensors to initiate inflammasome complex formation. Of these, NLRP3 is best characterized for its role in both immune and metabolic disorders.

The placenta expresses the cytosolic NLRP1, NLRP3, and NLRC4 [49], which respond to multiple factors associated with both pathogenic and sterile inflammation. Activation of inflammasomes in gestational tissues has been reported in a number of pregnancy complications including preterm birth [50–52], preeclampsia [53–55], and microbial infections [56]. The resulting release of mature IL-1β mediates a myriad of effects in gestational tissues including induction of IGFBP-1

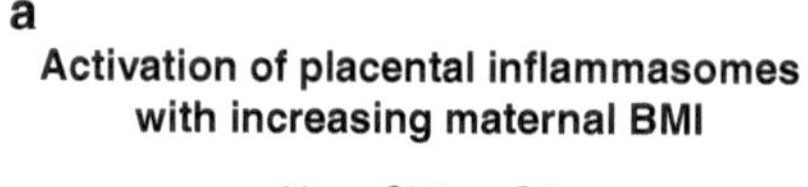

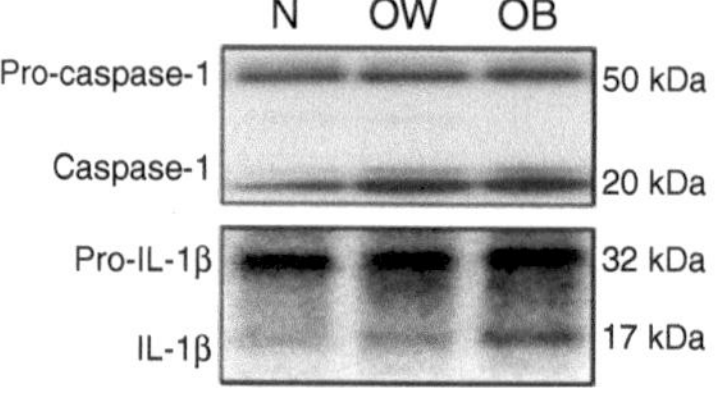

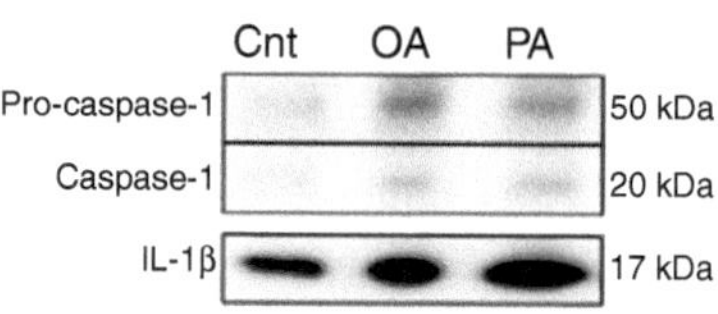

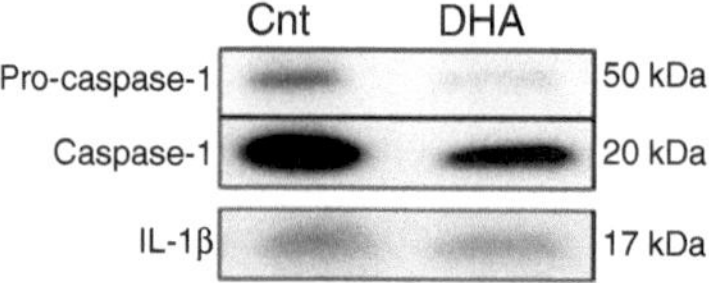

Fig. 6.2 Increased placental inflammasomes in maternal obesity – regulation by dietary fatty acids. (**a**) Representative immunoblot showing caspase-1 activation and increased IL-1β maturation with maternal adiposity. (**b**) Immunoblot demonstrating increased inflammasome activation by oleic and palmitic acid (100 μM) in primary human trophoblasts. (**c**) Immunoblot of decreased inflammasome activation by 50 μM DHA treatment in primary human trophoblasts. *BMI* body mass index, *DHA* docosahexaenoic acid, *N* normal, *OW* overweight, *OB* obese, *Cnt* BSA-control, *OA* oleic acid, *PA* palmitic acid

expression in decidual tissues thereby decreasing the bioavailability of IGF-I in the feto-maternal interface and in the maternal circulation [57] and stimulating placental production of progesterone [58], hCG [59], and activin-A [60]. Furthermore, IL-1β is a highly apoptotic agent in human gestational tissues [61]. Hence knowledge of the mechanisms governing IL-1β production in the placenta plays a critical role in understanding the pathogenesis of several pregnancy disorders.

We recently identified increased caspase-1 activation in placentas of women with high BMI ([62] and Fig. 6.2), despite no changes in placental NF-κB DNA-binding activity. Likewise, expression of the mature IL-1β protein (17 kDa) in placental tissues was also positively correlated with maternal BMI, whereas pro-IL-1β (32 kDa) was not significantly altered by maternal BMI. These findings indicate a novel mechanism in which IL-1β is regulated at the posttranslational level by maternal obesity. We further determined the impact of IL-1β on placental function and demonstrated that IL-1β inhibits insulin signaling and function (as measured by insulin-mediated amino acid transport) in primary human trophoblasts [46]. Inhibition of insulin signaling was mediated at the level of the insulin receptor substrate-1 (IRS-1), where IL-1β increased the inhibitory serine phosphorylation of IRS-1 (Ser307), decreased tyrosine phosphorylation-mediated activation of IRS-1 (Tyr612), and reduced total IRS-1 levels. Decreased IRS-1 activity led to inactivation of both the PI3K and GRB2 signaling pathways downstream of IRS-1. Taken together, these findings suggest that the increased inflammasome activation in placentas of high BMI mothers may lead to decreased placental insulin sensitivity. However, the signals activating inflammasomes in these placentas are currently unclear.

Because the classical inflammatory pathways associated with the microbial response (namely, NF-κB and JNK) were not altered in the placenta in pregnancies complicated by maternal obesity, we hypothesized that placental inflammasome activation is a result of DAMPs or nutritional and/or oxidative stress. Robust activation of the inflammasomes requires two signals: a first "priming" signal, which promotes NF-κB activity leading to pro-IL-1β expression, and a second "activating" signal that activates caspase-1. In the placenta, constitutive NF-κB activity is likely to contribute to pro-IL-1β expression, whereas caspase-1 activation requires a specific event. DAMPs including cholesterol crystals, ATP, potassium efflux, and ceramide initiate caspase-1 maturation in many cell types [63]. However, it is currently unclear if DAMPs provide the mechanistic link to placental inflammasome activation because these factors have not been implicated in maternal obesity. On the other hand, maternal obesity is associated with oxidative stress, which may provide the necessary signal required for caspase-1 activation [12, 14, 64]. Dietary SFAs activate inflammasomes in a cell-specific manner [65, 66]. In immune cells palmitic acid, but not oleic acid, triggered inflammasome activation [67]. In contrast, both these saturated fatty acids increased caspase-1 activity and IL-1β maturation in cultured primary human trophoblast cells (Fig. 6.2). This discrepancy is particularly relevant in pregnancy because obese mothers typically have high circulating levels of SFA, especially palmitic acid and monounsaturated fatty acid (MUFA) such as oleic acid [68]. Interestingly, both palmitic and oleic acids are capable of activating TLR4 [35, 69], suggesting that these fatty acids stimulate both the necessary pathways required for robust inflammasome activation. Moreover, most Western diets have low levels of

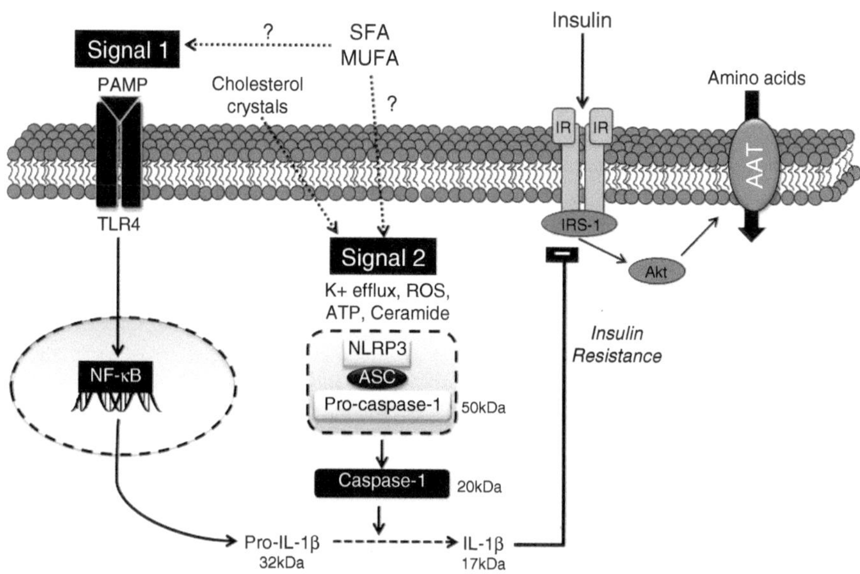

Fig. 6.3 Mechanisms linking dietary inflammasome activation to placental insulin resistance. Inflammasome-mediated IL-1β maturation requires a "priming" signal involving TLR4-NF-κB-mediated pro-IL-1β expression. A secondary "activation" signal in the form of DAMPs or dietary fatty acids promotes NLRP3-inflammasome complex formation resulting in caspase-1-mediated proteolytic cleavage of IL-1β. Mature IL-1β may function in an autocrine manner to degrade IRS-1 protein leading to decreased insulin signaling and insulin-mediated amino acid transport. *AAT* amino acid transport, *ASC* apoptosis-associated speck-like protein containing a CARD adaptor, *IR* insulin receptor, *IRS-1* insulin receptor substrate-1, *MUFA* monounsaturated fatty acid, *NF-κB* nuclear factor kappa B, *NLRP3* nod-like receptor 3, *PAMP* pathogen-associated molecular pattern, *ROS* reactive oxygen species, *SFA* saturated fatty acid, *TLR4* toll-like receptor 4

long-chain n-3 PUFA – in particular docosahexaenoic acid (DHA) [70], which has previously been shown to prevent inflammasome activation in macrophages [71–73]. Consistent with these reports, our preliminary data demonstrates that DHA decreases (pro-)caspase-1 expression thereby attenuating IL-1β maturation (Fig. 6.2). The high dietary SFA and MUFA combined with low n-3 PUFA may therefore favor inflammasome activation in the placentas of high BMI mothers (Fig. 6.3).

The clinical significance of increased inflammasome activation leading to IL-1β-mediated insulin resistance in the placenta may be substantial. Although, increased placental amino acid transport activity has been reported in obese [13] or diabetic mothers [74], other studies demonstrate either no changes [75] or reduced transport activity [76, 77]. The discrepancy between these reports may be due to the inflammatory status of these placentas. It is possible that an increased placental inflammatory response associated with maternal obesity [8, 10–12, 35] or diabetes [78–81] may limit placental insulin-mediated transport, featuring an adaptive mechanism to limit excessive fetal growth in the presence of maternal hyperinsulinemia. Providing circumstantial support for this concept are reports demonstrating that the inflammatory processes associated with fetal growth restriction also inhibit placental transport activity in pregnancies complicated by malaria, a condition which increases the risk of fetal growth restriction [48].

Glyburide is a sulfonylurea agent which stimulates insulin release in the pancreas. The use of glyburide in the management of gestational diabetes has been actively explored, due to its glucose-lowering effects. While generally considered a safe alternative to insulin treatment in gestational diabetes pregnancies [82], a recent meta-analysis demonstrated that glyburide use in pregnancy is associated with increased fetal growth [83]. Although it is currently unclear if the association represents a cause and effect, it is interesting to note that glyburide is a potent inhibitor of inflammasome activation [84]. Hence inhibition of inflammasomes by glyburide may reduce IL-1β maturation, resulting in unrestricted insulin signaling in the placenta. Because insulin stimulates placental amino acid transport [45, 85], this may result in increased nutrient transfer to the fetus. In vitro studies testing this hypothesis will establish a mechanistic link between glyburide use in pregnancy and fetal growth.

Conclusions

The incidence of maternal obesity and its comorbidities (diabetes and cardiovascular disease) continues to surge, with major public health ramifications. Maternal obesity not only affects newborn health, but it also impacts the long-term health of the child leading to increased risk of childhood obesity and diabetes. Given all the evidence for the critical role of the in utero environment for lifelong health, understanding the impact of obesity in pregnancy represents a significant challenge, but also an intriguing opportunity to improve the health of future generations. Obesity is associated with the triad of metabolic complications: insulin resistance, dyslipidemia, and inflammation. Studies in recent years have demonstrated intimate links between these metabolic pathways, for example, inflammation causes insulin resistance and dyslipidemia, and dyslipidemia causes inflammation and insulin resistance. Excess nutrients, in particular dietary fatty acids, have emerged as a common instigator of these metabolic complications influencing insulin signaling and inflammatory pathways. As an organ of exchange, the placenta is a critical mediator of fetal health and is highly responsive to maternal health and diet. We recently reported inflammasome activation in the placentas of high BMI mothers, which inhibits placental insulin signaling and nutrient transport function. In vitro data suggests that placental inflammasomes are highly responsive to dietary fatty acids, with SFA and MUFA promoting inflammasome activation and n-3 PUFA inhibiting its activity. Future clinical studies are warranted to determine whether dietary interventions during pregnancy can impact upon infant and placental health by altering placental inflammatory pathways.

References

1. Flegal KM, Carroll MD, Kit BK, Ogden CL. Prevalence of obesity and trends in the distribution of body mass index among US adults, 1999–2010. JAMA. 2012;307:491–7.
2. Catalano PM, Presley L, Minium J, Hauguel-de Mouzon S. Fetuses of obese mothers develop insulin resistance in utero. Diabetes Care. 2009;32:1076–80.

3. Drake AJ, Reynolds RM. Impact of maternal obesity on offspring obesity and cardiometabolic disease risk. Reproduction. 2010;140:387–98.
4. Kral JG, Biron S, Simard S, Hould FS, Lebel S, Marceau S, Marceau P. Large maternal weight loss from obesity surgery prevents transmission of obesity to children who were followed for 2 to 18 years. Pediatrics. 2006;118:e1644–9.
5. Hotamisligil GS. Inflammation and metabolic disorders. Nature. 2006;444:860–7.
6. Lumeng CN, Saltiel AR. Inflammatory links between obesity and metabolic disease. J Clin Invest. 2011;121:2111–7.
7. Basu S, Haghiac M, Surace P, Challier JC, Guerre-Millo M, Singh K, Waters T, Minium J, Presley L, Catalano PM, Hauguel-de Mouzon S. Pregravid obesity associates with increased maternal endotoxemia and metabolic inflammation. Obesity (Silver Spring). 2011; 19:476–82.
8. Aye IL, Lager S, Ramirez VI, Gaccioli F, Dudley DJ, Jansson T, Powell TL. Increasing maternal body mass index is associated with systemic inflammation in the mother and the activation of distinct placental inflammatory pathways. Biol Reprod. 2014;90:129.
9. Basu S, Leahy P, Challier JC, Minium J, Catalano P, Hauguel-de Mouzon S. Molecular phenotype of monocytes at the maternal-fetal interface. Am J Obstet Gynecol. 2011;205(265):e261–8.
10. Challier JC, Basu S, Bintein T, Minium J, Hotmire K, Catalano PM, Hauguel-de Mouzon S. Obesity in pregnancy stimulates macrophage accumulation and inflammation in the placenta. Placenta. 2008;29:274–81.
11. Roberts KA, Riley SC, Reynolds RM, Barr S, Evans M, Statham A, Hor K, Jabbour HN, Norman JE, Denison FC. Placental structure and inflammation in pregnancies associated with obesity. Placenta. 2011;32:247–54.
12. Saben J, Lindsey F, Zhong Y, Thakali K, Badger TM, Andres A, Gomez-Acevedo H, Shankar K. Maternal obesity is associated with a lipotoxic placental environment. Placenta. 2014;35: 171–7.
13. Jansson N, Rosario FJ, Gaccioli F, Lager S, Jones HN, Roos S, Jansson T, Powell TL. Activation of placental mTOR signaling and amino acid transporters in obese women giving birth to large babies. J Clin Endocrinol Metab. 2013;98:105–13.
14. Mele J, Muralimanoharan S, Maloyan A, Myatt L. Impaired mitochondrial function in human placenta with increased maternal adiposity. Am J Physiol Endocrinol Metab. 2014;307(5): E419–25.
15. DuBois BN, O'Tierney-Ginn P, Pearson J, Friedman JE, Thornburg K, Cherala G. Maternal obesity alters feto-placental cytochrome P4501A1 activity. Placenta. 2012;33:1045–51.
16. Higgins L, Mills TA, Greenwood SL, Cowley EJ, Sibley CP, Jones RL. Maternal obesity and its effect on placental cell turnover. J Matern Fetal Neonatal Med. 2013;26:783–8.
17. Hayward CE, Higgins L, Cowley EJ, Greenwood SL, Mills TA, Sibley CP, Wareing M. Chorionic plate arterial function is altered in maternal obesity. Placenta. 2013;34: 281–7.
18. Frias AE, Morgan TK, Evans AE, Rasanen J, Oh KY, Thornburg KL, Grove KL. Maternal high-fat diet disturbs uteroplacental hemodynamics and increases the frequency of stillbirth in a nonhuman primate model of excess nutrition. Endocrinology. 2011;152:2456–64.
19. Brass E, Hanson E, O'Tierney-Ginn PF. Placental oleic acid uptake is lower in male offspring of obese women. Placenta. 2013;34:503–9.
20. Desforges M, Ditchfield A, Hirst CR, Pegorie C, Martyn-Smith K, Sibley CP, Greenwood SL. Reduced placental taurine transporter (TauT) activity in pregnancies complicated by pre-eclampsia and maternal obesity. Adv Exp Med Biol. 2013;776:81–91.
21. Uysal KT, Wiesbrock SM, Marino MW, Hotamisligil GS. Protection from obesity-induced insulin resistance in mice lacking TNF-alpha function. Nature. 1997;389:610–4.
22. Walsh JM, McGowan CA, Byrne JA, Rath A, McAuliffe FM. The association between TNF-alpha and insulin resistance in euglycemic women. Cytokine. 2013;64:208–12.
23. Lee JY, Sohn KH, Rhee SH, Hwang D. Saturated fatty acids, but not unsaturated fatty acids, induce the expression of cyclooxygenase-2 mediated through Toll-like receptor 4. J Biol Chem. 2001;276:16683–9.

24. Huang S, Rutkowsky JM, Snodgrass RG, Ono-Moore KD, Schneider DA, Newman JW, Adams SH, Hwang DH. Saturated fatty acids activate TLR-mediated proinflammatory signaling pathways. J Lipid Res. 2012;53:2002–13.
25. Beg AA. Endogenous ligands of Toll-like receptors: implications for regulating inflammatory and immune responses. Trends Immunol. 2002;23:509–12.
26. Erridge C, Kennedy S, Spickett CM, Webb DJ. Oxidized phospholipid inhibition of toll-like receptor (TLR) signaling is restricted to TLR2 and TLR4: roles for CD14, LPS-binding protein, and MD2 as targets for specificity of inhibition. J Biol Chem. 2008;283:24748–59.
27. Tsan MF, Gao B. Endogenous ligands of Toll-like receptors. J Leukoc Biol. 2004;76:514–9.
28. Fujioka S, Niu J, Schmidt C, Sclabas GM, Peng B, Uwagawa T, Li Z, Evans DB, Abbruzzese JL, Chiao PJ. NF-kappaB and AP-1 connection: mechanism of NF-kappaB-dependent regulation of AP-1 activity. Mol Cell Biol. 2004;24:7806–19.
29. Udalova IA, Kwiatkowski D. Interaction of AP-1 with a cluster of NF-kappa B binding elements in the human TNF promoter region. Biochem Biophys Res Commun. 2001;289: 25–33.
30. Baker RG, Hayden MS, Ghosh S. NF-kappaB, inflammation, and metabolic disease. Cell Metab. 2011;13:11–22.
31. Vallerie SN, Hotamisligil GS. The role of JNK proteins in metabolism. Sci Transl Med. 2010;2:60rv65.
32. Rebholz SL, Jones T, Burke KT, Jaeschke A, Tso P, D'Alessio DA, Woollett LA. Multiparity leads to obesity and inflammation in mothers and obesity in male offspring. Am J Physiol Endocrinol Metab. 2012;302:E449–57.
33. Li HP, Chen X, Li MQ. Gestational diabetes induces chronic hypoxia stress and excessive inflammatory response in murine placenta. Int J Clin Exp Pathol. 2013;6:650–9.
34. Heerwagen MJ, Stewart MS, de la Houssaye BA, Janssen RC, Friedman JE. Transgenic increase in N-3/n-6 Fatty Acid ratio reduces maternal obesity-associated inflammation and limits adverse developmental programming in mice. PLoS One. 2013;8:e67791.
35. Saben J, Zhong Y, Gomez-Acevedo H, Thakali KM, Borengasser SJ, Andres A, Shankar K. Early growth response protein-1 mediates lipotoxicity-associated placental inflammation: role in maternal obesity. Am J Physiol Endocrinol Metab. 2013;305:E1–14.
36. Lappas M. Cellular inhibitors of apoptosis (cIAP) 1 and 2 are increased in placenta from obese pregnant women. Placenta. 2014;35:831–8.
37. Cnattingius S, Villamor E, Johansson S, Edstedt Bonamy AK, Persson M, Wikstrom AK, Granath F. Maternal obesity and risk of preterm delivery. JAMA. 2013;309:2362–70.
38. Metzger BE, Lowe LP, Dyer AR, Trimble ER, Chaovarindr U, Coustan DR, Hadden DR, McCance DR, Hod M, McIntyre HD, Oats JJ, Persson B, Rogers MS, Sacks DA. Hyperglycemia and adverse pregnancy outcomes. N Engl J Med. 2008;358:1991–2002.
39. Stewart FM, Freeman DJ, Ramsay JE, Greer IA, Caslake M, Ferrell WR. Longitudinal assessment of maternal endothelial function and markers of inflammation and placental function throughout pregnancy in lean and obese mothers. J Clin Endocrinol Metab. 2007;92:969–75.
40. Thornburg KL, Louey S. Uteroplacental circulation and fetal vascular function and development. Curr Vasc Pharmacol. 2013;11:748–57.
41. Jones HN, Jansson T, Powell TL. IL-6 stimulates system A amino acid transporter activity in trophoblast cells through STAT3 and increased expression of SNAT2. Am J Physiol Cell Physiol. 2009;297:C1228–35.
42. Lager S, Jansson N, Olsson AL, Wennergren M, Jansson T, Powell TL. Effect of IL-6 and TNF-alpha on fatty acid uptake in cultured human primary trophoblast cells. Placenta. 2011;32(2):121–7.
43. von Versen-Hoynck F, Rajakumar A, Parrott MS, Powers RW. Leptin affects system A amino acid transport activity in the human placenta: evidence for STAT3 dependent mechanisms. Placenta. 2009;30:361–7.
44. Jansson N, Greenwood SL, Johansson BR, Powell TL, Jansson T. Leptin stimulates the activity of the system A amino acid transporter in human placental villous fragments. J Clin Endocrinol Metab. 2003;88:1205–11.

45. Jones HN, Jansson T, Powell TL. Full-length adiponectin attenuates insulin signaling and inhibits insulin-stimulated amino Acid transport in human primary trophoblast cells. Diabetes. 2010;59:1161–70.
46. Aye IL, Jansson T, Powell TL. Interleukin-1beta inhibits insulin signaling and prevents insulin-stimulated system A amino acid transport in primary human trophoblasts. Mol Cell Endocrinol. 2013;381:46–55.
47. Thongsong B, Subramanian RK, Ganapathy V, Prasad PD. Inhibition of amino acid transport system a by interleukin-1beta in trophoblasts. J Soc Gynecol Investig. 2005;12:495–503.
48. Boeuf P, Aitken EH, Chandrasiri U, Chua CL, McInerney B, McQuade L, Duffy M, Molyneux M, Brown G, Glazier J, Rogerson SJ. Plasmodium falciparum malaria elicits inflammatory responses that dysregulate placental amino acid transport. PLoS Pathog. 2013;9:e1003153.
49. Pontillo A, Girardelli M, Agostinis C, Masat E, Bulla R, Crovella S. Bacterial LPS differently modulates inflammasome gene expression and IL-1beta secretion in trophoblast cells, decidual stromal cells, and decidual endothelial cells. Reprod Sci. 2013;20:563–6.
50. Ammala M, Nyman T, Salmi A, Rutanen EM. The interleukin-1 system in gestational tissues at term: effect of labour. Placenta. 1997;18:717–23.
51. Gotsch F, Romero R, Chaiworapongsa T, Erez O, Vaisbuch E, Espinoza J, Kusanovic JP, Mittal P, Mazaki-Tovi S, Kim CJ, Kim JS, Edwin S, Nhan-Chang CL, Hamill N, Friel L, Than NG, Mazor M, Yoon BH, Hassan SS. Evidence of the involvement of caspase-1 under physiologic and pathologic cellular stress during human pregnancy: a link between the inflammasome and parturition. J Maternal Fetal Neonatal Med. 2008;21:605–16.
52. Jaiswal MK, Agrawal V, Mallers T, Gilman-Sachs A, Hirsch E, Beaman KD. Regulation of apoptosis and innate immune stimuli in inflammation-induced preterm labor. J Immunol. 2013;191:5702–13.
53. Mulla MJ, Myrtolli K, Potter J, Boeras C, Kavathas PB, Sfakianaki AK, Tadesse S, Norwitz ER, Guller S, Abrahams VM. Uric acid induces trophoblast IL-1beta production via the inflammasome: implications for the pathogenesis of preeclampsia. Am J Reprod Immunol. 2011;65:542–8.
54. Mulla MJ, Salmon JE, Chamley LW, Brosens JJ, Boeras CM, Kavathas PB, Abrahams VM. A role for uric acid and the Nalp3 inflammasome in antiphospholipid antibody-induced IL-1beta production by human first trimester trophoblast. PLoS One. 2013;8:e65237.
55. Shen F, Wei J, Snowise S, DeSousa J, Stone P, Viall C, Chen Q, Chamley L. Trophoblast debris extruded from preeclamptic placentae activates endothelial cells: a mechanism by which the placenta communicates with the maternal endothelium. Placenta. 2014;35(10):839–47.
56. Kavathas PB, Boeras CM, Mulla MJ, Abrahams VM. Nod1, but not the ASC inflammasome, contributes to induction of IL-1beta secretion in human trophoblasts after sensing of Chlamydia trachomatis. Mucosal Immunol. 2013;6:235–43.
57. Strakova Z, Srisuparp S, Fazleabas AT. Interleukin-1beta induces the expression of insulin-like growth factor binding protein-1 during decidualization in the primate. Endocrinology. 2000;141:4664–70.
58. Seki H, Zosmer A, Elder MG, Sullivan MH. The regulation of progesterone and hCG production from placental cells by interleukin-1beta. Biochim Biophys Acta. 1997;1336:342–8.
59. Tsukihara S, Harada T, Deura I, Mitsunari M, Yoshida S, Iwabe T, Terakawa N. Interleukin-1beta-induced expression of IL-6 and production of human chorionic gonadotropin in human trophoblast cells via nuclear factor-kappaB activation. Am J Reprod Immunol. 2004;52:218–23.
60. Keelan JA, Groome NP, Mitchell MD. Regulation of activin-A production by human amnion, decidua and placenta in vitro by pro-inflammatory cytokines. Placenta. 1998;19:429–34.
61. Fortunato SJ, Menon R. IL-1 beta is a better inducer of apoptosis in human fetal membranes than IL-6. Placenta. 2003;24:922–8.
62. Aye IL, Ramirez VI, Gaccioli F, Lager S, Jansson T, Powell T. Activation of placental inflammasomes in pregnant women with high BMI. Reprod Sci. 2013;20(S3):73A–73A.

63. Stutz A, Golenbock DT, Latz E. Inflammasomes: too big to miss. J Clin Invest. 2009;119:3502–11.
64. Hastie R, Lappas M. The effect of pre-existing maternal obesity and diabetes on placental mitochondrial content and electron transport chain activity. Placenta. 2014;35(9):673–83.
65. Luo X, Yang Y, Shen T, Tang X, Xiao Y, Zou T, Xia M, Ling W. Docosahexaenoic acid ameliorates palmitate-induced lipid accumulation and inflammation through repressing NLRC4 inflammasome activation in HepG2 cells. Nutr Metab. 2012;9:34.
66. Wen H, Gris D, Lei Y, Jha S, Zhang L, Huang MT, Brickey WJ, Ting JP. Fatty acid-induced NLRP3-ASC inflammasome activation interferes with insulin signaling. Nat Immunol. 2011;12:408–15.
67. L'Homme L, Esser N, Riva L, Scheen A, Paquot N, Piette J, Legrand-Poels S. Unsaturated fatty acids prevent activation of NLRP3 inflammasome in human monocytes/macrophages. J Lipid Res. 2013;54:2998–3008.
68. Chen X, Scholl TO, Leskiw M, Savaille J, Stein TP. Differences in maternal circulating fatty acid composition and dietary fat intake in women with gestational diabetes mellitus or mild gestational hyperglycemia. Diabetes Care. 2010;33:2049–54.
69. Lager S, Gaccioli F, Ramirez VI, Jones HN, Jansson T, Powell TL. Oleic acid stimulates system A amino acid transport in primary human trophoblast cells mediated by toll-like receptor 4. J Lipid Res. 2013;54:725–33.
70. Grant WF, Gillingham MB, Batra AK, Fewkes NM, Comstock SM, Takahashi D, Braun TP, Grove KL, Friedman JE, Marks DL. Maternal high fat diet is associated with decreased plasma n-3 fatty acids and fetal hepatic apoptosis in nonhuman primates. PLoS One. 2011; 6:e17261.
71. Snodgrass RG, Huang S, Choi IW, Rutledge JC, Hwang DH. Inflammasome-mediated secretion of IL-1beta in human monocytes through TLR2 activation; modulation by dietary fatty acids. J Immunol. 2013;191:4337–47.
72. Williams-Bey Y, Boularan C, Vural A, Huang NN, Hwang IY, Shan-Shi C, Kehrl JH. Omega-3 free fatty acids suppress macrophage inflammasome activation by inhibiting NF-kappaB activation and enhancing autophagy. PLoS One. 2014;9:e97957.
73. Yan Y, Jiang W, Spinetti T, Tardivel A, Castillo R, Bourquin C, Guarda G, Tian Z, Tschopp J, Zhou R. Omega-3 fatty acids prevent inflammation and metabolic disorder through inhibition of NLRP3 inflammasome activation. Immunity. 2013;38:1154–63.
74. Jansson T, Ekstrand Y, Bjorn C, Wennergren M, Powell TL. Alterations in the activity of placental amino acid transporters in pregnancies complicated by diabetes. Diabetes. 2002;51: 2214–9.
75. Dicke JM, Henderson GI. Placental amino acid uptake in normal and complicated pregnancies. Am J Med Sci. 1988;295:223–7.
76. Farley DM, Choi J, Dudley DJ, Li C, Jenkins SL, Myatt L, Nathanielsz PW. Placental amino acid transport and placental leptin resistance in pregnancies complicated by maternal obesity. Placenta. 2010;31:718–24.
77. Kuruvilla AG, D'Souza SW, Glazier JD, Mahendran D, Maresh MJ, Sibley CP. Altered activity of the system A amino acid transporter in microvillous membrane vesicles from placentas of macrosomic babies born to diabetic women. J Clin Invest. 1994;94:689–95.
78. Mrizak I, Grissa O, Henault B, Fekih M, Bouslema A, Boumaiza I, Zaouali M, Tabka Z, Khan NA. Placental infiltration of inflammatory markers in gestational diabetic women. Gen Physiol Biophys. 2014;33:169–76.
79. Radaelli T, Varastehpour A, Catalano P, Hauguel-de Mouzon S. Gestational diabetes induces placental genes for chronic stress and inflammatory pathways. Diabetes. 2003;52:2951–8.
80. Sisino G, Bouckenooghe T, Aurientis S, Fontaine P, Storme L, Vambergue A. Diabetes during pregnancy influences Hofbauer cells, a subtype of placental macrophages, to acquire a pro-inflammatory phenotype. Biochim Biophys Acta. 2013;1832:1959–68.

81. Yu J, Zhou Y, Gui J, Li AZ, Su XL, Feng L. Assessment of the number and function of macrophages in the placenta of gestational diabetes mellitus patients. J Huazhong Univ Sci Technolog Med Sci. 2013;33:725–9.
82. Langer O, Conway DL, Berkus MD, Xenakis EM, Gonzales O. A comparison of glyburide and insulin in women with gestational diabetes mellitus. N Engl J Med. 2000;343:1134–8.
83. Zeng YC, Li MJ, Chen Y, Jiang L, Wang SM, Mo XL, Li BY. The use of glyburide in the management of gestational diabetes mellitus: a meta-analysis. Adv Med Sci. 2014;59: 95–101.
84. Lamkanfi M, Mueller JL, Vitari AC, Misaghi S, Fedorova A, Deshayes K, Lee WP, Hoffman HM, Dixit VM. Glyburide inhibits the Cryopyrin/Nalp3 inflammasome. J Cell Biol. 2009;187:61–70.
85. Aye IL, Gao X, Weintraub ST, Jansson T, Powell TL. Adiponectin inhibits insulin function in primary trophoblasts by PPARalpha-mediated ceramide synthesis. Mol Endocrinol. 2014;28: 512–24.

PCOS and Pregnancy: Impact of Endocrine and Metabolic Factors

7

Felice Petraglia, Cinzia Orlandini, Silvia Vannuccini, and Vicki L. Clifton

Contents

7.1 Introduction

Polycystic ovary syndrome (PCOS) is one of the most common endocrine–metabolic disorders, affecting 4–7 % of women in reproductive age with significant racial and ethnic variations. PCOS is characterized by both gynecological and endocrine symptoms, and it is defined by an international consensus definition that includes at least two of three component criteria: ovarian dysfunction, hyperandrogenism, and polycystic ovaries by ultrasound [32]. The Excess Androgen Society

F. Petraglia (✉) • C. Orlandini • S. Vannuccini
Department of Molecular and Developmental Medicine, Obstetrics and Gynecology, University of Siena, Siena, Italy
e-mail: felice.petraglia@unisi.it

V.L. Clifton
Robinson Research Institute, University of Adelaide, Adelaide, Australia

E. Ferrazzi, B. Sears (eds.), *Metabolic Syndrome and Complications of Pregnancy: The Potential Preventive Role of Nutrition*,
DOI 10.1007/978-3-319-16853-1_7

uses an alternate criteria and includes only hyperandrogenism and ultrasound features. Even though 50 % of women with PCOS are overweight or obese [28] and a high proportion (30–70 %) have reduced insulin sensitivity, featuring core aspects of metabolic syndrome, these are not prerequisites for the diagnosis of the syndrome and vary significantly among phenotypes and among subjects with the same phenotype [7]. However, the variability in phenotype expression continues to render the clinical care and research of these women challenging. Besides metabolic abnormalities, the endocrine dysfunction of PCOS has complex effects on the endometrium, contributing to infertility and adverse pregnancy outcome, observed in women with this syndrome ([13] Amsterdam ESHRE/ASRM-Sponsored PCOS Consensus Workshop Group).

7.2 Origin of PCOS

The origin of PCOS includes genetic factors and lifestyle influences [15]. The PCOS phenotype may be found from early infancy to puberty, based on predisposing genetic factors. PCOS is unlikely to be driven by a single gene defect and is more likely to be a polygenic or oligogenic syndrome (Fig. 7.1). The intrauterine environment may also influence the programming of genes associated with the development of PCOS in adult life. The current hypothesis for a developmental origin of PCOS suggests an epigenetic phenomenon induced by fetal androgen excess. One possible pathway could be the enhancement of transforming growth factor (TGF)-β-regulated extracellular matrix protein production which would disrupt ovarian differentiation causing a polycystic phenotype. This possibility is particularly attractive as androgen exposure increases the expression of these proteins and, additionally, other TGF-β family members, including anti-Mullerian hormone (AMH), regulate the expression of CYP17, the main androgen-producing enzyme [23].

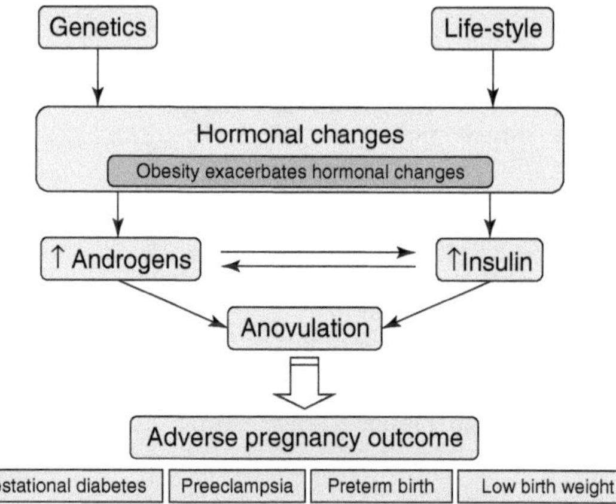

Fig. 7.1 The etiological, hormonal, and obstetric clinical outcomes of PCOS (Modified from Teede et al. [38])

7.3 PCOS: Infertility and Early Pregnancy Loss

The reproductive dysfunction in women with PCOS relates both to anovulation and to early pregnancy loss. Anovulation is the cause of infertility in about one third of couples seeking infertility treatment, and PCOS accounts for 90 % of those cases [1]. To conceive many of PCOS women require assisted reproductive techniques, such as ovulation induction or IVF [12].

Complications associated with PCOS such as hyperandrogenemia, hyperinsulinemia, and obesity have a major impact on ovulation and pregnancy outcome (Fig. 7.1). Miscarriage rate is high in PCOS women and varies between 15 and 35 % of all conceptions. This may be explained by the negative effect of the whole array of cofactors associated with PCOS, metabolic dysfunction, low-grade inflammation, endocrine abnormalities on ovulatory function, oocyte quality, and endometrial receptivity. Ovarian hyperandrogenism and hyperinsulinemia may promote premature granulosa cell luteinization, and paracrine dysregulation of growth factors may disrupt the intrafollicular environment and impair cytoplasmic and nuclear maturation of oocytes ([13] Amsterdam ESHRE/ASRM-Sponsored PCOS Consensus Workshop Group). Endometrial receptivity is disrupted by a number of altered mechanisms. The overexpression of androgen receptors in the endometrium and reduced biomarkers of endometrial receptivity to embryonic implantation contribute to lower implantation rates in women with PCOS. Elevated estrogen, low levels of progesterone, no ovulation, and hyperinsulinemia with elevated free IGFs all contribute to abnormal decidualization and increased miscarriage rate [18].

These features are not universal to all women with PCOS, as oocyte quality, fertilization, and implantation rates can be normal in some women with PCOS [32]. Diverse differences in fertility and pregnancy outcome between women with PCOS are clinically challenging, and risk factors need to be identified in this group of women to improve management of reproduction.

7.4 PCOS and Adverse Pregnancy Outcome

Several studies suggest that PCOS has a negative impact on pregnancy outcomes with an increased risk of gestational diabetes, pregnancy-induced hypertension, preeclampsia, preterm birth PTB, and need of cesarean section, even in the absence of obesity [2, 3, 26, 31]. A greater risk of neonatal complications has been reported and includes higher neonatal intensive care admissions; neonates were shown to have significantly increased risk of meconium aspiration, lower birth weights, and a low Apgar score (<7 at 5 min) [31]. In addition, multiple pregnancy contributes to increased risk of perinatal morbidity observed following fertility treatments of PCOS women [12].

PCOS pregnancies are further complicated by hyperinsulinemia and an increased risk of gestational diabetes. Normal pregnancy induces a state of insulin resistance which may result in impaired glucose tolerance or gestational diabetes mellitus. Since women with PCOS are predisposed to glucose intolerance, they are at increased risk of developing gestational diabetes. In addition obesity affects 5–40 % of pregnant women with PCOS [39] which can also increase the risk of gestational diabetes. Mexican women with a history of infertility and PCOS have 2.8 times greater risk of developing gestational diabetes when compared to Caucasians [30].

The prevalence of gestational hypertension and preeclampsia is estimated at 10–30 and 8–15 %, respectively, in women with PCOS. This prevalence may be even higher when PCOS women are obese and hyperinsulinemic.

Preterm delivery complicates 6–15 % of pregnancies in women with PCOS [41]. However, PCOS by itself is not an independent risk factor because these patients have more assisted reproductive technologies, more chance of multiple pregnancies, and pregnancy-induced hypertension contributing to more preterm deliveries [17]. A high frequency of cervical insufficiency was found in PCOS, with a prevalence in the range of 3 % and incidence rate of 18 per 1,000 births, particularly in South Asian and Black women [14]. Indeed, the increased risk of preterm birth is confined to hyperandrogenic women with PCOS who had a twofold increased risk of preterm delivery and preeclampsia compared to non-hyperandrogenic ones.

7.5 PCOS and Adverse Pregnancy Outcome: Pathogenetic Mechanisms

The spectrum of pregnancy complications associated with PCOS may be driven by impaired decidual trophoblast invasion and defects in placentation, related to hormonal and metabolic dysfunction. Alterations in the endovascular trophoblast invasion and in the macroscopic and microscopic structure of the placenta have been reported [29].

The alterations in early trophoblast invasion and placentation detected in PCOS patients vary among PCOS phenotypes. In particular, a higher rate of abnormalities in relation to trophoblastic invasion and placental development was observed in patients with hyperandrogenism and ovarian dysfunction regardless of whether they were diagnosed with PCOS or not. PCOS patients who had a complicated pregnancy were reported to have more severe serum androgen concentrations and insulin sensitivity indexes in comparison to subjects without any pregnancy and/or neonatal complications [11]. However, the exact mechanisms by which hyperandrogenemia and insulin resistance/compensatory hyperinsulinemia affect endovascular trophoblast invasion and induce placental alterations are unknown. Furthermore, the comorbidity of obesity may increase the risk of adverse pregnancy outcome in PCOS through enhanced hyperandrogenism, hyperinsulinemia, and, since excess adipose tissue acts as an endocrine and inflammatory organ, altered concentrations in leptin, TNF-α, and IL-6 [23] (Fig. 7.2). This obese phenotype of PCOS adds to possible abnormal trophoblastic invasion the preexisting endothelial dysfunction that might damage women affected by metabolic syndrome [9].

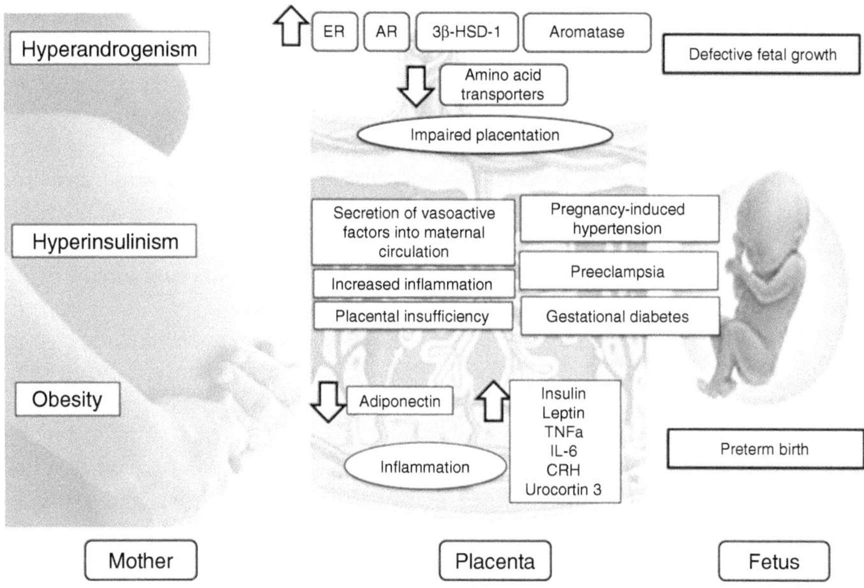

Fig. 7.2 Pathogenetic mechanisms of obstetric complications in PCOS

7.6 Hyperandrogenism

Ovarian hyperandrogenism is a cardinal feature of PCOS. Intrinsic amplified steroidogenetic capacity of theca cells results in increased ovarian androgen secretion. Several endocrine mechanisms may contribute to hyperandrogenism, and these include pituitary LH hypersecretion, relative FSH insufficiency, and high levels of insulin and AMH inhibiting aromatase activity. Obesity also amplifies hyperandrogenism in PCOS resulting in increased total testosterone, free androgen index, and decreased sex hormone-binding globulin (SHBG). Obese women with PCOS exhibit a higher degree of insulin resistance and compensatory hyperinsulinemia which contributes to androgen excess.

A number of studies have reported elevated levels of some, but not all, circulating androgens during normal pregnancy from the first trimester and toward term. In contrast, maternal circulating dehydroepiandrostenedione sulfate (DHEAS) levels fall across gestation to 50 % of the nonpregnant levels, and SHBG levels increase during the first trimester of pregnancy and continue to increase dramatically throughout mid- and late gestation. In the fetus, levels of some androgens are dependent on fetal sex; in fact in fetal blood, testosterone levels are higher in males, whereas dihydrotestosterone levels are similar in both sexes. Although testosterone levels are higher in the fetal compartment of male fetuses, there is no association between fetal sex and maternal serum concentrations of any androgen [23].

Elevated androgen levels during pregnancy are associated with low birth weight in humans and animals, and women experiencing hyperandrogenism associated with PCOS and preeclampsia have a higher than normal prevalence of small for gestational age newborn babies at delivery. Increased maternal testosterone concentrations do not cross the placenta to directly suppress fetal growth but affects amino acid nutrient delivery to the fetus by downregulating specific amino acid transporter activity. Thus, the fetus appears to be protected from excess maternal androgen perhaps due to effective enzymatic inactivation by the placenta, and in the absence of these protective mechanisms, high levels of androgens would cause hirsutism and virilization of both mother and female fetus.

Maternal mechanisms that protect the fetus from androgens include the physiological increase of maternal circulating SHBG and the pregnancy-induced rapid elevation of progesterone and androstenedione resulting in an inhibition of the conversion of testosterone to dihydrotestosterone. The fetus is further protected by the placenta which metabolizes androgens; in particular the placental aromatase complex rapidly converts testosterone or androstenedione to estrone and estradiol, respectively [23].

Fetal growth restriction may arise in the presence of hyperandrogenism by the specific downregulation of amino acid transporters within the placenta which results in a decrease of available nutrients to the fetus [34]. A rat model of excess maternal androgen reported a decrease in placental size, increased circulating androgens and increased circulating estradiol concentrations, and increased expression of androgen and estrogen receptors, potentially affecting the ability of the placenta to deliver nutrients to the fetus [36].

Other testosterone-induced alterations in endometrial, stromal, decidual, and placental function could influence fetal growth and pregnancy outcome in PCOS pregnancies. Testosterone regulates the endometrial expression of homeobox A10 (HOXA10) [5], and it is proposed that hyperandrogenism could impair the cell–cell and cell–extracellular matrix interactions during the first phases of pregnancy, thereby reducing HOXA10 expression. Furthermore, dihydrotestosterone exerts a direct effect on the ultrastructural changes associated with decidual transformation in human endometrial stromal cells. These early pregnancy events induced by androgens could reduce implantation success and increase the risk of miscarriage. Later in gestation testosterone can promote placental macrophage- and trophoblast-mediated low-density lipoprotein oxidation and cytotoxicity which could affect fetal development. Finally, the human placenta expresses CYP17 and produces androgens de novo, and a higher 3β-hydroxysteroid dehydrogenase type 1 activity and a lower P450 aromatase activity were detected in the placental tissue of PCOS patients, suggesting that the steroidogenic function of the placenta in PCOS women is altered per se, contributing to a higher androgen concentration observed in maternal blood of PCOS patients and therefore increasing the effects of hyperandrogenism in pregnancy [24].

7.7 Hyperinsulinism

Hyperinsulinemia can have multiple effects on fertility, pregnancy success, and fetal growth and well-being. PCOS-related secondary hyperinsulinemia may interfere with paracrine, and perhaps autocrine, signaling in the endometrium, causing inadequate cell differentiation during the first phases of pregnancy. In addition, the reduction in IGFBP-1 could increase the mitotic effect of insulin-like growth factor (IGF)-I on the endometrium [4], whereas the reduction of glycodelin could decrease the physiological immune suppression observed during the early phases of gestation and alter the modulation of trophoblast invasiveness. In the endometria of hyperinsulinemic hyperandrogenic PCOS patients, there is a reduced insulin-related expression of the transmembrane glucose transporter 4 (GLUT4) reducing the glucose uptake, with subsequent alterations in the metabolism of the endometrial cells.

During pregnancy, PCOS women are predisposed to peripheral tissue resistance to insulin, with consequent hyperinsulinism and fetal hyperglycemia. Moreover, hyperandrogenemia and hyperinsulinemia observed during pregnancy in PCOS women result in an abnormal lipid profile and a decrease in adiponectin concentrations, predisposing women to the onset of gestational diabetes [35].

Hyperinsulinemia in PCOS women is also associated with having low levels of insulin-like growth factor binding globulin-1 (IGFBP-1), a regulator of the activity of IGF-1, which may be implicated as a cause of higher incidence of growth abnormalities of the fetus and increased risk of preeclampsia.

7.8 Inflammation and Obesity

Clinical data demonstrated that hyperandrogenic and/or hyperinsulinemic PCOS patients are characterized by an abnormal pattern of low-grade chronic inflammation that may be responsible for abnormal immune regulation during pregnancy in PCOS patients, thereby increasing the frequency and the extent of immune-mediated placental pathologies [33] and possibly increasing the risk of preterm birth in women with PCOS.

PCOS has been characterized by chronic low-grade inflammation, with complex associations to insulin resistance, visceral adiposity, hyperandrogenism, and resultant increased production of specific cytokines and chemokines including TNF-alpha, IL-6 and IL-1, adhesion molecules, follistatin, and C-reactive protein. Furthermore, a panel of six proteomic biomarkers was similarly expressed in women with preterm birth and women with PCOS compared to their respective controls, including pyruvate kinase M1/M2, vimentin, fructose bisphosphonate aldolase A, heat-shock protein beta-1, peroxiredoxin-1, and transferrin, which could be potentially used to better understand the pathophysiological mechanisms linking PCOS and preterm birth [16].

Molecular and biochemical findings support the theory that in some situations, labor may be viewed as part of an inflammatory cascade model, including pathways involving specific leukocyte subsets and proinflammatory mediators. As such, underlying inflammatory mediators associated with PCOS may also contribute to predisposition for preterm delivery. This is an area that requires further investigation.

7.9 Long-Term Effects of PCOS

It is now well established that women with PCOS are at increased risk for developing diabetes mellitus, glucose intolerance, hypertension, hyperlipidemia, the metabolic syndrome, and cardiovascular disease. Although the high prevalence of insulin resistance in women with PCOS, especially those who are also obese, has been largely held accountable for these long-term sequelae, there is now emerging evidence for a role of androgen excess in these processes which is more than merely permissive [20]. There is a strong association between hyperandrogenemia, an increased free androgen index, and the metabolic syndrome in premenopausal women with or without PCOS ([13] Amsterdam ESHRE/ASRM-Sponsored PCOS Consensus Workshop Group). Moreover, among obese hyperandrogenic adolescents, hyperandrogenemia was found to be a significant predictor of the metabolic syndrome, independent of obesity and insulin resistance.

The association of androgen excess, abdominal adiposity, insulin resistance, and metabolic derangements in women with PCOS is a vicious cycle [21] that may start during early stages of life or even prenatally, whereby androgen excess regulates abdominal deposition of fat which further facilitates androgen secretion by the ovaries and adrenals in PCOS patients [10].

If the exposure to androgen excess starts during intrauterine life of the female fetus and is perpetuated and maintained by a series of feed forward mechanisms, then since PCOS is clearly a familial syndrome, the pregnant woman with PCOS closes the androgen cycle by either passing on her "PCOS genes" or exposing her female fetus to androgen excess, thus commencing another cycle and another generation of PCOS women. Acceptance of this concept may lead to more direct treatment of PCOS throughout a woman's life cycle with it being a major focus on women's health.

Lifestyle modification in PCOS is a reasonable approach to the management of obesity and hyperinsulinemia, which would include dietary modifications and exercise interventions with a focus on caloric restrictions and psychological support. All interventions would be targeted to improving biochemical and endocrinological parameters including body composition, insulin resistance, and hyperandrogenism, preventing progression to type 2 diabetes and cardiovascular diseases.

7.10 Nutritional Interventions

The metabolic background of PCOS itself involves a possible therapeutic intervention by using an appropriate nutritional profile. Randomized studies in overweight or obese PCOS patients proved that a reduction of carbohydrates in diet improves in

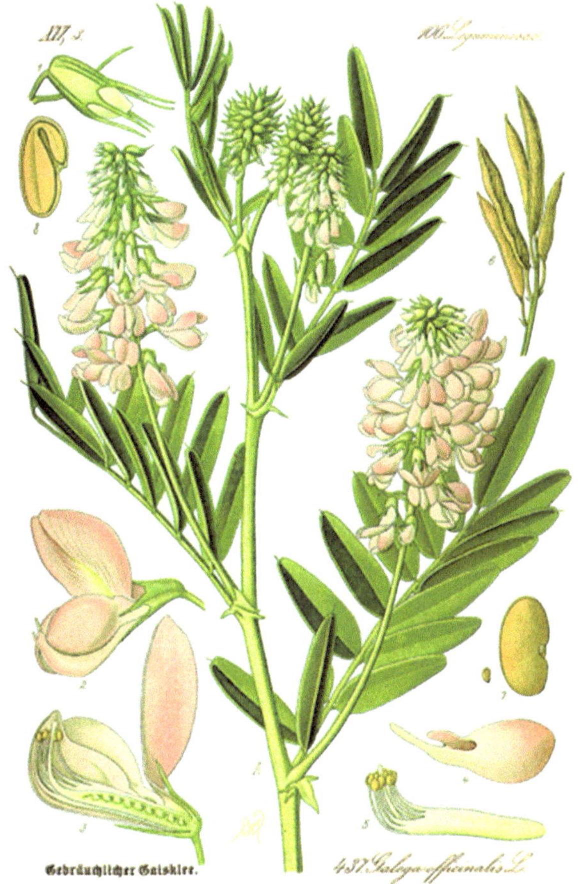

Fig. 7.3 *Galega officinalis* has been known since the Middle Ages for relieving the symptoms of diabetes mellitus. It contains guanidine compounds that decrease blood sugar by improving insulin resistance. Georges Tanret identified an alkaloid from this plant, galegine, that by further chemical processes led ultimately to the discovery of metformin

fasting insulin, fasting glucose, HOMA-IR, total testosterone, and all cholesterol measures, with a significant increase of insulin sensitivity and dynamic ("first-phase") β-cell response [[8], [19]]. Besides moderate decrease in carbohydrate, these isocaloric diets included higher levels of polyunsaturated fatty acids and lower cholesterol. A nutritional approach based on a low glycemic index carbohydrate isocaloric iso-carbohydrate diet was compared to a healthy diet and achieved a better metabolic result and a better glucose challenge test profile [25].

Metformin has a more significant impact on women on low glycemic index diet as regards insulin sensitivity (Fig. 7.3).

This finding brings into the debate on metformin its role in women with PCOS (who have type 2 diabetes or impaired glucose tolerance test) who fail lifestyle modification or in PCOS women with menstrual disorders who cannot take or do not tolerate HCs [22]. The role of metformin with lifestyle modifications and oral contraceptives ranged first (33 %) among the most common treatments reported by a recent European survey of the European Society of Endocrinology [6]. Metformin is a natural molecule (originally extracted and modified from the French lilac *Galega officinalis*), with insulin-lowering effects by improving insulin sensitivity and, in turn, decreases circulating androgen levels. A recent systematic review showed a significant reduction of IL-6 by metformin in agreement with its role in improving insulin receptors damaged by low-grade inflammation in overweight–obese women affected by PCOS [40].

Among other possible therapeutical molecules (rosiglitazone, pioglitazone, D-chiro-inositol), D-chiro-inositol deserves to be sorted out. A randomized study on D-chiro-inositol vs placebo on a small cohort of 44 PCOS overweight or obese women [27] showed a significant reduction of serum LH concentration paralleled by a significant increase of ovulation rate after 6–8 weeks of treatment by D-chiro-inositol (1,200 mg/day). In spite of a large number of prospective interventional studies on this nutraceutical approach, only a randomized study, of moderate quality, proved a possible effect of D-chiro-inositol in PCOS on ovulation (OR 5.39; CI 0.7–41.3) [37]. Like all nutraceutical interventions with moderate efficacy, this molecule risks to become a fashionable "remedy" before any requested prospective randomized study. D-chiro-inositol is a member of the inositol family that encompasses several isomers and may play a role in insulin signal transduction, a role that deserves additional prospective randomized studies.

Additional dietary suggestions might be derived by the prevalence of PCOS in different macro-ethnicities, whose affected women increase when moving into a Western-style diet, and in these cases a significant change in lifestyle and nutrition to prevent the vicious cycle of polygenic predisposition and ongoing damage of sedentary lifestyle and refined carbohydrate-rich Western-style diet is recommended.

References

1. Balen AH, Rutherford AJ. Managing anovulatory infertility and polycystic ovary syndrome. BMJ. 2007;335:663–6. Review.
2. Bjercke S, Dale PO, Tanbo T, Storeng R, Ertzeid G, Abyholm T. Impact of insulin resistance on pregnancy complications and outcome in women with polycystic ovary syndrome. Gynecol Obstet Invest. 2002;54:94–8.
3. Boomsma CM, Hughes EG, Visser GH, Fauser BC, Macklon NS. A meta-analysis of pregnancy outcomes in women with polycystic ovary syndrome. Hum Reprod Update. 2006;12:673–83.
4. Cakmak H, Taylor HS. Implantation failure: molecular mechanisms and clinical treatment. Hum Reprod Update. 2011;17:242–53.
5. Cermik D, Selam B, Taylor HS. Regulation of HOXA-10 expression by testosterone in vitro and in the endometrium of patients with polycystic ovary syndrome. J Clin Endocrinol Metab. 2003;88:238–43.
6. Conway G, Dewailly D, Diamanti-Kandarakis E, Escobar-Morreale HF, Franks S, Gambineri A, Kelestimur F, Macut D, Micic D, Pasquali R, et al. European survey of diagnosis and management of the polycystic ovary syndrome: results of the ESE PCOs Special Interest Group's Questionnaire. Eur J Endocrinol. 2014;171(4):489–98.
7. Diamanti-Kandarakis E, Dunaif A. Insulin resistance and the polycystic ovary syndrome revisited: an update on mechanisms and implications. Endocr Rev. 2012;33:981–1030.
8. Douglas CC, Gower BA, Darnell BE, Ovalle F, Oster RA, Azziz R. Role of diet in the treatment of polycystic ovary syndrome. Fertil Steril. 2006;85:679–88.
9. Duleba AJ, Dokras A. Is PCOs an inflammatory process? Fertil Steril. 2012;97:7–12.

10. Escobar-Morreale HF, San Millán JL. Abdominal adiposity and the polycystic ovary syndrome. Trends Endocrinol Metab. 2007;18:266–72. Review.
11. Falbo A, Rocca M, Russo T, D'Ettore A, Tolino A, Zullo F, Orio F, Palomba S. Changes in androgens and insulin sensitivity indexes throughout pregnancy in women with polycystic ovary syndrome (PCOs): relationships with adverse outcomes. J Ovarian Res. 2010;3:23.
12. Fauser BC, Devroey P, Macklon NS. Multiple birth resulting from ovarian stimulation for subfertility treatment. Lancet. 2005;365:1807–16.
13. Fauser BC, Tarlatzis BC, Rebar RW, Legro RS, Balen AH, Lobo R, Carmina E, Chang J, Yildiz BO, Laven JS, Boivin J, Petraglia F, Wijeyeratne CN, Norman RJ, Dunaif A, Franks S, Wild RA, Dumesic D, Barnhart K. Consensus on women's health aspects of polycystic ovary syndrome (PCOs): the Amsterdam ESHRE/ASRM-Sponsored 3rd PCOs Consensus Workshop Group. Fertil Steril. 2012;97:28–38.
14. Feigenbaum SL, Crites Y, Hararah MK, Yamamoto MP, Yang J, Lo JC. Prevalence of cervical insufficiency in polycystic ovarian syndrome. Hum Reprod. 2012;27:2837–42.
15. Franks S, Berga SL. Does PCOs have developmental origins? Fertil Steril. 2012;97:2–6.
16. Galazis N, Docheva N, Nicolaides KH, Atiomo W. Proteomic biomarkers of preterm birth risk in women with polycystic ovary syndrome (PCOs): a systematic review and biomarker database integration. PLoS One. 2013;8:e53801.
17. Ghazeeri GS, Nassar AH, Younes Z, Awwad JT. Pregnancy outcomes and the effect of metformin treatment in women with polycystic ovary syndrome: an overview. Acta Obstet Gynecol Scand. 2012;91:658–78.
18. Giudice LC. Endometrium in PCOs: implantation and predisposition to endocrine CA. Best Pract Res Clin Endocrinol Metab. 2006;202:235–44. Review.
19. Gower BA, Chandler-Laney PC, Ovalle F, Goree LL, Azziz R, Desmond RA, Granger WM, Goss AM, Bates GW. Favourable metabolic effects of a eucaloric lower-carbohydrate diet in women with PCOs. Clin Endocrinol (Oxf). 2013;79:550–7.
20. Homburg R. Androgen circle of polycystic ovary syndrome. Hum Reprod. 2009;24:1548–55.
21. Insenser M, Montes-Nieto R, Murri M, Escobar-Morreale HF. Proteomic and metabolomic approaches to the study of polycystic ovary syndrome. Mol Cell Endocrinol. 2013;370:65–77.
22. Legro RS, Arslanian SA, Ehrmann DA, Hoeger KM, Murad MH, Pasquali R, Welt CK, Endocrine Society. Diagnosis and treatment of polycystic ovary syndrome: an Endocrine Society clinical practice guideline. J ClinEndocrinol Metab. 2013;98:4565–92.
23. Makieva S, Saunders PT, Norman JE. Androgens in pregnancy: roles in parturition. Hum Reprod Update. 2014;204:542–59. Review.
24. Maliqueo M, Lara HE, Sánchez F, Echiburú B, Crisosto N, Sir-Petermann T. Placental steroidogenesis in pregnant women with polycystic ovary syndrome. Eur J Obstet Gynecol Reprod Biol. 2013;166:151–5.
25. Marsh KA, Steinbeck KS, Atkinson FS, Petocz P, Brand-Miller JC. Effect of a low glycemic index compared with a conventional healthy diet on polycystic ovary syndrome. Am J Clin Nutr. 2010;92:83–92.
26. Mikola M, Hiilesmaa V, Halttunen M, Suhonen L, Tiitinen A. Obstetric outcome in women with polycystic ovarian syndrome. Hum Reprod. 2001;16:226–9.
27. Nestler JE, Jakubowicz DJ, Reamer P, Gunn RD, Allan G. Ovulatory and metabolic effects of D-chiro-inositol in the polycystic ovary syndrome. N Engl J Med. 1999;340:1314–20.
28. Norman RJ, Noakes M, Wu R, Davies MJ, Moran L, Wang JX. Improving reproductive performance in overweight/obese women with effective weight management. Hum Reprod Update. 2004;10:267–80.
29. Palomba S, Russo T, Falbo A, Di Cello A, Tolino A, Tucci L, La Sala GB, Zullo F. Macroscopic and microscopic findings of the placenta in women with polycystic ovary syndrome. Hum Reprod. 2013;28:2838–47.
30. Reyes-Muñoz E, Castellanos-Barroso G, Ramírez-Eugenio BY, Ortega-González C, Parra A, Castillo-Mora A, De la Jara-Díaz JF. The risk of gestational diabetes mellitus among Mexican women with a history of infertility and polycystic ovary syndrome. Fertil Steril. 2012;97: 1467–71.

31. Roos N, Kieler H, Sahlin L, Ekman-Ordeberg G, Falconer H, Stephansson O. Risk of adverse pregnancy outcomes in women with polycystic ovary syndrome: population based cohort study. BMJ. 2011;343:d6309.
32. Rotterdam ESHRE/ASRM-Sponsored PCOs consensus workshop group. Revised 2003 consensus on diagnostic criteria and long-term health risks related to polycystic ovary syndrome (PCOs). Hum Reprod. 2004;191:41–7. Review.
33. Samy N, Hashim M, Sayed M, Said M. Clinical significance of inflammatory markers in polycystic ovary syndrome: their relationship to insulin resistance and body mass index. Dis Markers. 2009;26:163–70.
34. Sathishkumar K, Elkins R, Chinnathambi V, Gao H, Hankins GD, Yallampalli C. Prenatal testosterone-induced fetal growth restriction is associated with down-regulation of rat placental amino acid transport. Reprod Biol Endocrinol. 2011;9:110.
35. Sir-Petermann T, Echiburú B, Maliqueo MM, Crisosto N, Sánchez F, Hitschfeld C, Cárcamo M, Amigo P, Pérez-Bravo F. Serum adiponectin and lipid concentrations in pregnant women with polycystic ovary syndrome. Hum Reprod. 2007;22:1830–6. Seppala et al., 2002.
36. Sun M, Maliqueo M, Benrick A, Johansson J, Shao R, Hou L, Jansson T, Wu X, Stener-Victorin E. Maternal androgen excess reduces placental and fetal weights, increases placental steroidogenesis, and leads to long-term health effects in their female offspring. Am J Physiol Endocrinol Metab. 2012;303:E1373–85.
37. Tang T, Lord JM, Norman RJ, Yasmin E, Balen AH. Insulin-sensitising drugs (metformin, rosiglitazone, pioglitazone, D chiro-inositol) for women with polycystic ovary syndrome, oligoamenorrhoea and subfertility. Cochrane Database Syst Rev. 2012;(5):CD003053.
38. Teede HJ, Misso ML, Deeks AA, Moran LJ, Stuckey BG, Wong JL, Norman RJ, Costello MF. Guideline Development Groups. Assessment and management of polycystic ovary syndrome: summary of an evidence-based guideline. Med J Aust. 2011;195:S65–112.
39. Toulis KA, Goulis DG, Kolibianakis EM, Venetis CA, Tarlatzis BC, Papadimas I. Risk of gestational diabetes mellitus in women with polycystic ovary syndrome: a systematic review and a meta-analysis. Fertil Steril. 2009;92:667–77.
40. Xu X, Du C, Zheng Q, Peng L, Sun Y. Effect of metformin on serum interleukin-6 levels in polycystic ovary syndrome: a systematic review. BMC Womens Health. 2014;14:93–100.
41. Yamamoto M, Feigenbaum SL, Crites Y, Escobar GJ, Yang J, Ferrara A, Lo JC. Risk of preterm delivery in non-diabetic women with polycystic ovarian syndrome. J Perinatol. 2012; 32:770–6.

Part III

The Potential Value of Nutrition and Nutriceutical Supplementation to Prevent Obstetrical Complications

Gastrointestinal Symptoms and Nutritional Profile During Pregnancy

8

Carlo Selmi, Maria De Santis, Luigi Laghi, and Elena Generali

Contents

8.1 Introduction

Gastrointestinal disturbances are common complaints during pregnancy and are generally of mild intensity, even if associated to significant subjective discomfort. Previous gastrointestinal diseases can worsen during pregnancy, or a new

C. Selmi (✉) • M. De Santis
Rheumatology and Clinical Immunology, Humanitas Research Hospital, Rozzano, Milan, Italy

Biometra Department, University of Milan, Milan, Italy
e-mail: carlo.selmi@unimi.it

L. Laghi
Gastroenterology, Humanitas Research Hospital, Rozzano, Milan, Italy

E. Generali
Rheumatology and Clinical Immunology, Humanitas Research Hospital, Rozzano, Milan, Italy

E. Ferrazzi, B. Sears (eds.), *Metabolic Syndrome and Complications of Pregnancy: The Potential Preventive Role of Nutrition*,
DOI 10.1007/978-3-319-16853-1_8

onset of gastrointestinal diseases can be observed. Many factors are involved in the pathogenesis of these disturbances among which pregnancy itself, weight gain, and nutrition are of particular importance albeit overlooked by most gynecologists. In some cases, nutritional deficits may cause gastrointestinal symptoms, but this is a very rare occurrence in Western countries. In general terms, a careful nutritional evaluation using validated questionnaires and diaries [1, 2] should be part of the workup dedicated to all pregnant women, particularly if nutritionally at risk, because recommended dietary allowances change during pregnancy. We are now becoming more aware that nutritional impairment has a significant impact on the offspring [3–5]. Human interventional studies on nutrition are limited to few studies in developing countries [6]. Opposite to this, excess weight gain during pregnancy represents a major challenge for healthcare providers in high-income countries. This condition exposes both the mother and fetus at high-risk conditions in pregnancy, exposes the children to a higher risk of metabolic syndrome in the future [3, 7], and identifies women at risk of metabolic syndrome in the fifth decade.

8.2 Nausea and Vomiting

Nausea and vomiting are very common symptoms during pregnancy, affecting 50–90 % of pregnant women, more often during the first trimester and, in up to 15 % of the cases, beyond 15 weeks [8–13]. The severity of nausea and vomiting during pregnancy can vary significantly from mild to severe or even unremitting in the form coined *hyperemesis gravidarum* [8–13] for which an etiology is still unknown, but an interaction of genetic, biological, and psychological factors is likely [14]. Weight loss or electrolyte imbalance due to nausea and vomiting represents also the first cause of hospitalization in the first half of pregnancy [15, 16]. Risk factors include young age, obesity, first pregnancy, smoking [17], and vitamin B6 deficiency [18]. Adequate tests to rule out possible vitamin deficiencies are encouraged in the case of clinical suspicion. In the pathophysiology of nausea and vomiting during pregnancy, changes in gastric motility, pregnancy-associated alterations of the vestibular system, taste and smell, and behavioral and psychological factors seem to have a role [11, 17]. Moreover, a complex metabolic and hormonal background seems to be implicated as increased human chorionic gonadotropin (HCG), low levels of prolactin, and high levels of estradiol are observed [19–21]. Recent reports have suggested an association between HCG and *Helicobacter pylori* infection [22] and with increased concentrations of cell-free fetal deoxyribonucleic acid (DNA) and activation of natural killer and cytotoxic T cells in women with *hyperemesis gravidarum* [23]. This special repulsion toward foods might represent also an intricate evolutionary protective mechanism, an adaptation to protect the embryo from phytotoxins and other environmental hazards [24] in the 1st weeks of embryogenesis and of placental development.

8.3 Food-Related Causes of Nausea and Vomiting

In some cases, nausea and vomiting are directly triggered by food or food manipulation [25]. Bacterial toxins or whole bacteria and fungi grown in leftovers from previous meals can induce nausea or vomiting, such as *Salmonella, Aspergillus, Fusarium, Claviceps, Penicillium*, or *Stachybotrys.*

Moderate coffee intake may increase intestinal peristalsis, while high amounts cause nausea in selected individuals [25], similar to the paradoxical effects of coffee withdrawal [26]. Monosodium glutamate, primarily used in Chinese cooking, but also commonly used as a flavor enhancer in industrial food products, fast food, and sweets, is thought to be responsible for the "Chinese restaurant syndrome," characterized by nausea, headaches, and vomiting [27].

Polycyclic aromatic carbohydrates (PAC) can also cause nausea [25] as they enter food products through the atmosphere and accumulate in small quantities during baking. PAC can be found mainly in smoked and grilled foods, breakfast cereals, root vegetables, and especially in olive trester oil, i.e., olive pomace oil, olive residue oil, refined olive residue oil, and olive oil, obviously not in extra virgin olive oil [28].

Other causes of nausea and vomiting are heavy metals typically found in food boiled in copper pots and cans, which can cause also pronounced diarrhea as a spontaneous reaction. These metals are also found in drinking water delivered via lead pipes, in native beer and juices served from some lead-glazed pottery (as in Mexico), in wines served from pewter goblets in Italy and other European countries, and in coffee or alcohol from "tin" cups in Norway [25]. In the case of single metals, lead (Pb) is more specifically found in milk, beef, or cereals; cadmium (Cd) in kidney, mussels, and soybean; and mercury (Hg) in fish, especially tuna, swordfish, and mackerel, so pregnant women should be aware of the mercury levels present in fish, particularly farm-raised or big-size fish like swordfish, if consumed more than three times per week [25].

8.4 Immune-Mediated Mechanisms

Specific nutrients may cause nausea and vomiting in almost all individuals depending on the nutrient dosage, whereas other nutrients cause adverse reactions such as nausea and vomiting only in sensitive individuals because of specific immune-mediated allergies or most likely because of nonallergic food hypersensitivity [25]. As such is the most frequent case, a dedicated food diary is encouraged to determine which cluster of similar nutrients may cause nausea and vomiting, for instance, an excess of gluten, an excess of caseins, etc. About 20–30 % of the adult population in the UK, USA, and Germany suffer from adverse reactions to food [25]. Only in a quarter of children and a tenth of adults are these reactions caused by IgE-mediated allergic mechanisms; all other forms are broadly considered food intolerances, now more properly defined by some authors as food antigen hypersensitivity [29]. The latter induces immune cell activation by antigens of food clusters or by additives such as salicylates, benzoates

Table 8.1 Synoptic list of toxic substances, active compounds, and immune mechanisms that can activate nausea and vomiting

Direct toxic substances	
Bacterial and fungal toxins	Meal leftovers or "fast food"
Coffee	Excess
Glutamate	Chinese food
Polycyclic aromatic hydrocarbon	Grilled meat and vegetables
Heavy metals	Big fish, lead-covered pipes, glasses
Pharmacologically active compounds	
Histamine	Cheese, white wine, tuna, and salmon
Tyramine	Chocolate, cheese, red wine
Sulfites	Wine
Immune mechanisms	
IgE allergy mechanisms	IgE-mediated mast cell reactions
IgG-mediated food hypersensitivity	Excess of similar food active antigens in weekly diet (caseins, gluten, nickel compounds, etc.)
Celiac disease	Acquired antibodies to epithelial cells, negative IgE, villous damage – atrophy
Nonceliac gluten sensitivity	Excess submucosal lymphocytes
Genetics	
Lactose nontolerant genotype	Lactase gene progressively switched off after weaning
Fructose nontolerant genotype	Rare mutation of the aldolase B gene

and tartrazine. These reactions differ and may superimpose pharmacological reactions (e.g., to histamines found in cheeses, white wine, and scombroid fish such as tuna and salmon; tyramine, found in chocolate, herrings, tinned fish, brewer's yeast, red wine, and cheese such as *Roquefort* and cheddar; and additives such as sulfites, tartrazine, monosodium glutamate, and other amines) (Table 8.1) [25].

Some major genetic-based phenotypes are largely ignored by healthcare providers. Thirty percent of southern Europeans and a little less of northern Europeans are nonlactose tolerant. This percentage sums up to 80 % in Amerinds and 90 % of the Chinese Hun population. After weaning, like in all other mothers in these human phenotypes, the lactase gene progressively is switched off (Fig. 8.1). As a result of the lack of lactase, lactose cannot be split in its two composing sugars in the small intestine; as a cosequence, lactose acts either as an irritant molecule attracting fluids into the small intestine, determining immediate bowel emptying after consumption (subjects with chronic constipation that assume glasses of milk in the morning to evacuate thus making GI inflammation worse), or proceeds into the colon to feed otherwise marginal bacterial populations, which take advantage of lactose presence and produce hydrogen and finally cause the complex dysbiosis.

We also note rare inherited genetic carbohydrate intolerance (e.g., fructose intolerance, glucose or galactose intolerance) or protein intolerance (e.g., tryptophan intolerance or methionine intolerance) [25].

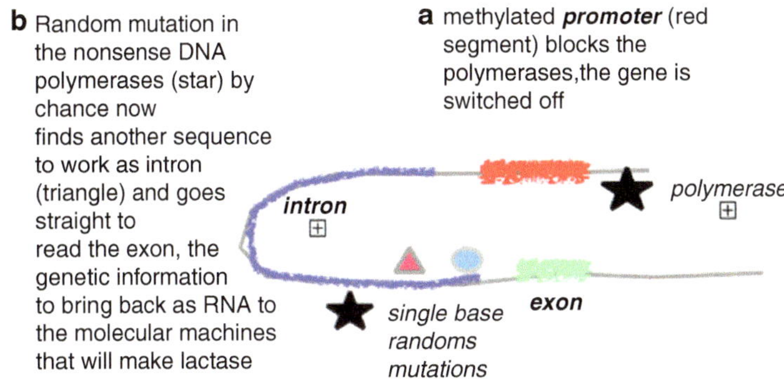

Fig. 8.1 Schematic representation of the typical switching of the lactase gene in mammalians. In some macro-ethnicities a relevant percentage of the population became lactose tolerant thanks to random mutations in the intron that allowed the polymerases to read the exon even in methylated gene. These random mutations are widespread among population that adopted cattle raising in the last 10,000 years. This allowed these lucky individuals to win the selective pressure given the advantage of being able to exploit cattle raising not only for meat but also for the reproducible rich source of protein, fat, and sugars provided by milk and dairy products. Unfortunately, this advantage is not universal among humans, and the introduction of dairy product in lactose-intolerant individual is a source of chronic disease

Spectrum of related gluten disorders

Investigation	Coeliac disease* (adaptive immune response)	Wheat allergy† (allergic immune response)	Non-coeliac gluten sensitivity‡ (innate immune response)
Coeliac serology (endomysial and tissue transglutaminase antibodies)	Positive	Negative	Negative
Duodenal biopsies	Villous atrophy	Normal	Normal or near normal with raised intraepithelial lymphocytes
IgE serology or skin prick test to wheat	Negative	Positive	Negative

Fig. 8.2 Simplified criteria to identify the possible clinical conditions based on gluten interactions with the digestive system. Unfortunately the present selected wheat esaploid species are far more rich in gluten, up to 14 % net weight, than the ancestral tetraploid species

Celiac disease is considered as a separate nosological entity, but its paradigms and continuity with other immune-mediated gluten sensitivity are still under investigation (Fig. 8.2).

Approximately 2–8 % of children and 1–2 % of adults suffer from food allergies. Typically, nausea and vomiting are predominant symptoms if the site of allergy is in the upper gastrointestinal tract. The food allergens that most frequently trigger nausea and vomiting are those inducing the oral allergy syndrome consisting of swelling and reddening of the lips and the buccal, pharyngeal, and laryngeal mucosa. These allergens are most frequently the pollen-associated food allergens such as pipfruits, drupes, nuts [25], and shellfish.

8.5 Miscellaneous Causes of Nausea and Vomiting

Finally, additional causes of nausea and vomiting include acute pancreatitis, obstetric cholestasis, acute fatty liver of pregnancy and HELLP (hemolysis, elevated liver enzymes, low platelets) syndrome, as well as intestinal conditions such as appendicitis, and these apparently rare conditions need to be ruled out in the presence of a strong suspicion [19].

8.6 Gastroesophageal Reflux

The percentage of women who experience symptoms associated with GERD at any time during pregnancy range from 30 to 80 %, being highest in the third trimester [30]. The clinical features of pregnancy-associated GERD do not differ from those seen in the general population, with predominant symptoms being heartburn and regurgitation, that aggravate following meals and when lying in a supine position. For women already diagnosed with GERD prior to pregnancy, symptoms often worsen as pregnancy progresses [17]. There are a number of functional and structural alterations that occur at the gastroesophageal junction during pregnancy that may at least explain the high prevalence of reflux symptoms in this population. Reflux is due to a combination of factors that may be worsened in late pregnancy by the enlarging uterus, including an increase in gastric pressure, reduction in lower esophageal sphincter tone, decrease in gastric peristalsis, delayed gastric emptying, and a reduction in pyloric sphincter competence. Both estrogen and progesterone may relax the lower esophageal sphincter, which is also under the control of a variety of humoral agents including motilin, acetylcholine, noradrenaline, histamine, 5-HT, and prostaglandins [31].

Overall, available evidence indicates that *H. pylori* status does not have any effect on severity of or recurrence of symptoms in GERD, nor impact treatment efficacy, and that the eradication of *H. pylori* is not associated with development or exacerbation of GERD [32, 33]. Antacids taken before meals and at bedtime, together with the avoidance of late-night meals; excluding some foods, as chocolate; and sometimes raising the head of the bed, can help in controlling GERD symptoms. However, when a therapy is necessary, symptomatic treatments include alginate-based formulations, which create a foamy raft over the gastric walls, and do not account for adverse effects both for the mother and baby [34], and H2-receptor antagonists, as ranitidine, which are commonly used in pregnancy to control reflux symptoms and seem to have no adverse effects on the fetus [35]. Conversely, there are concerns about proton pump inhibitor use during pregnancy and their effects on the fetus, especially regarding the risk of asthma [36]. Generally speaking, H2-receptor antagonist and proton pump inhibitors use should be discouraged because they may alter the digestive functions of the stomach if assumed for several months in a row. When heartburns and reflux become evident, lifestyle changes should be encouraged as regards composition of meals (check for food hypersensitivity), time from meal to bedtime, and moderate exercise after eating.

8.7 Constipation

The reported prevalence of constipation in pregnant women varies between 11 and 38 % and occurs mostly during the second and third trimester, although symptoms can also be present since the 12th week of gestation [37] and last until 3 months after delivery [38, 39]. The pathophysiology of constipation is multifactorial and not yet well clarified but recognized primarily as a functional basis. Progressively rising progesterone and estrogen levels have been suggested as cause of constipation during pregnancy that inhibits gut smooth muscle function [40]. Other factors involved in pregnancy constipation are decreased colon motility, oral iron supplements, poor fluid intake as a consequence of nausea, and pressure on the rectosigmoid colon by the gravid uterus in the third trimester, as well as functional bowel disorders [41]. Management usually involves reassurance and advice about increasing fluid and fiber intake, while laxatives are rarely required [17].

Moreover, dietary supplements of fibers, as bran or wheat fiber, are likely to help pregnant women experiencing constipation [37]. Fiber intake is usually well below the standard recommendations in the daily health plate and thus is frequently forgotten by healthcare providers. Five to six hundred grams of vegetables and fruit per day is far above the common daily plate in most Western-style nutritional profile. No fiber means inadequate microbiota, possibly a critical immune cross talk with the intestinal immune system and low-grade inflammation, and decreased motility; for sure it means less hydrophilic stools, all summed up to create a chronic constipation, just made worse by pregnancy hormones and abdominal "mass." Most women consider minor constipation and minor irritable colon a "normal condition" that just turns "unpleasant" in pregnancy, to be treated by drugs as it is common practice nowadays when doctors are confronted with lifestyle problems. Figure 8.3 could represent an interesting standard of counseling for women suffering from obstetrical constipation.

8.8 Probiotics in Pregnancy

Probiotics are defined as live microorganisms which when administered in adequate amounts confer a health benefit on the host [42]. Probiotics probably have at least two modes of action in improving constipation: firstly improving dysbiosis that is assumed to play a role in constipation [43, 44] and secondly lowering the colon pH by producing lactic, acetic, and other short-chain fatty acids and consequently enhancing colonic peristalsis and subsequently decreasing colonic transit time [43, 44]. Pilot studies have shown the beneficial use of probiotic mixtures for the treatment of constipation in pregnancy [39], as Ecologic®Relief (a mixture of *Bifidobacterium bifidum* W23, *Bifidobacterium lactis* W52, *Bifidobacterium longum* W108, *Lactobacillus casei* W79*nn*, *Lactobacillus plantarum* W62, and *Lactobacillus rhamnosus* W71) [39]. Probiotics might also reduce the risk of developing gestational diabetes [45]. In case of failure in resolving the constipation with both dietary supplements and probiotics, polyethylene glycol-based laxatives represent the ideal treatment for pregnant women [46] due to their very limited absorption.

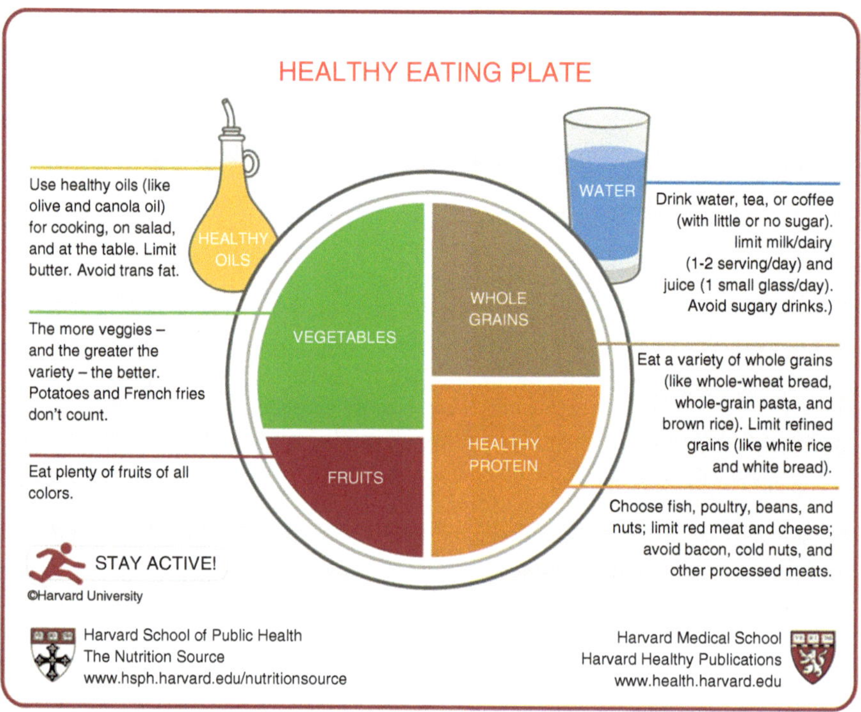

Fig. 8.3 The healthy eating plate as reported by the Harvard School of Nutrition considers that half of the daily plate is made up of veggies and fruits. A special note should include the additional concepts of "whole grains" (most of wheat products are now "refined") and of "healthy proteins" that limit red meat, as in Mediterranean, Asian, and South American food pyramids, to one portion per week, far below the present nutritional profile in most countries where meat and meat products and derivates are part of each meal for each day

8.9 Diarrhea

Together with the causes previously described for nausea and vomiting, irritable bowel disease, inflammatory bowel disease, and enteric infection have to be considered in case of diarrhea appearing or worsening during pregnancy.

The incidence of gastrointestinal infections in pregnancy is not increased. *Salmonella enteritidis* and *Campylobacter jejuni* infections have been associated with fetal mortality due to the transplacental passage of microorganisms [47, 48]. Infection with *Listeria monocytogenes* is a well-recognized very rare cause of intrauterine infection and perinatal death. The infection is acquired through eating foods contaminated with the organism, and appropriate dietary advice should be given to all pregnant women about the avoidance of foods such as *pâtés* and soft and blue-veined cheese [19]. Pregnancy has little effect on symptoms associated with inflammatory bowel disease [17], but, similar to other chronic inflammatory conditions, most guidelines advise optimizing lifestyle during pregnancy, such as dietary changes.

These include increasing fiber and water intake for those with predominant constipation, and reduced fat and dairy consumption for patients diagnosed with predominant diarrhea, and relaxation therapy [17, 19]. Symptoms of irritable bowel disease may be exacerbated by pregnancy, especially if constipation is the prominent feature [19], and also in this case careful reduction of food antigens that might determine food hypersensitivity and immune inflammatory response, a high-fiber diet, and a reduction of unhealthy proteins and animal fats might be helpful. Stool-bulking agents may be helpful for short courses as well as the prescription of high dosages of probiotics.

8.10 Concluding Remarks

Pregnancies in Westernized countries are seldom burdened by malnutrition, but evidences on the impact of nutritional factors on the offspring [49] are rapidly becoming available and encourage all physicians to carefully assess the nutritional status and micronutrient intake in women potentially at risk. Nutritional questionnaires [50] could help to figure out unhealthy habits compared to typical food pyramids (Fig. 8.3).

As we have shown the frequency of gastrointestinal disturbances in pregnancy is frequent, but mainly represented by mild symptoms that can be treated with education of the patient, diet adjustment, and possibly the introduction of specific dietary supplements as fiber and probiotics [39, 40]. Sometimes though, serious conditions underlie these symptoms, for example, appendicitis, gallbladder disease [51], and *hyperemesis gravidarum*, and so it is crucially important that the physician recognizes the importance of these symptoms to address the patient.

8.11 Summary

Gastrointestinal disturbances are common complaints during pregnancy and are generally of mild intensity, though leading to significant subjective discomfort. Nutritional factors including micronutrient deficiencies or malnutrition have not been fully addressed in adequate studies. Preexisting gastrointestinal diseases can worsen during pregnancy, or a new onset of gastrointestinal diseases can be observed. The main gastrointestinal symptoms found during pregnancy include nausea and vomiting (most commonly during the first trimester), gastroesophageal reflux, constipation (especially in the third trimester), and finally diarrhea, which is likely the least common than other symptoms. During pregnancy it may be difficult to assess if a specific symptom is an expression of a gastrointestinal disease or if it is caused by the pregnancy itself that simply adds on the preexisting subclinical gastrointestinal abnormalities. The aim of every healthcare provider is to identify gastrointestinal symptoms during pregnancy, refuse the idea that all of them are simple "normal" side effects of being pregnant, and, through them, identify pre-pregnancy subclinical conditions and to address the best treatment options, focusing particularly on nutritional mechanisms.

References

1. Sartorelli DS, Barbieri P, Perdona GC. Fried food intake estimated by the multiple source method is associated with gestational weight gain. Nutr Res. 2014;34(8):667–73.
2. Mathews F, Yudkin P, Neil A. Influence of maternal nutrition on outcome of pregnancy: prospective cohort study. BMJ. 1999;319(7206):339–43.
3. Arentson-Lantz EJ, et al. Excess pregnancy weight gain leads to early indications of metabolic syndrome in a swine model of fetal programming. Nutr Res. 2014;34(3):241–9.
4. Alkerwi A, et al. No significant independent relationships with cardiometabolic biomarkers were detected in the Observation of Cardiovascular Risk Factors in Luxembourg study population. Nutr Res. 2014;34(12):1058–65.
5. McGaughy JA, et al. Prenatal malnutrition leads to deficits in attentional set shifting and decreases metabolic activity in prefrontal subregions that control executive function. Dev Neurosci. 2014;36(6):532–41.
6. Salam RA, Das JK, Bhutta ZA. Multiple micronutrient supplementation during pregnancy and lactation in low-to-middle-income developing country settings: impact on pregnancy outcomes. Ann Nutr Metab. 2014;65(1):4–12.
7. Triunfo S, Lanzone A. Impact of overweight and obesity on obstetric outcomes. J Endocrinol Invest. 2014;37(4):323–9.
8. Baron TH, Ramirez B, Richter JE. Gastrointestinal motility disorders during pregnancy. Ann Intern Med. 1993;118(5):366–75.
9. Goodwin TM. Nausea and vomiting of pregnancy: an obstetric syndrome. Am J Obstet Gynecol. 2002;186(5 Suppl Understanding):S184–9.
10. Jarvis S, Nelson-Piercy C. Management of nausea and vomiting in pregnancy. BMJ. 2011;342:d3606.
11. Keller J, Frederking D, Layer P. The spectrum and treatment of gastrointestinal disorders during pregnancy. Nat Clin Pract Gastroenterol Hepatol. 2008;5(8):430–43.
12. Knudsen A, Lebech M, Hansen M. Upper gastrointestinal symptoms in the third trimester of the normal pregnancy. Eur J Obstet Gynecol Reprod Biol. 1995;60(1):29–33.
13. Koch KL. Gastrointestinal factors in nausea and vomiting of pregnancy. Am J Obstet Gynecol. 2002;186(5 Suppl Understanding):S198–203.
14. McCarthy FP, Lutomski JE, Greene RA. Hyperemesis gravidarum: current perspectives. Int J Womens Health. 2014;6:719–25.
15. Sanu O, Lamont RF. Hyperemesis gravidarum: pathogenesis and the use of antiemetic agents. Expert Opin Pharmacother. 2011;12(5):737–48.
16. Matthews A, et al. Interventions for nausea and vomiting in early pregnancy. Cochrane Database Syst Rev. 2014;(3):CD007575.
17. van der Woude CJ, Metselaar HJ, Danese S. Management of gastrointestinal and liver diseases during pregnancy. Gut. 2014;63(6):1014–23.
18. Hovdenak N, Haram K. Influence of mineral and vitamin supplements on pregnancy outcome. Eur J Obstet Gynecol Reprod Biol. 2012;164(2):127–32.
19. Boregowda G, Shehata HA. Gastrointestinal and liver disease in pregnancy. Best Pract Res Clin Obstet Gynaecol. 2013;27(6):835–53.
20. Tsuruta E, et al. Pathogenic role of asialo human chorionic gonadotropin in gestational thyrotoxicosis. J Clin Endocrinol Metab. 1995;80(2):350–5.
21. Lagiou P, et al. Nausea and vomiting in pregnancy in relation to prolactin, estrogens, and progesterone: a prospective study. Obstet Gynecol. 2003;101(4):639–44.
22. Sandven I, et al. Helicobacter pylori infection and hyperemesis gravidarum: a systematic review and meta-analysis of case-control studies. Acta Obstet Gynecol Scand. 2009;88(11):1190–200.
23. Sugito Y, et al. Relationship between severity of hyperemesis gravidarum and fetal DNA concentration in maternal plasma. Clin Chem. 2003;49(10):1667–9.
24. Cardwell MS. Pregnancy sickness: a biopsychological perspective. Obstet Gynecol Surv. 2012;67(10):645–52.
25. Bischoff SC, Renzer C. Nausea and nutrition. Auton Neurosci. 2006;129(1–2):22–7.

26. Griffiths RR, et al. Low-dose caffeine discrimination in humans. J Pharmacol Exp Ther. 1990;252(3):970–8.
27. De Francisci G, Parisi N, Magalini SI. The Chinese restaurant syndrome. Recenti Prog Med. 1981;70(4):353–7.
28. Garcia-Falcon MS, Simal-Gandara J, Carril-Gonzalez-Barros ST. Analysis of benzo[a]pyrene in spiked fatty foods by second derivative synchronous spectrofluorimetry after microwave-assisted treatment of samples. Food Addit Contam. 2000;17(12):957–64.
29. Pereira B, et al. Prevalence of sensitization to food allergens, reported adverse reaction to foods, food avoidance, and food hypersensitivity among teenagers. J Allergy Clin Immunol. 2005;116(4):884–92.
30. Richter JE. Gastroesophageal reflux disease during pregnancy. Gastroenterol Clin North Am. 2003;32(1):235–61.
31. Welsh T, et al. Prostaglandin H2 synthase-1 and −2 expression in guinea pig gestational tissues during late pregnancy and parturition. J Physiol. 2005;569(Pt 3):903–12.
32. Moayyedi P, et al. Helicobacter pylori eradication does not exacerbate reflux symptoms in gastroesophageal reflux disease. Gastroenterology. 2001;121(5):1120–6.
33. Cardaropoli S, Rolfo A, Todros T. Helicobacter pylori and pregnancy-related disorders. World J Gastroenterol. 2014;20(3):654–64.
34. Quartarone G. Gastroesophageal reflux in pregnancy: a systematic review on the benefit of raft forming agents. Minerva Ginecol. 2013;65(5):541–9.
35. Magee LA, et al. Safety of first trimester exposure to histamine H2 blockers. A prospective cohort study. Dig Dis Sci. 1996;41(6):1145–9.
36. Gill SK, et al. The safety of proton pump inhibitors (PPIs) in pregnancy: a meta-analysis. Am J Gastroenterol. 2009;104(6):1541–5; quiz 1540, 1546.
37. Jewell DJ, Young G. Interventions for treating constipation in pregnancy. Cochrane Database Syst Rev. 2001;(2):CD001142.
38. Bradley CS, et al. Constipation in pregnancy: prevalence, symptoms, and risk factors. Obstet Gynecol. 2007;110(6):1351–7.
39. de Milliano I, et al. Is a multispecies probiotic mixture effective in constipation during pregnancy? 'A pilot study'. Nutr J. 2012;11:80.
40. West L, Warren J, Cutts T. Diagnosis and management of irritable bowel syndrome, constipation, and diarrhea in pregnancy. Gastroenterol Clin North Am. 1992;21(4):793–802.
41. Johnson P, Mount K, Graziano S. Functional bowel disorders in pregnancy: effect on quality of life, evaluation and management. Acta Obstet Gynecol Scand. 2014;93(9):874–9.
42. Gill HS, Guarner F. Probiotics and human health: a clinical perspective. Postgrad Med J. 2004;80(947):516–26.
43. Picard C, et al. Review article: bifidobacteria as probiotic agents – physiological effects and clinical benefits. Aliment Pharmacol Ther. 2005;22(6):495–512.
44. Szajewska H, Ruszczynski M, Radzikowski A. Probiotics in the prevention of antibiotic-associated diarrhea in children: a meta-analysis of randomized controlled trials. J Pediatr. 2006;149(3):367–72.
45. Barrett HL, et al. Probiotics for preventing gestational diabetes. Cochrane Database Syst Rev. 2014;(2):CD009951.
46. Tytgat GN, et al. Contemporary understanding and management of reflux and constipation in the general population and pregnancy: a consensus meeting. Aliment Pharmacol Ther. 2003;18(3):291–301.
47. Roll C, et al. Fatal Salmonella enteritidis sepsis acquired prenatally in a premature infant. Obstet Gynecol. 1996;88(4 Pt 2):692–3.
48. Meyer A, et al. Lethal maternal sepsis caused by Campylobacter jejuni: pathogen preserved in placenta and identified by molecular methods. Mod Pathol. 1997;10(12):1253–6.
49. Triunfo S, Lanzone A. Impact of maternal under nutrition on obstetric outcomes. J Endocrinol Invest. 2014;38:31–8.
50. Maruyama K, et al. The reasonable reliability of a self-administered food frequency questionnaire for an urban, Japanese, middle-aged population: the Suita study. Nutr Res. 2014;35:14–22.
51. Parangi S, et al. Surgical gastrointestinal disorders during pregnancy. Am J Surg. 2007;193(2):223–32.

Micronutrients and the Obstetrical Syndromes

9

Irene Cetin and Maddalena Massari

Contents

9.1 Introduction

During recent years, awareness has increased that a healthy balanced diet provides the best basis for optimal pregnancy outcome. Nutritional status is an important aspect of health and wellness before and during pregnancy: as the foundations for a healthy life are already laid in the womb, adequate nutrition in this period is of great

I. Cetin, MD (✉) • M. Massari, MD
Mother-Child Department, Obstetrics and Gynecology Unit,
Biomedical and Clinical Sciences, L.Sacco-University of Milan, Milan, Italy
e-mail: irene.cetin@unimi.it

E. Ferrazzi, B. Sears (eds.), *Metabolic Syndrome and Complications of Pregnancy: The Potential Preventive Role of Nutrition*,
DOI 10.1007/978-3-319-16853-1_9

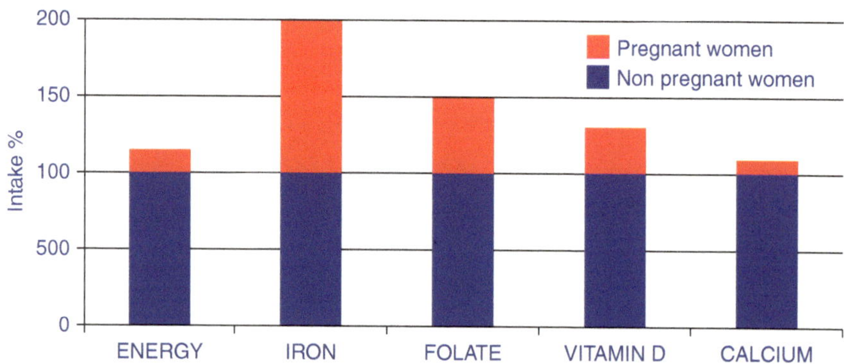

Fig. 9.1 Recommended intakes for pregnant women expressed as percentages of the reference intake values for nonpregnant women. The recommended intakes of iron and folate show great increases of 100 and 50 %, respectively, compared with those for the nonpregnant state, while energy needs, calcium, and vitamin D show a smaller change (Adapted from Koletzko et al. [26])

importance. Adequate nutrition is very important for adequate intake not only of macronutrients like proteins, carbohydrates, and fats but also of micronutrients for which we may more easily incur into deficiencies or inadequacies.

Micronutrients are vitamins and minerals required in minute amounts for metabolism and normal organism functioning. With their numerous functions in the body, micronutrients are essential for growth and development. Their requirements increase exponentially during pregnancy *in order to meet the growing demands of the fetoplacental unit*. Moreover, nutritional needs for micronutrients are increased during pregnancy not only for support of fetal growth and development but also for adaptations occurring in maternal tissues and metabolism. Energy needs increase only slightly during the course of pregnancy: indeed energy needs during the final months of pregnancy are only about 10 % higher than before pregnancy. So, compared to the increase in energy needs, the need for certain vitamins and minerals in pregnancy shows a much greater increase [26] (Fig. 9.1).

Micronutrient deficiencies have been associated with significantly high reproductive risks, ranging from infertility to fetal structural defects and long-term diseases. On the other side, healthy dietary patterns and micronutrient supplementation, particularly during the periconceptional period, are related to improved birth outcomes, probably through alterations in maternal and fetal metabolism due to micronutrient role/involvement in enzymes, signal transduction, transcription pathways, oxidative stress, and epigenetic modifications [11]. Since different pregnancy stages represent a continuum, from the preconception to the postpartum period, an injury acting before conception or in early pregnancy may have long-lasting effects on the well-being of the mother and the fetus and may further influence the health of the baby at a later age.

It has been estimated that more than two billion people in the world today suffer from micronutrient deficiencies caused largely by a dietary deficiency of vitamins and minerals. Nutritional deficiencies are known to lead to adverse pregnancy outcomes involving the great obstetrical syndromes such as preterm delivery, small for gestational age (SGA) offspring, and maternal hypertensive disorders as well as to long-term effects in the offspring. The chapter will focus primarily on the following outcomes: intrauterine growth restriction, preeclampsia, and preterm delivery.

9.2 Micronutrient Malnutrition

Contrary to previous thinking, micronutrient malnutrition is not uniquely the concern of poor countries. While micronutrient deficiencies are certainly more frequent and severe among disadvantaged populations, they do represent a public health problem also in most industrialized countries where obesogenic unbalanced diets have a major impact on macro- and micronutrients. Worldwide micronutrient intakes do not fit pregnancy requirements.

Since 1989 it has been shown that dietary surveys of pregnant women in industrialized countries consistently demonstrate Fe intake well below current recommendations. A recent review [6] summarizes the best available evidence related to the food-derived vitamin and mineral intakes of pregnant women in developed countries demonstrating that *folate, iron, and vitamin D intakes are consistently below nutrient recommendations in each geographical region.* In particular, despite folate recommendations varying across geographical regions, average folate intakes in all regions were between 13 and 63 % lower than recommendations. Similarly, iron intakes reported by pregnant women were below nutrient recommendations in almost all developed regions. However, these results underestimate the number of pregnant women who met national pregnancy micronutrient targets on the basis of combined food and supplement intakes.

Moreover, many micronutrients with important roles during pregnancy (e.g., iodine) were not commonly reported within the included studies, and thus, nutritional adequacy could not be evaluated. In the last 10 years, median urinary iodine below the recommended values has been reported in pregnant women of many countries in the world (Argentina, Greece, Italy, Wales, Ireland). However, there are no studies about a potential role of iodine in the great obstetrical syndromes.

In fact, although a balanced diet is generally accessible in industrialized countries, a switch to highly processed energy-dense but micronutrient-poor foods is likely to adversely affect micronutrient intake and status.

9.3 From Requirements to Recommendations: The Strange Case of Pregnancy

The ideal definition of a physiological requirement is the amount and chemical form of a nutrient that is needed systematically to maintain normal health and development without disturbing metabolism of any other nutrient. The physiological requirement is very difficult to be estimated, and for this reason micronutrient requirement is defined as the minimum amount needed by an individual to avoid deficiency.. However, micronutrient recommendations are designed for populations or subgroups of populations, and they are defined as intakes of micronutrients sufficient to meet the requirements of the majority of healthy individuals (generally 97.5 %) of that population or group.

Many countries have developed recommendations for intake of micronutrients in the normal diet. However, there is considerable variation in the recommended micronutrient intakes used by countries in particular within Europe, partly due to different methodologies and concepts used to determine requirements and different approaches used to express the recommendations. The EURRECA Project was designed in Europe. Specifically, the EURopean micronutrient RECommendations Aligned (EURRECA) Network of Excellence has worked to provide an evidence-based framework for establishing micronutrient requirements. EURRECA is a network of excellence funded by the European Commission and established to address the problem of differences between countries in micronutrient recommendations [15].

First of all the EURRECA network developed a selection process to identify a list of micronutrients to focus on. The prioritization of micronutrients was based on the availability of new scientific evidence, the public health relevance, and the heterogeneity of the recommendations [10]. Ten micronutrients were identified as most urgently in need of review: vitamin D, iron, folate, vitamin B12, zinc, calcium, vitamin C, selenium, iodine, and copper. Of these, vitamin C, vitamin D, folate, calcium, selenium, and iodine were the nutrients showing a higher prevalence of inadequate intakes in Europe. In particular, a lack of harmonized and evidence-based recommendations was found for the supply of vitamin D, folate, and iron during pregnancy, lactation, and infancy [21].

9.3.1 Identification and Reference Values of Micronutrients

Once the most important micronutrients are identified, valid information on micronutrient intakes and status of a population (Fig. 9.2) is fundamental for deriving micronutrient reference values.

For this purpose, biomarkers of micronutrient status need to be identified for each micronutrient. Examples of types of status biomarkers include plasma concentrations, the size of body pools, enzyme levels and activities, urinary excretion, and

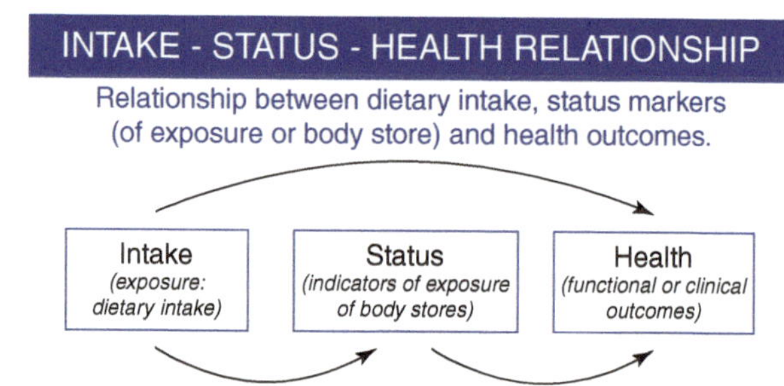

Fig. 9.2 Intake–status–health relationship

Table 9.1 The reliable biomarkers or indicators of status of the main micronutrients

Micronutrient	Biomarkers
Folate	Erythrocyte folate
	Serum/plasma folate
	Serum/plasma total homocysteine
Vitamin B12	Serum/plasma vitamin B12
	Serum/plasma methylmalonic acid (MMA)
Iron	Hemoglobin
	Serum ferritin
	Serum transferrin receptor
Vitamin D	Plasma 25-hydroxyvitamin-D [25(OH)D]
Iodine	Urinary iodine excretion in 24 h
	Serum thyroid-stimulating hormone (TSH)

a range of other biochemical and/or functional indicators which have varying degrees of specificity and sensitivity (Table 9.1). Indeed, nutritional status, when applied to specific micronutrients, reflects a continuum, from short-term (hours) exposure (to long-term (months/years) effects. Moreover, a rigorous selection process needs to be carried out also for identifying health outcomes of interest for each micronutrient: for example, EURRECA identified the most relevant health outcomes by determining the number of hits that emerged in preliminary searches of the literature combined with the opinion of scientific nutritional experts [17].

Finally, there are different approaches for deriving reference dietary values. The association approach addresses the dose–response relationship between dietary micronutrient intake and body status or health outcomes. The factorial approach addresses micronutrient losses and maintenance, absorption/bioavailability, and additional requirements for specific life stages. Currently, most of the available studies evaluate the role of different nutrients such as micronutrients in pathologies and health outcomes. However, foods are not consumed in isolation. An overall dietary pattern might have a greater effect on health than a single food or nutrient. Methods most often used to characterize diet and dietary pattern have been based either on a priori knowledge (hypothesis-oriented DP) or derived from food frequency questionnaires using data-driven dimension reduction techniques, such as principal components analysis (PCA) (empirically derived DP).

9.3.2 Genetics and Individualization

It is important to recognize the multiple ways by which a nutritional deficiency may arise. First, a deficiency can occur as a consequence of an inadequate dietary intake of an essential nutrient. But a secondary deficiency may occur even if the dietary content of the essential nutrient appears to be adequate. Conditioned deficiencies can arise through several mechanisms as genetic factors, nutritional interactions, effects of drugs or chemicals, or diseases (as diabetes or hypertension).

Fig. 9.3 Nutritional phenotype of pregnancy

Nutritional phenotype of pregnancy

- **Dynamic state**: adjustments in nutrient metabolism evolve continuously as the mother switches from an ***anabolic condition*** during early pregnancy to a ***catabolic state*** during late pregnancy

- **Three compartments model**, i.e., ***mother/placenta/fetus***, each of them has different metabolism - fetal growth regulated by the balance between fetal nutrient demand and maternal-placental nutrient supply

Critical to this consideration will be the need for a better understanding of the influence of maternal and conceptus genotype on their susceptibility to the toxicity as well as the deficiency of essential micronutrients.

In addition, a new reference intake, the tolerable upper intake level (UL), has also been established to assist an individual in knowing how much is "too much" of a nutrient. Where adequate scientific data are available, determining tolerable upper intake levels for each micronutrient in specific population subgroups should be a primary goal.

9.3.3 Vulnerable Groups: Pregnant Women

A critical step is also to identify vulnerable population groups who are at greater nutritional risk: i.e., population groups in a healthy population having a higher requirement. Pregnant women are considered a "vulnerable group," as their nutritional requirements increase significantly to support fetal and infant growth and development as well as maternal metabolism and tissue accretion.

From a nutritional point of view, pregnancy can be simplified by a three-compartment model, i.e., mother/placenta/fetus. Each of them has a different metabolism and they interact. Apart from maternal diet and from metabolism of the various organs, placenta transport function determines the composition of the umbilical cord blood providing nutrients and oxygen to the fetus. Fetal growth is regulated by the balance between fetal nutrient demand and maternal–placental nutrient supply. Maternal nutrition and metabolism, uteroplacental blood flow, size, and transfer capabilities of the placenta all determine the maternal–placental supply of nutrients. On the other hand, pregnancy is a dynamic state, during which adjustments in nutrient metabolism evolve continuously as the mother switches from an anabolic condition during early pregnancy to a catabolic state during late pregnancy. Consequently, qualitative differences in dietary requirements exist during early and late pregnancy [3] (Fig. 9.3).

Dietary assessment using food frequency questionnaire (FFQ) during pregnancy may be complex. Some recommendations should be applied when dietary patterns during pregnancy are analyzed: (1) to employ a validated food frequency questionnaire designed for use in pregnancy, (2) to consider the special role exerted by mineral and vitamin supplements in this particular population group, (3) to adequately select the time in which dietary data are collected, and (4) to adjust the results for lifestyle and educational characteristics [34].

9.4 Preeclampsia

Preeclampsia is one of the leading causes of maternal morbidity and mortality and preterm delivery in the world. Nutritional interventional studies to prevent hypertension and different end-organ diseases grouped under the same syndrome are biased by the different prevalence of clinical phenotypes that are the results of various pathological process. Abnormal placentation with release of anti-angiogenetic factors in the maternal circulation, together with a predisposed maternal phenotype, seems to be involved. In particular, preeclampsia is associated with an increased inflammatory state, but the role of maternal nutrition in influencing the risk of developing preeclampsia is unclear.

9.5 Preterm Delivery

Low body mass index (BMI) before pregnancy and inadequate body weight gain of pregnant women in the second and third trimesters have been shown to be significantly associated with spontaneous preterm delivery in the USA and in Europe. Moreover, recent data obtained in 66,000 women in Norway showed that high scores on the "prudent" dietary pattern in the first months of pregnancy are associated with significantly reduced risk of preterm delivery hazard ratio [16]. This dietary pattern is characterized by intake of vegetables, fruit, whole grains, fish, and water, suggesting higher intake of micronutrients.

In this context, several studies suggest that multivitamin and mineral use before and during pregnancy may potentially prevent preterm birth. However, there is still not enough evidence to support multivitamin supplementation for reduction of preterm delivery.

A trial by Catov et al. [8] demonstrates a reduced risk of preterm delivery and small for gestational age in a cohort of 1,823 women who reported periconceptional multivitamin use, even if this finding was limited to women with a BMI <30. In 2011 data from more than 35,000 women in the Danish National Birth Cohort [9] confirmed that women who reported periconceptional multivitamin use had a reduced risk of preterm birth and a reduced risk of SGA (<5th percentile). The risk of an SGA birth was reduced in multivitamin users regardless of their prepregnancy BMI, with the strongest association in regular users in the post-conception period. However, these findings should be interpreted with caution because multivitamin use also correlated strongly with other lifestyle factors.

Although mechanisms that may link periconceptional multivitamin use to preterm delivery are not understood, impaired placentation seems to be implicated. Placentation is characterized by vascular remodeling, oxidative stress, inflammation, and rapid cell division, all of which may be affected by nutritional status. During pregnancy, oxidative stress has been implicated not only in the pathophysiology of preeclampsia but also of preterm birth leading to poor birth outcome. Moreover, hyperhomocysteinemia, as a consequence of altered micronutrients like folic acid and vitamin B12, is associated with increased production of reactive oxygen species that generate oxidative stress. One case–control study related the preconception sufficiency of vitamins B6 and B12 in maternal serum to a 50–60 % reduced risk of a PTB. Nevertheless a large prospective national birth cohort study in Norway did not find a protective effect of dietary folate intake or folic acid supplementation on spontaneous preterm delivery in uncomplicated pregnancies [33].

9.6 Low Birth Weight and Intrauterine Growth Restriction

Mothers in low-income countries frequently have inadequate micronutrient intakes. They often consume inadequate levels of micronutrients due to limited intake of animal products, fruits, vegetables, and fortified foods. Low birth weight (LBW) is common in undernourished populations in low- and middle-income countries, predominantly because of intrauterine growth restriction. Micronutrient supplementation and fortification are currently being used as strategies to improve nutrition even in resource-poor settings since many girls and women are chronically undernourished. Many trials have assessed the effect on birth weight of giving women of low socioeconomic status micronutrient supplements during pregnancy.

In 2001 the Pune (India) Maternal Nutrition Study showed the lack of association between size at birth and maternal energy and protein intake but strong associations with folate status and with intakes of foods rich in micronutrients that suggested that micronutrients may be important limiting factors for fetal growth in this undernourished community [30]. However, in another trial performed in the Indian population, a daily snack providing additional green leafy vegetables, fruit, and milk before conception and throughout pregnancy had no overall effect on birth weight. Subgroup analyses indicated a possible increase in birth weight if the mother was supplemented >3 months before conception and was not underweight.

In the USA a prospective cohort study of 1,116 low-income and minority pregnant women showed that suboptimal maternal calcium intake and vitamin D status might affect fetal growth [32]. Studies in India have shown a low dietary consumption of vitamin B12 due to dietary pattern of vegetarianism and poor consumption of milk and milk products. In vegetarian Indians, deficiency of vitamin B12 is commonly seen, while concentrations of folate are adequate. Together with folic acid, vitamin B12 is also an important determinant of fetal growth and development. During pregnancy, the increased requirement of folic acid is met with supplementation, while vitamin B12 remains untreated and possibly deficient. In addition to vitamin B12 and folate deficiencies alone, there may be adverse birth outcomes associated with unbalanced vitamin B12 and folate intakes or status during pregnancy. Folate to vitamin B12 ratio was correlated to neonatal anthropometric measures. Imbalance in the maternal micronutrients with increasing ratios of folate to vitamin B12 was associated with an increase in plasma homocysteine and lowering of neonatal birth weight, birth length, head circumference, and chest circumference, while no significant association to other anthropometrics was observed.

In 2009 a meta-analysis on original data from 12 randomized, controlled trials concluded that compared with iron–folic acid supplementation alone, maternal supplementation with multiple micronutrients during pregnancy in low-income countries resulted in a small increase in birth weight and a reduction in the prevalence of LBW of about 10 %. The effect was greater among women with higher BMI [18].

A recent meta-analysis of 21 randomized controlled trials on the effects of multiple supplementation on pregnancy outcome found that low-/middle-income women who received multiple supplements had a significant reduction in the risk of SGA offspring compared with women who received iron/folate supplements alone also in developing countries [19]. However, this study failed to show a significant impact on any of the other outcomes of pregnancy. The Generation R Study in Rotterdam provided evidence that low adherence to the Mediterranean diet in the periconceptional period significantly increased the risk of intrauterine growth restriction [37].

9.6.1 Iron Requirements in Pregnancy and Small Fetuses

Indeed, current studies indicate that micronutrient deficiencies might increase the risk of preterm delivery and impair fetal growth also in industrialized countries. Specifically, iron depletion in pregnancy has been associated with maternal anemia, reduced fetal and neonatal iron stores, increased risk of SGA offspring, and preterm delivery. Placental iron transport against a concentration gradient firstly allows to minimize the effect of fetal deficiencies by upregulating the proteins involved in iron transfer.

Iron deficiency is one of the most prevalent nutritional deficiencies worldwide and often leads to iron deficiency anemia (IDA). An inadequate dietary intake is the leading cause of IDA development, although other physiological and pathologic conditions, including impaired absorption or transport of iron, physiological losses, or chronic blood loss secondary to disease, could contribute as well. Worldwide, the prevalence of anemia (defined as a hemoglobin level <11 g/dl) has recently been estimated around 38 % in pregnancy, translating into 32 million pregnant women (Nutrition Impact Model Study 1995–2011) [36], with a small reduction compared with the 1990s. Even in high-income countries, it is estimated that approximately 45 % of women have serum ferritin <30 μg/l, indicating small or absent iron reserves, while only 15–20 % have ferritin >70 μg/l, which nearly balances the net iron loss during pregnancy.

From the meta-analysis of Blumfield et al. [6], iron intakes reported by pregnant women in developed countries were below the nutrient recommendations in all regions except the UK.

Another reason for risk of IDA is that the major fraction of dietary iron (about 90 %) is nonheme iron, which, in the average European diet, has a bioavailability of only 10–15 %. Although iron status is strongly dependent on adequate iron intake, it is still unclear whether prophylactic iron supplementation can reduce the rates of preterm delivery or LBW. Potentially harmful effects of routine iron supplementation during pregnancy in iron-sufficient women are still a matter of discussion because results related to clinical endpoints are conflicting.

The WHO recommends to supplement the diet of all pregnant women with 60 mg of iron plus 400 μg of folic acid/day for at least 6 months even in countries with a low anemia prevalence (<40 %) [40]. Intermittent iron supplementation (one to three times/week) appears to be as effective as daily supplementation for preventing anemia at term, and it is better tolerated [28].

However, due to the possibility of adverse side effects and to the potential placental oxidative stress in supplemented women, the European trend is that of an individualized supplementation, as opposed to general supplementation in the USA. Individualized supplementation should be based on the periconceptional ferritin value, with a cutoff of 70 μg/l to decide on supplementation [27].

In a 2013 systematic review including 48 randomized trials (17,793 women) and 44 cohort studies (1,851,682 women), daily prenatal iron supplementation/fortification with or without folic acid increased the mean maternal hemoglobin and significantly reduced the risk of anemia, iron deficiency, and iron deficiency anemia compared with controls [20]. Preterm birth was not significantly reduced, but for each 1 g/l increase in mean hemoglobin level, the birth weight increased by 14.0 g and the risk of low birth weight was significantly reduced. The results were confirmed even in the subgroup analysis separating trials from high-income and from low-to-middle-income countries.

9.6.2 Calcium

An inverse relationship between calcium intake and hypertensive disorders of pregnancy was first described in 1980s. This was based on the observation that populations where diet contained high levels of calcium had a very low prevalence of preeclampsia.

Low calcium intake may cause high blood pressure by stimulating either parathyroid hormone or renin release, thereby increasing intracellular calcium in vascular smooth muscle and leading to vasoconstriction. Calcium supplementation reduces parathyroid release and intracellular calcium and so reduces smooth muscle contractility. Calcium might also have an indirect effect on smooth muscle function by increasing magnesium levels. In fact magnesium deficiency has been linked with preeclampsia and preterm delivery. Moreover, recent evidence indicates that calcium supplementation affects uteroplacental blood flow and may be lowering the resistance index in uterine and umbilical arteries.

Calcium supplementation was tested in several randomized trials: some studies suggest that supplementation with calcium have beneficial effects in the treatment of preeclampsia. On the other hand, other studies suggest that dietary supplementation with calcium and dietary intake of magnesium do not aid in reducing the risk of preeclampsia.

In 2014 a Cochrane review reported that calcium supplementation with at least 1 g of calcium reduces by 50 % the risk of preeclampsia, but it does not appear to be effective for healthy nulliparous women in whom the baseline dietary calcium intake is adequate. This review also presented a 35 % reduction in the risk of gestational hypertension, with the greatest effect also among women at high risk and those with low-calcium diets [22]. Based on evidence included in the previous version of this review, which was limited to high-dose calcium supplementation, the WHO recommends supplementation with 1.5–2.0 g/day in case of low calcium intake and for preeclampsia prevention in high-risk populations. In settings in which the recommended dosage of 1.5–2 g daily is not feasible, using a lower dose, rather than nothing, seems to be a reasonable approach.

9.6.3 Antioxidants

Oxidative stress has also been implicated in the pathophysiology of preeclampsia. Oxidative stress is a condition of overabundance of reactive oxygen species (nitric oxide, superoxide anion, and hydrogen peroxide (H_2O_2)) versus antioxidants. The consequence of this unbalanced condition can be observed as increased levels of markers of oxidative stress, such as lipid peroxides. Abnormal placentation leads in fact to placental ischemia, resulting in generation of placental oxidative stress and increased levels of lipid peroxidation. Trophoblastic oxidative stress might also be the result of the mismatch in term, otherwise normal, placentas between terminal villi overgrowth and reduced intervillous space [31]. Throphoblastic oxidative stress might be worsened in dyslipidemic pregnant women that might suffer of diffuse acute decidual atherothrombosis [35].

The use of antioxidants could theoretically be useful to reduce the damage on placenta, thereby the risk of preeclampsia, especially because of its limited antioxidant enzyme capacity in the first trimester. The pathogenesis of adverse pregnancy outcomes including preeclampsia and intrauterine growth restriction (IUGR) and a number of neonatal outcomes have been shown to be associated with oxidative stress.

Although the concentrations of these vitamins remain significantly reduced in women with preeclampsia, supplementation with higher doses of vitamin C and E has not been shown to prevent development of preeclampsia in either high-risk or lower-risk women [12]. This was confirmed by Vadillo-Ortega et al. [38] who found a 50 % reduction of preeclampsia recurrence in overweight/obese women who suffered late preeclampsia in their previous history. In 2014 similar to this a review by Dean et al. [14], pooling two cohort studies, found a significant 27 % reduction in the risk of preeclampsia obtained by maternal periconceptional multivitamin supplementation.

9.6.4 Folate

Maternal folate status has also been associated with adverse pregnancy outcomes such as preeclampsia, fetal growth restriction, and preterm delivery, although these results still remain inconclusive. Higher risk of preeclampsia in women with higher homocysteine and lower folate concentrations and vitamin B12 levels has been reported.

Some "placenta events" are postulated to arise from deficiencies of either folate and/or vitamin B12 or defects within the methionine–homocysteine metabolic pathways. In this context, hyperhomocysteinemia has been shown to provoke vascular inflammation and to decrease the bioavailability of nitric oxide that is an important endothelium vasodilatator and seems to be associated with the production of reactive oxygen species. This means that folate deficiency or hyperhomocysteinemia may underlie endothelian dysfunction and therefore placental endovasculature, a theory supported by the observation that elevated serum homocysteine concentrations have been associated with an increased risk of diseases, such as atherosclerotic, thromboembolic, and neurodegenerative disorders. Hyperhomocysteinemia has been implicated in other adverse pregnancy outcomes such as placental abruption or infarction. In contrast, other studies indicate no association of vitamin B12 with preeclampsia. Further, folic acid supplementation studies are inconsistent with some indicating beneficial effects and others indicating no benefits.

9.6.5 Vitamin D

It has been hypothesized that dysregulated vitamin D action in uteroplacental tissues disrupts extravillous trophoblast invasion leading to abnormal placentation. Maternal vitamin D deficiency early in pregnancy, defined as 25(OH)D <30 nmol/l, may therefore represent an independent risk factor for preeclampsia [1]. For this reason, vitamin D supplementation for women of childbearing age should be a strategy for reducing preeclampsia.

Previous recommendations to protect from vitamin D deficiency report a recommended daily intake of 400 IU (10 μg), derived from the observation that this amount of vitamin D was sufficient to prevent rickets. However, nowadays the Food and Drug Administration recommends a daily vitamin D intake during pregnancy of 600 IU (15 μg).

Classic vitamin D deficiency is rare in developed countries; however, there is evidence, based on plasma levels, that the recommendations do not meet the individual requirements of 97.5 % of healthy individuals. The meta-analysis by Blumfield et al. [6] showed vitamin D intakes below the recommendations for all developed regions except Europe, which reported an intake within the acceptable range of intake (ARI) compared with European recommendations (ARI: 0–10 μg/day). However, obviously these recommendations are not appropriate since they are starting from a value of 0. A recent study by Johnson et al. [25] showed that 97 % of African-American, 81 % of Hispanic, and 67 % of Caucasian pregnant women were vitamin D deficient or insufficient based on 25(OH)D levels. Data from the German National Nutrition Survey (2008) showed that the mean intake of vitamin D from food of pregnant and lactating females was 3.1 μg/day, an amount far below the recommended. Therefore, recently, the German Nutrition Society indicated that pregnant women with an increased risk of vitamin D deficiency for lack of exposure to sunlight should be provided with supplements of 20 μg (800 IU)/day [26].

Even if there is no evidence of a benefit with general supplementation and screening of deficiency during pregnancy, given the low intake and maternal vitamin D status, the IOM [24] and the US Endocrine Task Force on Vitamin D [23] commented that 600 IU/day may not be sufficient to correct vitamin D deficiency in pregnant and lactating women, increasing the recommendation to 1,500–2,000 IU/day of vitamin D for pregnant and lactating women with vitamin D deficiency [5].

9.7 Supplementation: What Is the Evidence?

It is now well recognized that the frequency and severity of pregnancy complications may be reduced through an improvement in the micronutrient status of the mothers. The best way of preventing micronutrient malnutrition is to ensure consumption of a balanced diet that is adequate in every nutrient. Unfortunately, this is far from being achievable everywhere since it requires universal access to adequate food and appropriate dietary habits. Supplementation and/or fortification can make a contribution when the high demands for growth and development are difficult to be met through food alone.

Nutritional counseling for pregnant women should be a public health priority. Many women are still unaware of how much their nutritional status impacts their pregnancy outcomes, and improving women's nutrition and weight-related behaviors should therefore begin during their earlier reproductive years. Dietary recommendations for women of childbearing age should promote greater consumption of green leafy vegetables, whole-grain breads/cereals, oily fish, eggs, and fortified food products. Furthermore, each woman, who does not avoid a pregnancy, should be advised to use folic acid supplements during the periconceptional period.

However, there is no clear consensus on need of other supplements. In general, studies show that multiple micronutrient supplementation improves outcomes as far as low birth weight, preterm delivery, and preeclampsia. On the other hand, in medium- to high-income countries, there is currently insufficient evidence to support a routine supplementation at the population level, except for periconceptional folate supplementation. Therefore, for most pregnant women, a more individualized approach is recommended with a specific focus on iron, calcium, and vitamin D status (Table 9.2).

In general, there is growing interest in multiple micronutrient supplementation in at-risk populations in whom multiple deficiencies often coexist. In the USA, the Institute of Medicine (IOM) and the Centers for Disease Control and Prevention (CDC) recommend multivitamin supplements for pregnant women who do not consume an adequate diet. Women considered at higher risk of dietary deficiencies include also those who are carrying a multiple gestation as well as heavy smokers, adolescents, vegetarians, substance abusers, and those with a short inter-pregnancy interval. Women at extremes of BMI like underweight or obesity should also be considered at risk for micronutrient deficiencies.

Table 9.2 Adequate intakes during pregnancy for the main micronutrients

	Adequate intake during pregnancy
Folic acid	600 μg/day
Iron	27 mg/day
Iodine	220 μg/day
Vitamin D	15 μg/day–600 UI/day
Calcium	1,000 mg/day

The adequate intake is a recommended average daily nutrient intake level based on observed or experimentally determined approximations or estimates of nutrient intake by a group (or groups) of apparently healthy people who are assumed to be maintaining an adequate nutritional state. AI is derived for a nutrient if sufficient scientific evidence is not available to set a Recommended Dietary Allowance (RDA)

9.7.1 Folate: Is Current Supplementation Adequate?

Folic acid supplementation is recommended worldwide in the periconceptional period for the prevention of neural tube defects. Since 1990s, internationally, women are advised to use folic acid supplements during the periconceptional period. The US Preventive Services Task Force (USPSTF) recommends supplementation containing 0.4–0.8 mg of folic acid for all women 1 month before and for the first 2–3 months after conception to reduce the risk of NTDs. The current recommendation to supplement 400 μg folic acid daily starting at least 4 weeks before conception is likely inadequate to achieve optimal red cell folate levels within 4 weeks, because this requires at least 8–12 weeks of daily intake. In fact Daly et al. [13] found that red cell folate levels higher than 906 nmol/l are associated with maximal risk reduction of NTDs. In 1998 the German Nutritional Survey evaluated folate concentrations in serum and in red cells of women of childbearing age. Only 13 % of the women showed a red cell folate level higher than 906 nmol/l. With a daily dosage of 800 mg folic acid, the preventive red blood cell level of 906 nmol/l is reached within an average 4 weeks after the start of supplementation [2] (Table 9.3).

The biologically active derivate [6S]-5-methyltetrahydrofolate ([6S]-5-MTHF) has been found to be more effective than folic acid supplementation in improving folate status, and since it represents the main folate form in cord blood (mean 89.4 % of total folate), it may be hypothesized that 5-MTHF can provide an immediate source for folate to be transported to the fetus.

Folate intake and status has been consistently reported to be related to birth weight, and recently the periconceptional folate status has been also related to embryonic growth in the first trimester. However, lowest embryonic growth was found both in the lowest and in the highest quartiles of red blood cell folate levels [39].

Although major health organizations promote the use of folic acid by women of reproductive age and the prevalence of folic acid use is reportedly high in the prenatal period, most women do not take folate supplements in the periconceptional period, even if they are aware of its benefits.

A recent study among 1,296 pregnant women sampled in the NHANES demonstrated that only 55–60 % of the women reported taking folic acid-containing supplementation in their first trimester, with red blood cell folate showing the lowest

Table 9.3 Dietary and supplementation advices during pregnancy

Advice	When?
General population	
Prudent diet	Always
Folate supplementation	All women periconceptionally
At-risk populations	
Prudent Mediterranean diet	Always
Folate supplementation	All women periconceptionally
	Higher intake for previous NTD, diabetes, epilepsy, etc.
Iron supplementation	Based on ferritin level
Calcium supplementation	In case of low-calcium-intake diet
	To prevent preeclampsia in women at risk
Vitamin D supplementation	People with darker skin, people who have low or no sun exposure, obese women, risk of preeclampsia
Iodine supplementation	In iodine-deficient areas

level in the first trimester compared with the last part of pregnancy [7]. Even in most European countries, pregnant and childbearing-aged women showed a folate intake of less than half the recommended amount of 600 μg/day. Recent trials carried out in Italy and the UK found that only 11.3 % of the Italian and 45.1 % of the British reached the optimal dietary folate intake of 400 μg/day. Of the women, all at childbearing age, almost 70 % of Italian women had inadequate folate serum levels [29]. A recent English study on 466,860 women showed that the proportion of women taking folic acid supplements before pregnancy declined from 35 % in 1999–2001 to 31 % in 2011–2012, with an increase in supplementation use with maternal age [4]. All these data show that the policy of folic acid supplementation is failing in industrialized countries. It is necessary to improve awareness and use folic acid supplements among all women of reproductive age so that even women with unplanned pregnancies are protected. Moreover, it is likely that public health policy cannot rely on prepregnancy folic acid supplementation alone, and programs of food fortification and social education need to be promoted.

References

1. Achkar M, Dodds L, Giguère Y, Forest J, Armson BA, Woolcott C, Agellon S, Spencer A, Weiler HA. Vitamin D status in early pregnancy and risk of preeclampsia. Am J Obstet Gynecol. 2014. doi:10.1016/j.ajog.2014.11.009.
2. Berti C, Biesalski HK, Gärtner R, Lapillonne A, Pietrzik K, Poston L, Redman C, Koletzko B, Cetin I. Micronutrients in pregnancy: current knowledge and unresolved questions. Clin Nutr. 2011;30(6):689–701. doi:10.1016/j.clnu.2011.08.004.
3. Berti C, Decsi T, Dykes F, Hermoso M, Koletzko B, Massari M, Moreno LA, Serra-Majem L, Cetin I. Critical issues in setting micronutrient recommendations for pregnant women: an insight. Matern Child Nutr. 2010;6 Suppl 2:5–22. doi:10.1111/j.1740-8709.2010.00269.
4. Bestwick JP, Huttly WJ, Morris JK, Wald NJ. Prevention of neural tube defects: a cross-sectional study of the uptake of folic acid supplementation in nearly half a million women. PLoS One. 2014;9:e89354.

5. Biesalski HK. Vitamin D, recommendations: beyond deficiency. Ann Nutr Metab. 2011;59:10–6.
6. Blumfield ML, Hure AJ, Macdonald-Wicks L, Smith R, Collins CE. A systematic review and meta-analysis of micronutrient intakes during pregnancy in developed countries. Nutr Rev. 2013;71:118–32.
7. Branum AM, Bailey R, Singer BJ. Dietary supplement use and folate status during pregnancy in the United States. J Nutr. 2013;143:486–92.
8. Catov JM, Bodnar LM, Ness RB, Markovic N, Roberts JM. Association of periconceptional multivitamin use and risk of preterm or small-for-gestational-age births. Am J Epidemiol. 2007;166(3):296–303.
9. Catov JM, Bodnar LM, Olsen J, Olsen S, Nohr EA. Periconceptional multivitamin use and risk of preterm or small-for-gestational-age births in the Danish National Birth Cohort. Am J Clin Nutr. 2011;94(3):906–12. doi:10.3945/ajcn.111.012393.
10. Cavelaars AE, Doets EL, Dhonukshe-Rutten RA, Hermoso M, Fairweather-Tait SJ, Koletzko B, Gurinović M, Moreno LA, Cetin I, Matthys C, van't Veer P, Ashwell M, de Groot CP. Prioritizing micronutrients for the purpose of reviewing their requirements: a protocol developed by EURRECA. Eur J Clin Nutr. 2010;64 Suppl 2:S19–30. doi:10.1038/ejcn.2010.57.
11. Cetin I, Berti C, Calabrese S. Role of micronutrients in the periconceptional period. Hum Reprod Update. 2010;16:80–95.
12. Conde-Agudelo A, Romero R, Kusanovic JP, Hassan SS. Supplementation with vitamins C and E during pregnancy for the prevention of preeclampsia and other adverse maternal and perinatal outcomes: a systematic review and metaanalysis. Am J Obstet Gynecol. 2011;204:503.e1–12.
13. Daly LE, Kirke PN, Molloy A, Weir DG, Scott JM. Folate levels and neural tube defects. Implications for prevention. JAMA. 1995;274:1698–702.
14. Dean SV, Lassi ZS, Imam AM, Bhutta ZA. Preconception care: nutritional risks and interventions. Reprod Health. 2014;11 Suppl 3:S3.
15. Dhonukshe-Rutten RA, Bouwman J, Brown KA, Cavelaars AE, Collings R, Grammatikaki E, de Groot LC, Gurinovic M, Harvey LJ, Hermoso M, Hurst R, Kremer B, Ngo J, Novakovic R, Raats MM, Rollin F, Serra-Majem L, Souverein OW, Timotijevic L, Van't Veer P. EURRECA-evidence-based methodology for deriving micronutrient recommendations. Crit Rev Food Sci Nutr. 2013;53(10):999–1040. doi:10.1080/10408398.2012.749209.
16. Englund-Ögge L, Brantsæter AL, Sengpiel V, Haugen M, Birgisdottir BE, Myhre R, Meltzer HM, Jacobsson B. Maternal dietary patterns and preterm delivery: results from large prospective cohort study. BMJ. 2014;348:g1446. doi:10.1136/bmj.g1446.
17. EURopean micronutrients RECommendations Aligned (EURRECA). 2014. Available from: http://www.eurreca.org/everyone).
18. Fall CH, Fisher DJ, Osmond C, Margetts BM, Maternal Micronutrient Supplementation Study Group. Multiple micronutrient supplementation during pregnancy in low-income countries: a meta-analysis of effects on birth size and length of gestation. Food Nutr Bull. 2009;30(4 Suppl):S533–46.
19. Haider BA, Bhutta ZA. Multiple-micronutrient supplementation for women during pregnancy. Cochrane Database Syst Rev. 2012;(11):CD004905. doi:10.1002/14651858.CD004905.
20. Haider BA, Olofin I, Wang M, Spiegelman D, Ezzati M, Fawzi WW, Nutrition Impact Model Study Group (anaemia). Anaemia, prenatal iron use, and risk of adverse pregnancy outcomes: systematic review and meta-analysis. BMJ. 2013;346:f3443.
21. Hermoso M, Vollhardt C, Bergmann K, Koletzko B. Critical micronutrients in pregnancy, lactation, and infancy: considerations on vitamin D, folic acid, and iron, and priorities for future research. Ann Nutr Metab. 2011;59(1):5–9. doi:10.1159/000332062.
22. Hofmeyr GJ, Lawrie TA, Atallah AN, Duley L, Torloni MR. Calcium supplementation during pregnancy for preventing hypertensive disorders and related problems. Cochrane Database Syst Rev. 2014;(6):CD001059. doi:10.1002/14651858.CD001059.
23. Holick MF, Binkley NC, Bischoff-Ferrari HA, Gordon CM, Hanley DA, Heaney RP, Murad MH, Weaver CM, Endocrine Society. Evaluation, treatment, and prevention of vitamin D deficiency: an Endocrine Society clinical practice guideline. J Clin Endocrinol Metab. 2011;96:1911–30.

24. IOM. Dietary reference intakes for calcium and vitamin D. 2010. http://www.iom.edu/vitamind.
25. Johnson DD, Wagner CL, Hulsey TC, Mc-Neil RB, Ebeling M, Hollis BW. Vitamin D deficiency and insufficiency is common during pregnancy. Am J Perinatol. 2011;28:7–12.
26. Koletzko B, Bauer CP, Bung P, Cremer M, Flothkötter M, Hellmers C, Kersting M, Krawinkel M, Przyrembel H, Rasenack R, Schäfer T, Vetter K, Wahn U, Weissenborn A, Wöckel A. German national consensus recommendations on nutrition and lifestyle in pregnancy by the 'Healthy Start – Young Family Network'. Ann Nutr Metab. 2013;63:311–22.
27. Milman N. Iron in pregnancy: how do we secure an appropriate iron status in the mother and child? Ann Nutr Metab. 2011;59:50–4.
28. Peña-Rosas JP, De-Regil LM, Dowswell T, Viteri FE. Intermittent oral iron supplementation during pregnancy. Cochrane Database Syst Rev. 2012;(7):CD009997.
29. Pounis G, Di Castelnuovo AF, de Lorgeril M, Krogh V, Siani A, Arnout J, Cappuccio FP, van Dongen M, Zappacosta B, Donati MB, de Gaetano G, Iacoviello L, European Collaborative Group of the IMMIDIET Project. Folate intake and folate serum levels in men and women from two European populations: The IMMIDIET project. Nutrition. 2014;30(7–8):822–30. doi:10.1016/j.nut.2013.11.014.
30. Rao S, Yajnik CS, Kanade A, Fall CH, Margetts BM, Jackson AA, Shier R, Joshi S, Rege S, Lubree H, Desai B. Intake of micronutrient-rich foods in rural Indian mothers is associated with the size of their babies at birth: Pune Maternal Nutrition Study. J Nutr. 2001;131(4):1217–24.
31. Redman CW, Sargent IL, Staff AC. IFPA Senior Award Lecture: making sense of pre-eclampsia – two placental causes of preeclampsia? Placenta. 2014;35(Suppl):S20–5.
32. Scholl TO, Chen X, Stein TP. Maternal calcium metabolic stress and fetal growth. Am J Clin Nutr. 2014;99(4):918–25. doi:10.3945/ajcn.113.076034.
33. Sengpiel V, Bacelis J, Myhre R, Myking S, Pay AD, Haugen M, Brantsæter AL, Meltzer HM, Nilsen RM, Magnus P, Vollset SE, Nilsson S, Jacobsson B. Folic acid supplementation, dietary folate intake during pregnancy and risk for spontaneous preterm delivery: a prospective observational cohort study. BMC Pregnancy Childbirth. 2013;13:160. doi:10.1186/1471-2393-13-160.
34. Serra-Majem L, Bes-Rastrollo M, Román-Viñas B, Pfrimer K, Sánchez-Villegas A, Martínez-González MA. Dietary patterns and nutritional adequacy in a Mediterranean country. Br J Nutr. 2009;101 Suppl 2:S21–8. doi:10.1017/S0007114509990559.
35. Staff AC, Redman CW. IFPA Award in Placentology Lecture: preeclampsia, the decidual battleground and future maternal cardiovascular disease. Placenta. 2014;35(Suppl):S26–31.
36. Stevens GA, Finucane MM, De-Regil LM, Paciorek CJ, Flaxman SR, Branca F, Peña-Rosas JP, Bhutta ZA, Ezzati M, Nutrition Impact Model Study Group (Anaemia). Global, regional, and national trends in haemoglobin concentration and prevalence of total and severe anaemia in children and pregnant and non-pregnant women for 1995–2011: a systematic analysis of population-representative data. Lancet Glob Health. 2013;1(1):e16–25. doi:10.1016/S2214-109X(13)70001-9.
37. Timmermans S, Jaddoe VW, Hofman A, Steegers-Theunissen RP, Steegers EA. Periconception folic acid supplementation, fetal growth and the risks of low birth weight and preterm birth: the Generation R Study. Br J Nutr. 2009;102(5):777–85. doi:10.1017/S0007114509288994.
38. Vadillo-Ortega F, Perichart-Perera O, Espino S, Avila-Vergara MA, Ibarra I, Ahued R, Godines M, Parry S, Macones G, Strauss JF. Effect of supplementation during pregnancy with L-arginine and antioxidant vitamins in medical food on pre-eclampsia in high risk population: randomised controlled trial. BMJ. 2011;342:d2901. doi:10.1136/bmj.d2901.
39. Van Uitert E, van Ginkel S, Willemsen S, Lindemans J, Koning A, Eilers P, Exalto N, Laven J, Steegers E, Steegers-Theunissen R. An optimal periconception maternal folate status for embryonic size: the Rotterdam Predict study. BJOG. 2014;121:821–9.
40. WHO. Micronutrient deficiencies: iron deficiency anaemia. 2014. http://www.who.int/nutrition/topics/ida/en/.

Gestational Diabetes and Maternogenic Preeclampsia: By-products of the Accelerated Metabolic Syndrome in Pregnancy

10

Enrico Ferrazzi, Valeria Mantegazza, Sara Zullino, and Tamara Stampaljia

Contents

E. Ferrazzi (✉) • V. Mantegazza • S. Zullino
Woman, Mother and Neonate Department, University of Milan,
Buzzi Children's Hospital, Milan, Italy
e-mail: enrico.ferrazzi@unimi.it

T. Stampaljia
Unit of Prenatal Diagnosis, Institute for Maternal and Child Health, IRCCS Burlo Garofolo, Trieste, Italy

E. Ferrazzi, B. Sears (eds.), *Metabolic Syndrome and Complications of Pregnancy: The Potential Preventive Role of Nutrition*,
DOI 10.1007/978-3-319-16853-1_10

10.1 Maternal Cardiovascular and Metabolic Adaptation to Pregnancy in a Nutshell

Pregnancy, actually the changes driven by feto-placental unit in maternal organism, tantamount to a cardiovascular and metabolic stress test.

10.1.1 Cardiovascular Stress

In a few weeks from the beginning of pregnancy, plasma volume is increased by 30 % with a net increase of the visceral venous reservoir. Cardiac output is increased through higher heart rate frequency and diastolic function improvements.

The complex inflammatory balance plays a major role as well. The TH1 pro-inflammatory state of early pregnancy and placental development soon leaves the stage for a long period of balanced anti-inflammatory TH2 milieu. In late gestation, TH1 returns to be prevalent.

This latter process favours the expression of a new array of genes among which the expression of decoy progesterone receptors that in humans block the progesterone function and lead to functional changes in the myometrium and eventually to labour and delivery. This immune process in late gestation is favoured or paralleled by a possible increasing oxidative stress of the syncithiotrophoblast of the tertiary villi. These parts of the villi tree grow more than the volume of the intervillous space to the point of causing an imbalance of perfusion and the production of reactive oxygen species [1].

All these changes might be interpreted in the light of adaptative mechanisms of human pregnancy. The increase of plasma volume reservoir, together with pro-coagulatory changes, might have represented a survival advantage in epochs when postpartum haemorrhage was a real life-threatening event in human reproduction and was among of the strongest pressures in genomic selection. Similarly the unique "invention" of decoy receptors for progesterone allowed for "premature" onset of labour when bipedalism and cephalisation were conjuring against survival of our species for the high toll of lives lost in labour. The "solution" resulted in an altricial neonate, a neonate that needs weeks of gestation outside the uterus, in a manner totally different from his anthropoid relatives [2].

10.1.2 Metabolic Stress on Insulin, Glucose and Lipids

All these adaptive mechanism plus feto-placental growth itself require a profound "protected" adaptation of metabolism to meet energy requirements. During pregnancy, metabolic rates in human mothers quickly approach 2.5 times the basal metabolic rate (BMR), and by the sixth month BMR is twice the pre-pregnancy state. Only athletes can go much further than that and for a limited period of time (Fig. 10.1). Part of this increment is due to the oxidation of 20–25 g of glucose per day by the placenta and the fetus that evenly absorb this metabolic strain.

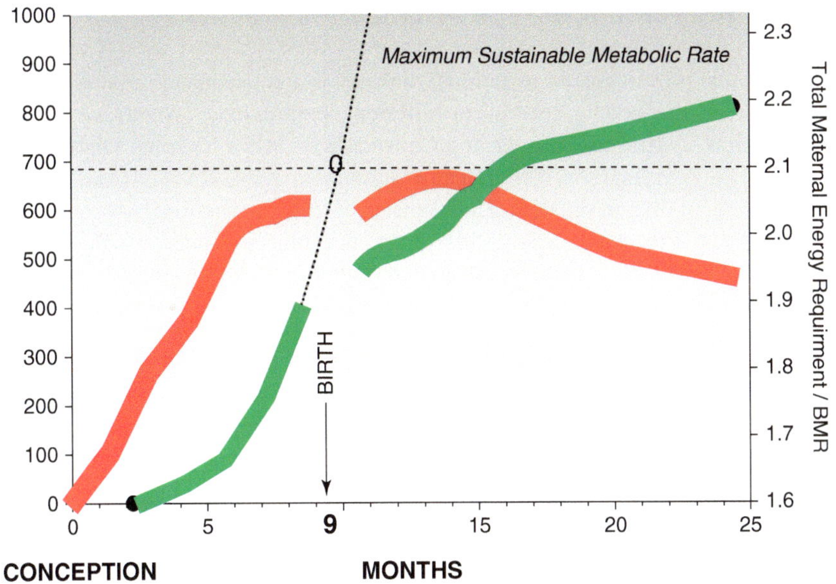

Fig. 10.1 Metabolic constraint on gestation length and fetal size. (*Y* axis). Fetal energy demands (*green line*, kcal/day) increase exponentially during gestation (*X* axis). Maternal energy expenditure (*red line*) rises during the first two trimesters but reaches a metabolic ceiling in the third, as total energy requirements approach 2.0× basal metabolic rate (4)

To summarise extensive reviews on pregnancy energy metabolism, among which one is by Nancy Butte [3], one can depict glucose and insulin changes as follows. In early pregnancy, basal glucose concentrations and hepatic basal glucose production do not differ significantly from pre-pregnancy values; muscle and hepatic sensitivity to insulin is normal. Insulin incretion is normal or even increased in its first minute response to glucose.

By the third trimester, basal glucose concentrations go 10–15 mg/dL below pre-pregnancy levels (0.56–0.83 mmol/L), and insulin is almost twice the concentration. Postprandial glucose concentrations are significantly elevated and the glucose peak is prolonged. These changes are paralleled by an increase of 16–30 % in basal endogenous hepatic glucose production to meet the increasing energy needs of the placenta and fetus. In late gestation these changes are driven by the combination of rising concentrations of human chorionic gonadotropin, prolactin, cortisol and glucagon that overall exert anti-insulinogenic and anti-lipolytic effects to achieve availability of alternative fuels, especially fatty acids, by peripheral tissues.

Changes in hepatic and adipose metabolism alter lipids profile as well. In pregnancy we observe a steady increase in triglycerides; cholesterol, with a higher LDL rise; fatty acids; lipoproteins; and phospholipids. The HDL triglycerides ratio goes up from 2 to 4–5, pretty in the range of dyslipidemia in non-pregnant women. These are good news for the fetus that can claim its share of glucose and amino acids while the mother diverts her energy metabolism with mobilisation of lipid store.

10.2 The Paradox of Type 2 Diabetes in Pregnancy

The variable prevalence of gestational diabetes is a consequence of mixed effects of different diagnostic criteria in different populations: American Diabetes Association, 2–19 %; Carpenter and Coustan, 3.6–38 %; National Diabetes Data Group, 1.4–50 %; and the World Health Organization, 2–24.5 % [4]. According to the criteria of the international consensus of the International Association of Diabetes and Pregnancy Study, this prevalence ranges around 16 % in a large mixed population of 23 thousand women recruited in different countries and ethnically diverse, with 48 % white Caucasians, 12 % black, 29 % Asian/Oriental and 8 % Hispanic/mestizos.

Indeed, this huge variability appears to be the obvious clinical result of two evidences: first, there is a continuous positive linear association between maternal glucose and increased fetal birthweight, as well as fetal hyperinsulinaemia [5] and eventually abnormal short-term and long-term outcome (Fig. 10.2); second, there is a strict association between lifestyle, macro-ethnicity and metabolic syndrome, altogether major risk factors for insulin resistance, and abnormal lipid and carbohydrate metabolism.

These aspects compose a puzzle where pieces of epidemiology and pieces of diagnostic tests are confronted with the objective to fit the final design of chronic diseases: changing thresholds in different or mixed populations might cause huge variations in prevalence estimates.

But why this puzzle should happen in the 9 months span of a pregnancy, not at all a chronic scenario?

A dominant party of Western medicine look at this phenomena from the point of view of higher prevalence of the disease (ICD-9, 648.83) therapy, health-care costs and hence insurance costs: thresholds are brought as high as decently possible, the prevalence of the disease reduced, and its costs cut [4]. Others, when faced with chronic degenerative diseases, favour prevention. Low screening thresholds yield the opportunity to intervene before the full-blown disease is established.

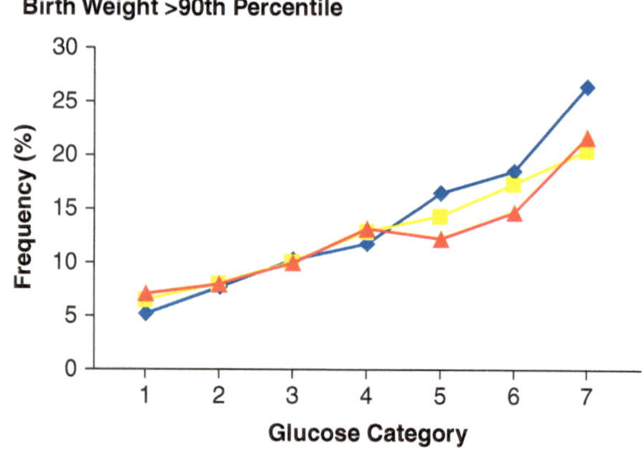

Fig. 10.2 Birthweight >90th percentile across glucose categories (mg/dL). Glucose category 1, <75; category 2, 75–79; category 3, 80–84; category 4, 85–89, category 5, 90–94, category 6, 95–99; category 7, > 100 mg/dL. *Blue line* = fasting glucose values; *yellow line* = 1 h glucose values; *red line* = 2 h glucose values (2)

We totally embrace the following vision of the Society of Maternal-Fetal Medicine: "There are three times during a woman's life that she accesses the health care system on a regular basis and is seen by a trained health-care provider: as an infant, for pregnancy and postpartum care and when she develops a chronic disease. Given that chronic diseases like cardiovascular disease are usually decades in development, for the majority of women of reproductive age, pregnancy and the postpartum provides a new early window of opportunity to identify risk factors and improve their long-term health".

10.3 Gestational Diabetes: A Clinical Phenotype of an Accelerated Metabolic Syndrome in Pregnancy

10.3.1 Anti-insulin Effects of Pregnancy

The anti-insulin effects of pregnancy are a well-known history. At the end of the day, a few weeks with high glycaemic values do not represent a health problem for the adult woman and a large baby can be safely delivered by caesarean section, and its possible neonatal metabolic disturbances might be safely treated in any hospital setting. So what? This first player in the unbalanced "metabolism" frequently covers in the clinical practice the more complex picture that is associated with maternal gestational diabetes and promotes a critical intrauterine environment.

10.3.2 Dyslipidaemia

The role of lipids has been frequently overlooked by obstetricians in gestational diabetes. Indeed, dyslipidaemia is a constitutional part of metabolic syndrome in adults and, more specifically, in type 2 diabetes in a way that resemble normal gestation: dense LDL and triglyceride increases versus low level of HDL. Elevated levels of free fatty acids (FFA) cause insulin resistance in muscle and liver cells. Saturated fatty acids are among the most detrimental of FFA, being the main culprit of insulin resistance and inflammation. On the other hand, FFAs act on the beta cell of the pancreas to stimulate insulin secretion, both directly improving the glucose-stimulated insulin secretion and potentiating glucose-stimulated insulin secretion. To some extent, this counterbalances peripheral insulin resistance.

10.3.3 The Microbiota

A third player comes on stage to promote an accelerated metabolic syndrome in pregnancy. The pregnant state modify the intestinal microbiome [6] in a way that faeces of third-trimester mothers showed increased signs of inflammation and energy loss. In a germ free mice, transplant of faeces of third trimester human

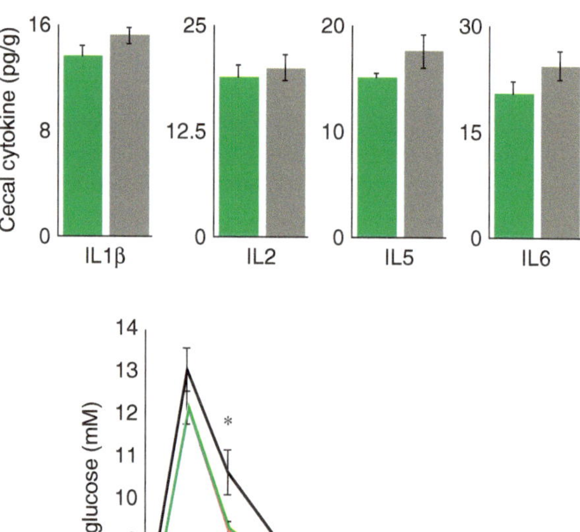

Fig. 10.3 Impact on inflammation and glucose metabolism on germ-free mice, of intragastrically administered inoculum of faeces from the first trimester (T1 – *green bars and line*) and third trimester (T3 – *grey bars and line*) human donors (6)

pregnant women, but not first trimester pregnant women, increased adiposity, insulin resistance and inflammation were determined (Fig. 10.3).

The higher prevalence of firmicutes over bacteroides observed by Koren et al. [6] in human pregnancy matches similar findings in obese adults [7].

10.3.4 Unbalanced Western Supermarket-Style Nutrition

The final fourth player of this picture introduces us to the substantial impact of lifestyle in nutrition in Western societies of lipid metabolism. The original balance of n-6 (linoleic acid metabolised to arachidonic acid) and n-3 (alfa linolenic metabolised to eicosapentaenoic acid (EPA) and docosahexaenoic acid (DHA)) essential fatty acid that at the best of our knowledge as qualified human diets for at least 160 thousand years in a 2:1 and 1:1 ratio has been dramatically changed in Western diets up to a ratio of 10:1 and 25:1. n-3 essential fatty acids are indeed essential in an array of positive human metabolic pathways [8]. Beyond this, it might be of relevant interest the recent association of n-3 essential fatty acid with the biosynthesis of a specialised family of pro-resolving mediators of inflammation [9] (resolvins, protectins and maresins). This is probably what is needed to soothe the strained insulin receptors and the endothelium.

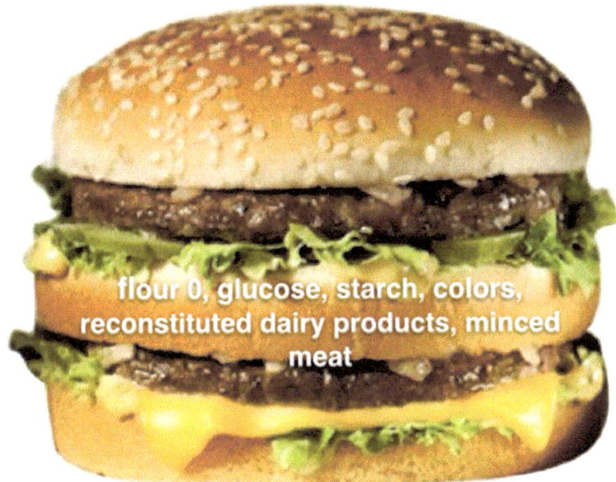

Fig. 10.4 More than 40 million people feed every day similar unbalanced food, frequently associated with a sugary carbonated drink and fried starch. The bread is usually made with wheat flour type 0, added with glucose, rapeseed oil, potato starch and chemical colours. The meat comes from intensive cattle raising, and the part of the cow from which it is minced is an "industrial secret". The cheese is a complex mix of reconstituted dairy products and artificial colours. A few human dishes are so far from a balanced nutritional profile. A touch of green, less than 20 g in weight, and here we go promoting the metabolic syndrome

10.3.5 Macro-Ethnicities

These two latter elements, microbiota and nutrition interact to lessen or increase the risk of the accelerated metabolic syndrome of pregnancy. What is not widely and properly acknowledged in nutritional counselling is the importance of the phenotype of different macro-ethnicities in which this interaction takes place. Asian, mestizos and AmerInds (sometimes defined as Hispanics in North American literature) and Native American women, as compared with white women of Caucasian ancestry, have an increased risk of GDM [10]. The large human migrations from Asia and South America [11] into Europe and the USA and the spread of Western-style diet (Fig. 10.4) have proved that the metabolic syndrome, originally a rare phenomenon in these macro-ethnicities, has become a major health problem both in Western countries and in these original countries [12, 13].

A special mention is deserved to slave trade from Western Africa and the fate of these macro-ethnicities in North America and the Caribbean. Agriculture and farming entered East Africa eight thousands years ago. We can trace its slowly spreading south in millennia, thanks to archaeological findings, and the prevalence of lactose persistence in micro-ethnicities of Eastern Africa [14]. When slave trade was started by "colonial powers", in the sixteenth century, farming products as we know them (protein-rich grains such as wheat, cow milk and dairy products; fat-rich meat from cattle raising) had not yet entered the nutritional profile of black ethnicities of West

Africa. The descendants of the forced migration exposed to Western-style diet are even more prone to obesity and abdominal obesity than populations of Caucasian ancestry in whom such a prevalence occurs only in areas of very low income (http://www.cdc.gov/obesity/data/prevalence see maps 2011–2013 of white adults - and maps of Black Adults).

Metabolic syndrome in these macro-ethnicities is not just eating too much but is an accelerated consequence of the mismatch between their genome and their nutritional profile that is even more alien to them than to population of Caucasian ancestry.

All these "players" conjure to make pregnancy a possible pray of an accelerated metabolic syndrome both igniting a trans-generational legacy of diabetes-causing diabetes [15] and signalling the future risk to develop a full-blown type 2 diabetes in the fifth decade [16] up to 11 times the risk of women who did not suffer of GDM.

10.4 The Magic Challenge of Prevention Through Food and Exercise

We all have, somewhere in a box, images of our grand grandparents, not necessarily during wartime: abdominal obesity was then a rare condition if ever existed in a family in two generation spans. That was the waistline then, not only for people of Caucasian ancestry in Europe and the USA but also for Afro-Americans, natives, first-generation Chinese and Asians. In 1950 the average BMI of white Americans was 22.4. In 2012 the average BMI was up to 27.8. Unfortunately Europe and Arabian countries are "catchin' up" this "Western inequality" very rapidly. Among all variables interwoven in the social fabric that lead to present epidemics of obesity, it is likely that industrial processing of food, food marketing, quantity vs. quality policy and fast food eateries bear the largest responsibility for the epidemics (Fig. 10.4).

Poor food, according to the Alternate Healthy Eating Index 2010 (AHE) adherence score, overweight and inactivity yield a risk of up to 45 % of developing gestational diabetes in future pregnancies [17]. According to the same study, based on a cohort of 14 thousand, mostly white Caucasian women, the risk of gestational diabetes was 83 % lower (RR 0.17) in women with normal weight, good diet, exercise and no cigarette smoking. This is a proof of principle that gestational diabetes could be preventable just by changing lifestyle and reverting it back to a more "human lifestyle", nothing more. To make it simple we can summarise the adherence to AHE under the name of prudent diet characterised by a high intake of fruits, green leafy vegetables, poultry and fish. A "poor" diet can be characterised by a high intake of red meat, processed meat, refined grain products, sweets, French fries, pizza, sugary beverages and sugary snacks or Western-pattern diet.

Unfortunately, lifestyle and nutrition cannot be changed at the snap of the fingers or just through a medical consultation. This is why pregnancy and the special compliance that can be nurtured in this delicate frame are a window of opportunity to win bad habits and introduce a healthier lifestyle and nutrition.

10.4.1 Healthy Diet or Healthy Diets?

Troubles begin when one has to enter the field of defining what a healthy diet is. For decades this has been defined just by relative amounts of protein, fats and carbohydrates. Such useless profile avoids to meet the real-world problems where governmental regulatory bodies live under tremendous pressure of the agro-industrial system. A huge amount of literature on dietary prevention and treatment of gestational diabetes came to almost no conclusions until a few years ago [18]. However some pillars can be deducted by good-quality pre-pregnancy studies [10] and by the few more recent studies [19, 20] .

According to these studies, the culprit of an increased incidence of gestational diabetes in pre-pregnancy studies are (a) insufficient consumption of vegetables and fruit; (b) refined cereal that deprives the organism of the natural fibre content of these nutrients; (c) sugar-sweetened beverages, sugary snacks and fruit juices; (d) products rich in cholesterol and other animal fats; and (e) overconsumption of red meat and processed meats. The latter item comes to a surprise and requires some explanatory notes. First of all, red meat from farm-raised cattle is rich in cholesterol that was pretty scarce in the game meat of our ancestors; nitrites used in processed meat might be transformed into nitrosamine that might damage the pancreatic beta cell; heating cholesterol-rich meat produced glycated compounds, excess of haem iron in women without iron deficiency, and eventually the pro-inflammatory role of the sialic acid of cell walls of mammalians (*N*-glycolylneuraminic acid) that differ from human sialic acid by one acetyl compound (*N*-acetylneuraminic acid) [21]. This latter unwanted interaction of mammalian red meat with our immune system is caused by a single gene mutation that sets human cell membrane apart from anthropoid monkeys and all other mammalians including cattle. This mutation makes the human red cell membrane free from the aggression of the lethal malaria agent, the *Plasmodium reichenowi* that infects monkeys [22]. However, the continued supplementation of this molecule through diet stimulates a low-grade immune reaction and eventually this alien immunogenic sialic acid might be incorporated in high turnover tissues, such as the endothelium [23].

One single aspect has been sorted out by many studies and requires a proper focus. We know that pregnancy in patients fed on a Western diet induces diabetogenic changes in the intestinal microbiota [6]. The intestinal microbiota modulates the immune system and this might balance the low-grade inflammation of visceral obesity and of term pregnancy. Obviously, negligible supplementation with one billion single-strain bacteria for a negligible number of weeks does not achieve any results in reducing risk factors [24]. Positive results were observed by single trials adopting proper dosage and length of administration [25–27]. In addition to this, preliminary data show how probiotic yogurt can reduce the inflammatory profile in pregnancy [20] as well as it has been proved in non-pregnant adults [28].

The nutritional prevention of gestational diabetes should then be tailored on each woman who requires the assistance of health-care providers.

Macro-ethnicity, cultural values, nutritional traditions and family habits, individual intolerance to food, lactose non-persistence and gastrointestinal signs and symptoms – all these elements should be investigated and become the background for nutritional advice. The healthy plate should accommodate all nutritional balances based on vegetable and fruit carbohydrate oligo elements and fibres, a variety of whole grains, healthy vegetable fats and healthy proteins including a prudent weekly share of fermented dairy products and red meat.

10.5 The Paradox of Hypertensive Diseases of Pregnancy: Preeclampsia

For almost 100 years preeclampsia had been defined by the coexistence of hypertension and proteinuria in a pregnant woman. Eventually, recently major scientific bodies such as the Royal College, the American College and The Canadian Society of Obstetricians and Gynaecologists picked out foamy urine – or proteinuria as more properly diagnosed by chemical reagents – from the definition of preeclampsia. This syndrome now accommodates a huge variety of signs, clinical conditions and laboratory abnormalities, and some guidelines even include fetal growth restriction to allow for a diagnosis of preeclampsia; others exclude this condition. A more generalized name could probably better fit the whole scenario: hypertensive diseases of pregnancy. Besides guidelines, or ahead of official scientific bodies, single scholars or international working groups, such as the Global Pregnancy CoLaboratory [29], proposed novel strategies to diagnose the different clinical phenotypes and possible different diseases, included unto the huge umbrella of preeclampsia.

For more than a scholar, this conflicting inclusive definition appears totally devoid of any explicatory pathogenesis, a criterion that is otherwise a paradigm in Western scientific medicine. We need to go back a few centuries to find such another big "clinical" vague definition articulated in a variety of signs and symptoms, some of them on the opposite site of pathophysiology: consider "dropsy". The Emperor Adriano suffered of dropsy and died of this disease in 138 AD. Was it a cardiac insufficiency, was it nephrosis, was it a pre-renal cause, or was it hepatic cirrhosis? The detailed array of clinical conditions, organ damages, criteria of severity, etc., included by recent guidelines without any attempt to reassemble clinical phenotypes on the ground of their "pathophysioloy" might appear alien to doctors not familiar with our specialty, a kind of modern "dropsy".

10.6 The Major Clinical Phenotypes of Preeclampsia

10.6.1 Early Preeclampsia or Preeclampsia Associated with Fetal Growth Restriction

A relatively rare, approximately less than 1 % of pregnancies, well-known cause of preeclampsia, if fetal growth restriction is allowed into the definition, is caused by shallow trophoblastic invasion and placental insufficiency [30]; this abnormal feto-maternal interface causes an early syncytiotrophoblastic oxidative stress that alters the balance of placental growth factors and its soluble blocking binding factors [31] and the development of villi and intervillous space. This condition starting in the first trimester later causes fetal growth restriction and in most of the cases subsequently determines a maternal endothelial dysfunction that results in high blood pressure and a possible variety of organ and function damages [32]. Approximately one in ten cases of preeclampsia adhere to this pathophysiological course, both in countries not affected by obesity epidemics [33] and in those affected [34]. Mothers do not adapt to pregnancy cardiovascular request developing a low cardiac output and high total vascular resistance from the early trimesters [35], just opposite to normal pregnancy physiology [36]. Its clinical differential diagnosis is centred on the finding of abnormal uterine Doppler velocimetry, abnormal PLGF/Sflit-1 ratio and poor fetal growth as assessed by abdominal circumference at ultrasound. In high-income or in Western countries, this condition is usually screened at prenatal visits and mothers and fetuses can be treated by antihypertensive drugs, fetal and maternal monitoring and timing of delivery.

For sure we cannot accept that the clinical phenotype of "early onset" preeclampsia ends at 33 weeks and 6 days, and that, 1 day later, it becomes a brand new disease under the name of "late-onset" preeclampsia, as one should assume according to present clinical practice guidelines. Placental insufficiency due to shallow trophoblastic invasion, and possible coexisting risk factors, varies in severity, clinical signs, and symptoms, obviously might appear at any gestational age and can be diagnosed with the same tools adopted in early gestation: uterine Doppler velocimetry fetal growth assessment and PLGF/Sflit-1 ratio. Hypertensive diseases associated with fetal growth restriction due to shallow trophoblastic invasion do become clinically evident also well after 33 weeks of gestation. Unfortunately, under present classifications, this disease remains nameless.

10.6.2 Maternal Preeclampsia Associated with Normal or Accelerated Fetal Growth

The clinical experience of each obstetrician recognises two main clinical phenotypes: the first, in which gestational hypertension is associated with fetal growth restriction (IUGR) as we briefly described in the previous paragraph, and the second, in which hypertension is associated with a fetus appropriate for gestational age, or sometimes even with large for gestational age fetuses, and a placenta that is normal for weight and number of primary villi. The latter occurs more commonly in the last weeks of pregnancy and even after birth and recognises the pre-existence of cardiovascular or metabolic risk factors related to the context of the metabolic syndrome [32, 37, 38] which is superimposed on the normal condition of pro-inflammatory normal placenta at term [39].

Total vascular resistance is decreased in the vast majority of preeclampsia occurring late in gestation, and cardiac output is increased, in an opposite fashion to preeclampsia, due to shallow trophoblastic invasion [36].

We have already discussed in previous paragraphs, as regards gestational diabetes, the common pathway of metabolic syndrome as a pro-inflammatory condition. The inflammatory endothelial dysfunction is the common pathway that merges this clinical phenotype of preeclampsia with the more "famous", but less frequent, phenotype caused by shallow trophoblastic invasion.

10.6.3 Oxidative Stress of the Trophoblast in Late Gestation

Unfortunately for the pregnant women, other partners of inflammation come on stage to add on their effects on metabolic syndrome in the late part of pregnancy. Recently, the appearance of macroscopically normal placenta has been redefined as a condition of overcrowding of the tertiary villi at the expense of the intervillous space [40], leading to conditions of hypoxia and oxidative stress on the syncytiotrophoblast [1]. This latter condition is similar to the oxidative stress of the syncytiotrophoblast caused by the growth-restricted placenta but occurs in normally developed placenta in late gestation.

10.6.4 Microbiota

A special recent focus has been put forward by the studies of Emry Koren on the changes and the role of intestinal microbiota in pregnancy [6]. As we have already described in previous paragraphs with the authors own words, "Third trimester stool is associated with greater inflammation and energy content".

10.6.5 Dyslipidaemia and Late Decidual Changes

The late histological abnormality of placental tissue is associated with inflammatory changes of the basal decidua [41] with a population of inflammatory immune cells that increases in the final stages of gestation, thereby contributing with other "partners", dyslipidemia, low-grade inflammation driven by visceral adipocytes, syncytiotrophoblastic oxidative stress, to acute atherosis at the level of spiral arteries [42].

The role of decidua as an "immune battleground" probably explains why preeclampsia is five to six times more frequent in pregnancies conceived from ovodonation [43], that is, a complete allograft for the maternal immune systems. In ovodonated mothers, unique and typical immune-adaptive changes are found in successful pregnancies, but not in those developing preeclampsia [44].

10.6.6 Abdominal Venous Pressure in Late Gestation

Finally a new area of investigation is focusing on venous pressure in the abdominal compartment. The post-glomerular venous pressure in kidneys is increased in late

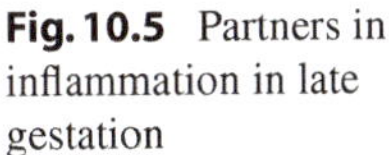

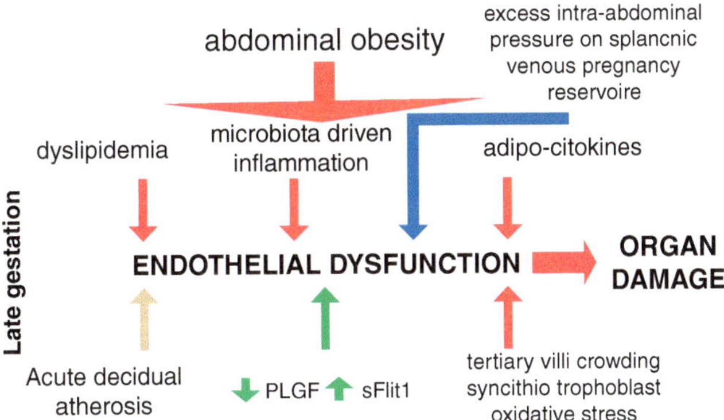

Fig. 10.5 Partners in inflammation in late gestation

preeclampsia. This decreased venous flow from the kidneys results in lower glomerular flow and filtration rate. This activates the local renin-angiotensin-aldosterone system in order to "increase" glomerular filtration rate [45] (Fig. 10.5).

There are other phenotypes of preeclampsia caused by predisposing conditions such as (1) immune damage that alters the development of the trophoblast (acquired autoimmune diseases), (2) severe chronic inflammatory diseases such as coeliac disease, (3) conditions such as some congenital thrombophilia, (4) the causes that lead to fetal hypoxic injury of the placenta (fetal heart failure, multi-fetal pregnancy) and (5) the conditions of peculiar disturbance of the immune decidual balance such as in oocyte donation.

10.7 Maternogenic Preeclampsia: Good News for a Possible Prevention

Good news for the possible prevention of maternogenic preeclampsia! So far, we have learned that the gestational age at which hypertensive disorder of pregnancy occurs is just a poor proxy of the different pathogenesis of hypertensive diseases of pregnancy, based on the more frequent epoch at which the clinical disease becomes apparent. Obviously when obesity and metabolic syndrome become epidemics, the overlapping of this cause with other causes of preeclampsia become more and more common so as to blur the information we can derive from epidemiology.

Indeed, the hard numbers are there; worldwide the major phenotype of preeclampsia is the one occurring late in gestation, in association with normal weight or large fetuses [46], in women affected by metabolic syndrome [47]. Contradictory reports as regards the risk of later cardiovascular risks are often retrospective studies based on regions with epidemics of obesity over 30 % of female population [48] or from studies in which the borders of "early preeclampsia" are moved up to 37 weeks of gestation [49]. In longitudinal prospective studies in regions where obesity is not making its disease toll on large shares of the female population, such as in Norway [37], maternogenic preeclampsia is significantly associated with a higher risk of developing cardiovascular disease in the fifth decade, due largely to pre-pregnancy risk factors.

From the point of view of those who believe that lifestyle might prevent at least part of this great obstetrical syndrome, these are good news. This allows drug regimen aimed at reducing endothelial dysfunction as nitric oxide donors [47], proper antihypertensive drugs that do not primarily reduce vascular peripheral resistance, or mainly action might and should be taken by tackling abdominal obesity since early gestation by adequate nutritional counselling and exercise promotion.

Smoke reduction has been more and more received by the general public when the perception of cancer later in life had become widespread; similarly changes in lifestyle during pregnancy might be better received and compliance improved when a more simple and lifelong perspective of health is envisioned to women since the very beginning of pregnancy.

References

1. Redman CW, Sargent IL, Staff AC. IFPA Senior Award Lecture: making sense of pre-eclampsia. Placenta. 2014;35(S):S20–5 Elsevier Ltd.
2. Dunsworth HM, Warrener AG, Deacon T, Ellison PT, Pontzer H. Metabolic hypothesis for human altriciality. Proc Natl Acad Sci U S A. 2012;109(38):15212–6.
3. Butte NF. Carbohydrate and lipid metabolism in pregnancy: normal compared with gestational diabetes mellitus. Am J Clin Nutr. 2000;71(5 Suppl):1256S–61.
4. Hartling L, Dryden DM, Guthrie A, Muise M, Vandermeer B, Aktary WM, Pasichnyk D, Seida JC, Donovan L. Screening and diagnosing gestational diabetes mellitus. Evid Rep Technol Assess (Full Rep). 2012;(210):1–327. Review.
5. Metzger BE, Lowe LP, Dyer AR, Trimble ER, Chaovarindr U, Coustan DR, et al. Hyperglycemia and adverse pregnancy outcomes. New Engl J Med. 2008;358(19):1991–2002.
6. Koren O, Goodrich JK, Cullender TC, Spor A, Laitinen K, Bäckhed HK, et al. Host remodeling of the gut microbiome and metabolic changes during pregnancy. Cell. 2012;150(3):470–80. Elsevier.
7. Nicholson JK, Holmes E, Kinross J, Burcelin R, Gibson G, Jia W, et al. Host-gut microbiota metabolic interactions. Science. 2012;336(6086):1262–7.
8. Cetin I, Koletzko B. Long-chain [omega]-3 fatty acid supply in pregnancy and lactation. Curr Opin Clin Nutr Metab Care. 2008;11(3):297–302.
9. Serhan CN. Pro-resolving lipid mediators are leads for resolution physiology. Nature. 2014;510(7503):92–101.
10. Zhang C, Ning Y. Effect of dietary and lifestyle factors on the risk of gestational diabetes: review of epidemiologic evidence. Am J Clin Nutr. 2011;94(6 Suppl):1975S–9.
11. Wood LEP. Obesity, waist-hip ratio and hunter-gatherers. BJOG: Br J Obstet Gynaecol. 2006;113(10):1110–6.
12. Song S, Lee JE, Song WO, Paik HY, Song Y. Carbohydrate intake and refined-grain consumption are associated with metabolic syndrome in the Korean adult population. J Acad Nutr Diet. 2014;114(1):54–62.
13. Odegaard AO, Koh WP, Butler LM, Duval S, Gross MD, Yu MC, Yuan JM, Pereira MA. Dietary patterns and incident Type 2 diabetes in Chinese men and women: the Singapore Chinese Health Study. Diabetes Care. 2011;34(4):880–5.
14. Tishkoff SA, Reed FA, Ranciaro A, Voight BF, Babbitt CC, Silverman JS, et al. Convergent adaptation of human lactase persistence in Africa and Europe. Nat Genet. 2006;39(1):31–40.

15. Hillier TA, Pedula KL, Schmidt MM, Mullen JA, Charles MA, Pettitt DJ. Childhood obesity and metabolic imprinting: the ongoing effects of maternal hyperglycemia. Diabetes Care. 2007;30(9):2287–92.
16. Bellamy L, Casas JP, Hingorani AD, Williams D. Type 2 diabetes mellitus after gestational diabetes: a systematic review and meta-analysis. Lancet. 2009;373(9677):1773–9.
17. Zhang C, Tobias DK, Chavarro JE, Bao W, Wang D, Ley SH, et al. Adherence to healthy lifestyle and risk of gestational diabetes mellitus: prospective cohort study. BMJ. 2014;349:g5450.
18. Han S, Crowther CA, Middleton P, Heatley E. Different types of dietary advice for women with gestational diabetes mellitus. Cochrane Database of Systematic Reviews 2013, Issue 3. Art. No.: CD009275. DOI: 10.1002/14651858.CD009275.pub2.
19. Asemi Z, Samimi M, Tabassi Z, Esmaillzadeh A. The effect of DASH diet on pregnancy outcomes in gestational diabetes: a randomized controlled clinical trial. Eur J Clin Nutr. 2014;68(4):490–5.
20. Asemi Z, Samimi M, Tabasi Z, Talebian P, Azarbad Z, Hydarzadeh Z, et al. Effect of daily consumption of probiotic yoghurt on lipid profiles in pregnant women: a randomized controlled clinical trial. J Matern Fetal Neonatal Med. 2012;25(9):1552–6.
21. Muchmore EA, Diaz S, Varki A. A structural difference between the cell surfaces of humans and the great apes. Am J Phys Anthropol. 1998;107(2):187–98.
22. Martin MJ, Rayner JC, Gagneux P, Barnwell JW, Varki A. Evolution of human-chimpanzee differences in malaria susceptibility: relationship to human genetic loss of N-glycolylneuraminic acid. Proc Natl Acad Sci U S A. 2005;102(36):12819–24.
23. Ajit V. Human evolution: details of being human. Nature. 2008;454(7200):21–3.
24. Lindsay KL, Walsh CA, Brennan L, McAuliffe FM. Probiotics in pregnancy and maternal outcomes: a systematic review. J Matern Fetal Neonatal Med. 2013;26(8):772–8.
25. Laitinen K, Poussa T, Isolauri E, the Nutrition, Allergy, Mucosal Immunology and Intestinal Microbiota Group. Probiotics and dietary counselling contribute to glucose regulation during and after pregnancy: a randomised controlled trial. Br J Nutr. 2008;101(11):1679.
26. Luoto R, Laitinen K, Nermes M, Isolauri E. Impact of maternal probiotic-supplemented dietary counseling during pregnancy on colostrum adiponectin concentration: a prospective, randomized, placebo-controlled study. Early Hum Dev. 2012;88(6):339–44.
27. Barrett HL, Dekker Nitert M, Conwell LS, Callaway LK. Probiotics for preventing gestational diabetes. Cochrane Database of Systematic Reviews 2014, Issue 2. Art. No.: CD009951. DOI: 10.1002/14651858.CD009951.pub2.
28. Bäckhed F, Ley RE, Sonnenburg JL, Peterson DA, Gordon JI. Host-bacterial mutualism in the human intestine. Science: Am Assoc Advan Sci. 2005;307(5717):1915–20.
29. Myatt L, Redman CW, Staff AC, Hansson S. Strategy for standardization of preeclampsia research study design. Hypertension. 2014;6332(6):1293–301.
30. Burton GJ, Woods AW, Jauniaux E, Kingdom JCP. Rheological and physiological consequences of conversion of the maternal spiral arteries for uteroplacental blood flow during human pregnancy. Placenta. 2010;30(6):473–82.
31. Romero R, Nien JK, Espinoza J, Todem D, Fu W, Chung H, et al. A longitudinal study of angiogenic (placental growth factor) and anti-angiogenic (soluble endoglin and soluble vascular endothelial growth factor receptor-1) factors in normal pregnancy and patients destined to develop preeclampsia and deliver a small for gestational age neonate. J Matern Fetal Neonatal Med. 2008;21(1):9–23.
32. Steegers EA, von Dadelszen P, Duvekot JJ, Pijnenborg R. Pre-eclampsia. Lancet. 2010; 376(9741):631–44.
33. Sohlberg S, Stephansson O, Cnattingius S, Wikström A-K. Maternal body mass index, height, and risks of preeclampsia. Am J Hypertens. 2010;25(1):120–5.
34. Mbah AK, Kornosky JL, Kristensen S, August EM, Alio AP, Marty PJ, et al. Super-obesity and risk for early and late pre-eclampsia. BJOG Br J Obstet Gynaecol. 2010;117(8):997–1004.
35. De Paco C, Kametas N, Rencoret G, Strobl I, Nicolaides KH. Maternal cardiac output between 11 and 13 weeks of gestation in the prediction of preeclampsia and small for gestational age. Obstet Gynecol. 2008;111(2 Pt 1):292–300.

36. Valensise H, Vasapollo B, Gagliardi G, Novelli GP. Early and late preeclampsia: two different maternal hemodynamic states in the latent phase of the disease. Hypertension. 2008;52(5): 873–80.
37. Romundstad PRP, Magnussen EBE, Smith GDG, Vatten LJL. Hypertension in pregnancy and later cardiovascular risk: common antecedents? Circulation. 2010;122(6):579–84.
38. Sara Z, Enrico F, Tamara S, Maria Luisa M, Eleonora R, Valeria M. Maternal and fetal phenotypes in hypertensive disorders of pregnancy are greater determinants of perinatal outcome than gestational age at onset of hypertension. Reproductive Sciences. 2014;1–2.
39. Borzychowski AM, Sargent IL, Redman CWG. Inflammation and pre-eclampsia. Semin Fetal Neonatal Med. 2006;11(5):309–16.
40. Egbor M, Ansari T, Morris N, Green CJ, Sibbons PD. Maternal medicine: morphometric placental villous and vascular abnormalities in early- and late-onset pre-eclampsia with and without fetal growth restriction. BJOG Br J Obstet Gynaecol. 2006;113(5):580–9.
41. Erlebacher A. Immunology of the maternal-fetal interface. Annu Rev Immunol. 2013;31(1):387–411.
42. Staff AC, Redman CWG. IFPA Award in Placentology Lecture: preeclampsia, the decidual battleground and future maternal cardiovascular disease. Placenta. 2014;35(S):S26–31, Elsevier Ltd.
43. Le Ray C, Scherier S, Anselem O, Marszalek A, Tsatsaris V, Cabrol D, et al. Association between oocyte donation and maternal and perinatal outcomes in women aged 43 years or older. Hum Reprod. 2012;27(3):896–901.
44. Schonkeren D, Swings G, Roberts D, Claas F, de Heer E, Scherjon S. Pregnancy close to the edge: an immunosuppressive infiltrate in the chorionic plate of placentas from uncomplicated egg cell donation. PLoS One. 2012;7(3):e32347. Veitia RA, editor.
45. Gyselaers W, Mullens W, Tomsin K, Mesens T, Peeters L. Role of dysfunctional maternal venous hemodynamics in the pathophysiology of pre-eclampsia: a review. Ultrasound Obstet Gynecol. 2011;38(2):123–9.
46. Conde-Agudelo A, Belizan JM. Risk factors for pre-eclampsia in a large cohort of Latin American and Caribbean women. Br J Obstetr Gynecol. 2000;107(1):75–83.
47. Vadillo-Ortega F, Perichart-Perera O, Espino S, Avila-Vergara MA, Ibarra I, Ahued R, et al. Effect of supplementation during pregnancy with L-arginine and antioxidant vitamins in medical food on pre-eclampsia in high risk population: randomised controlled trial. BMJ. 2011;342:d2901.
48. Lisonkova S, Joseph KS. Incidence of preeclampsia: risk factors and outcomes associated with early- versus late-onset disease. Am J Obstet Gynecol. 2013;209(6):544–e12.
49. Irgens HU, Reisaeter L, Irgens LM, Lie RT. Long term mortality of mothers and fathers after pre-eclampsia: population based cohort study. BMJ. 2001;323(7323):1213–7.

Nutrition, Immune System and Preeclampsia

11

Maria Teresa Gervasi and Gianna Bogana

Contents

11.1 Introduction

Hypertension represents the most common syndrome of pregnancy. Its diverse clinical phenotypes affect up to 7–15 % of pregnancies worldwide [1, 2]. Hypertensive disorders of pregnancy (HDP) include gestational hypertension, generally defined as new-onset hypertension (≥140 mmHg systolic or 90 mmHg diastolic blood pressure) arising after 20 week's gestation, and pre-eclampsia, defined as gestational hypertension accompanied by proteinuria (excretion of ≥300 mg protein every 24 h) and or other end organ diseases associated with hypertension [1, 3]. Less

M.T. Gervasi, MD (✉) • G. Bogana, MD
Obstetric and Gynecology Unit, Women's and Children's Health Department, Padova, Italy
e-mail: mtgervasi@gmail.com

E. Ferrazzi, B. Sears (eds.), *Metabolic Syndrome and Complications of Pregnancy: The Potential Preventive Role of Nutrition*,
DOI 10.1007/978-3-319-16853-1_11

frequent phenotypes include chronic hypertension, and chronic hypertension with superimposed pre-eclampsia.

The central hypothesis of HDPs is that these disorders might result either from shallow trophoblastic invasion in early gestation and utero-placental underpefusion and subsequent oxidative stress or from over-croweded terminal villi near term with abnormal intervillous perfusion, hypoxia and oxidatively stressed syncythiotrophoblast. Both these abnormal placental diseases release dysregulated vascular active proteins into the maternal circulation that are capable of inducing the clinical manifestation of the disease [4]. The former disease, with its typical early onset, has be defined in the last 10 years by many scholars as "placental pre-eclampsia" whereas the second phenotype, whose clinical severity is associated with preexixting or pregnancy-accelerated maternal metabolic syndrome and occurs usually later in pregnancy, might be defined as "maternal pre-eclampsia" [3, 4] assuming that pre-existing maternal subclinical endothelial dysfunction sums up to oxidatively stressed syncythiotrophoblast and maternal dyslipidemia facilitate the process of decidual arteries thrombosis near term.

Hypertension disorders of pregnancy are a major cause of maternal and perinatal morbidity and mortality [2], and result in an increased future risk for cardiovascular disease [5] and type 2 diabetes mellitus [6] for both mother and offspring. These lifelong and inter-generational adverse health consequences highlight the need for identification of preventive strategies.

Nutrition and systemic inflammation may play a role in the genesis of HDPs. In particular both placental and maternogenic preeclampsia are characterized by their impact on final pathways similar to those found in cardiovascular diseases, including endothelial dysfunction, inflammation, oxidative stress [4, 7]. A dysregulation of natural killer cells, activation of CD4_T lymphocytes, and the release of antiangiogenic and proinflammatory factors such as the soluble VEGF receptor-1 (sFlt-1) and s-endoglin, the angiotensin II type-1 receptor autoantibody (AT1-AA), and cytokines such as TNF-α and IL-6 and IL-17 [1, 2] have been described. Many of these pro-inflammatory factors are able to stimulate maternal endothelial dysfunction, circulating and local endothelin (ET-1), reactive oxygen species (ROS) and enhanced vascular sensitivity to angiotensin II, and consequently to hypertension in pregnancy.

Diet is a well-known risk factor for cardiovascular disease [8].

11.2 Nutrition and Placental Preclampsia

Unhealthy diets (such as elevated polyunsaturated fatty acids, and decreased vitamins C and E, zinc, and iron) have been associated with increased inflammation, oxidative stress, and dyslipidemia [9, 10]. Yet, current evidences from observational studies on the association between dietary factors and HDP is limited. Intervention trials have examined the effects of single nutrient supplementation in pregnant women on HDP risk, and recently several systematic reviews and meta-analyses have synthesized the results [11–15].

11.2.1 Total Energy Intake

Based on a review of the current literature maternal dietary intake of total energy was higher for preeclampsia cases compared with non-cases [9, 10].

Findings from cohort studies [19, 21, 23, 36, 39, 41–43, 48, 49] indicated that preeclampsia cases reported an energy intake of 87 kcal/day higher than women without pre-eclampsia (95 % CI 5.99 to 168.11; I2 = 0.0 %, P = 0.45). Results from a Norwegian prospective cohort study [39] showed higher odds for developing pre-eclampsia with higher early second trimester energy intake (OR = 3.7, 95 % CI 1.5–8.9, highest versus lowest quartile). Kazemian et al. [54] reported a positive association between higher energy intake and pre-eclampsia in a case–control study (OR = 1.33, 95 % CI 1.17–1.52, per 200 kcal).

Furthermore, data suggest that higher calcium and magnesium intake and a diet rich in fruit and vegetables may be beneficial for placental pre-eclampsia. In line with existing guidelines, pregnant women should be advised to avoid excessive energy intake and excessive weight gain during their pregnancy and an adequate calcium and magnesium intake may be achieved by increasing intake of low-fat dairy and fruit and vegetables [35, 38, 53].

11.2.2 Calcium

Calcium supplementation during pregnancy is recommended for prevention of pre-eclampsia in women with low dietary calcium intake and for those at high risk [16–18, 34]. Four case–control studies [20, 24, 26, 54] and two cohort studies [41, 42] reported adjusted estimates for the association between calcium intake and HDP. Calcium intake in the highest (>1,600 mg/day approximately) compared with the lowest (<1,000 mg/day approximately) quintile consistently showed lower odds for gestational hypertension (OR = 0.63, 95 % CI 0.41–0.97; I2 = 0.0 %, P = 0.53) and overall HDP (OR = 0.76, 95 % CI 0.57–1.01; I2 = 0.0 %, P = 0.79) [44, 45].

11.2.3 Magnesium

Two case–control studies [20, 54] and four cohort studies [21, 41, 42, 48] reported on insufficient magnesium intake in women with and without pre-eclampsia. Pooled results revealed statistically significantly lower mean magnesium intake of 8 mg/day for women with pre-eclampsia (95 % CI −13.99 to −1.38; I2 = 0.0 %, P = 0.41). Five studies [20, 41, 42, 48, 54] reported multivariate results for the association between magnesium intake and pre-eclampsia. Studies consistently trended towards an inverse association between magnesium intake and gestational hypertension [41, 42, 54] and pre-eclampsia [20, 41, 42, 48], although this was not statistically significant.

Magnesium may lower blood pressure by changing nitric oxide synthesis [60]. In addition, it has been suggested that lower magnesium intake may reduce the prostacyclin:thromboxane ratio, and thereby with a direct influence on HDP [61].

11.2.4 Associations Between Food Groups/Dietary Patterns and Pre-Eclampsia

Results for associations between food groups and overall dietary patterns and HDP suggested beneficial effects of fruit and vegetable consumption. Inflammation and endothelial dysfunction may play a role in the development of pre-eclampsia and lower concentrations of inflammatory markers have been found to be associated with consumption of a diet rich in fruit and vegetables. These aliments are low in fat and calories and are important sources of nutrient related to hypertension even in non pregnant population including dietary fiber, calcium, magnesium, potassium and vitamin C [47, 57, 58].

Six case–control [20, 22, 52, 55, 56, 59] and four cohort studies [25, 36, 39, 40] examined the association between fruit and/or vegetable consumption and pre-eclampsia. These studies consistently suggested a beneficial effect of higher fruit and/or vegetable consumption on pre-eclampsia, although they were not all statistically significant. Three studies reported on the associations between overall dietary patterns and HDP [37, 46, 50, 51]. In the MoBa study (23.423 women, including 1.267 pre-eclampsia cases) [37] inverse associations were found with development of pre-eclampsia in women with high scores on a dietary pattern characterized by vegetables, plant foods, and vegetable oils (third versus first tertile OR = 0.72, 95 % CI 0.62–0.85), and higher odds of pre-eclampsia were found in women with a dietary pattern characterized by processed meat, salty snacks, and sweet drinks (OR = 1.21, 95 % CI 1.03–1.42) [27–30].

In the Generation R study [50], an association was found between low adherence to a Mediterranean-style dietary pattern and high adherence to a traditional dietary style but these patterns were not associated with gestational hypertension or pre-eclampsia outcomes. In the US cohort study Project Viva [46], diet quality, as measured by the Alternate Healthy Eating Index slightly modified for pregnancy (AHEI-P), was not associated with pre-eclampsia (OR = 0.96, 95 % CI 0.84–1.10, 5 point increase) when assessed in the first trimester, but slightly lowered the odds of developing pre-eclampsia when assessed in the second trimester of pregnancy (OR = 0.87, 95 % CI 0.76–1.00).

Torjusen studied the potential health effects of eating organic food either in the general population or during pregnancy and his study shows that choosing organically grown vegetables during pregnancy is associated with reduced risk of pre-eclampsia. A possible explanations for an association between pre-eclampsia and use of organic vegetables could be that organic vegetables may change the exposure to pesticides, secondary plant metabolites and/or influence the composition of the gut microbiota [62]. Increased consumption of plant food, including vegetables, is recommended to all pregnant women, and this study shows that choosing organically grown vegetables may yield additional benefits.

Lindsay et al. systematically reviewed the literature on the use of probiotics in pregnancy and their impact on maternal outcomes. Results demonstrated that probiotic use in pregnancy can significantly reduce maternal fasting glucose, incidence of GDM and pre-eclampsia rates and levels of C-reactive protein. Probiotics hold potential as a safe therapeutic tool for the prevention of pre-eclampsia and adverse outcomes related to maternal metabolism [63].

11.3 Immune System and Placental Preclampsia

The partial failure of the maternal immune tolerance mechanisms precedes the development of placental oxidative stress and ischemia, which we know to be major players in the pathophysiology of placental pre-eclampsia. Maternal-fetal immune recognition during early trophoblastic invasion is controlled by two polymorphic gene system: HLA-C molecules of trophoblast and their receptors (killer cell immunoglobulin-like receptor of natural killer cells – KIRs). Two types of HLA-C (C1 e C2) are know: HLA-C2 interacts with KIRs more strongly than HLAC1. Promoters of trophoblast invasion as chemochine, angiogenic factors and cytokines are increased upon binding of HLA-C antigens to stimulatory KIRs, whereas they are reduced by antigen binding to KIRs. Mothers carrying HLA-C2 fetuses might have an increased susceptibility to placental pre-eclampsia [72].

During placentation fetal cells and maternal cells come into contact in the decidua; successful pregnancy requires that the maternal immune system does not reject the trophoblast; changes in the immune tolerance of the embryo, whose full genome is not concordant with the recipient's, is the principal explication of the more than threefold higher risk of hypertension and pre-eclampsia found in pregnancies following egg donation (Fig. 11.1) [73].

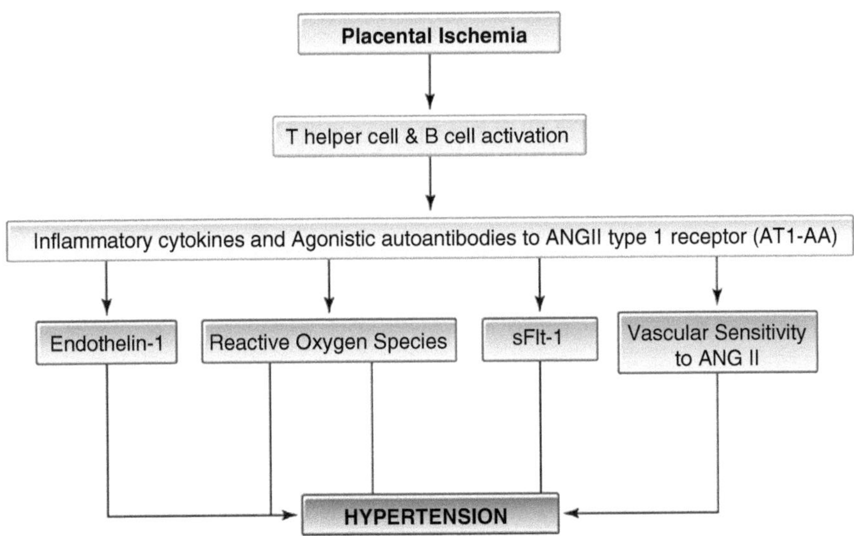

Fig. 11.1 Hypertension in response to placental ischemia: proceeds via immune activation, CD4+ T-cells mediating the release of angiotensin II type-1 receptor autoantibody (*AT1-AA*), and inflammatory cytokines that contribute to the increased vasoactive peptide ET-1 increased sensitivity to ANGII, oxidative stress, and sFlt-1, all known players in the pathophysiology of preeclampsia (Modified from La Marca et al. [75])

The following paragraphs will highlight the importance of inflammatory cells and products to cause the characteristic rise in blood pressure and decline in renal function that occur during placental pre-eclampsia.

11.3.1 Natural Killer Cells

Natural killer (NK) cells play an important role in the innate immune response providing viral protection and efficiently killing tumor cells by secreting granulosymes and cytotoxins.

NK cells compose a large portion of uterine lymphocytes from which they are distinguished by specific markers such as CD56 bright [64, 65]. These cells secrete angiogenic cytokines and proteins such as angiopoietin 1 and 2 and vascular endothelial growth factor (VEGF) and placenta growth factor (PlGF) [65]. Uterine NK cells prefer close association with the trophoblasts and secrete cytokines that play an important role in trophoblasts differentiation, growth, and spiral arteriole invasion during normal pregnancy and thus contribute to the success of trophoblasts invasion [64, 65].

Uterine NK cells can induce lysis of trophoblast cells lacking specific cellular surface antigens that would normally invade the spiral arteries. Incomplete loss of such cells results in the shallow trophoblast invasion and thus the deficient oxygen and nutrient supply to the developing placenta, which has been described as the genesis of placental pre-eclampsia. Furthermore, during pre-eclampsia inadequate vasculogensis of the placenta leads to hypoxia, thus stimulating production of the VEGF and PlGF antagonist sFlt, thereby stimulating a viscous cycle of events that worsens throughout the pregnancy. These data indicate the importance of the functional profile of the uterine NK cell to either maintain or compromise a potentially healthy pregnancy.

11.3.2 CD4_T Helper Lymphocytes

The maternal immune tolerance involves crucial interactions between regulatory CD4_T cells and uterine NK cells recognizing and accepting the fetal antigens and facilitating placental growth. Complete failure leads to poor placentation and dysfunctional placental perfusion and chronic immune activation originating from the placenta. Analysis of blood collected from preeclamptic women has demonstrated a decrease in the proportion of circulating regulatory CD4_ T cells [66, 67].

11.3.3 B Lymphocytes

An important function of CD4_ T cells is to facilitate the B lymphocyte memory immune response and specific antibody production toward a single antigen. This process is known as the T-cell-dependent antibody response [68].

Auto-antibodies are produced during pre-eclampsia, suggesting an important role for B lymphocytes in the pathogenesis of this disease. Moreover, Liao et al. demonstrated that the percentage of circulating memory B-lymphocytes were significantly greater in preeclamptic women than in the Non Preeclamptic (NP) cohort [69]. B-2 B lymphocytes are the conventional memory B cells that undergo antigen processing via recognition of MHC class II peptide complex with the activated CD4_T lymphocyte [68]. For B-cell maturation and IgG production, several co-stimulatory signals must occur between the antibody producing B lymphocyte and CD4_ T-helper cell [68]. One of these includes stimulation of the CD20 receptor on the surface of the B cell. This recognition stimulates the B cell to enter the circulation and produce antigen-specific immunoglobulin. Another necessary co-stimulatory molecule for B-cell maturation is the CD40 on the surface of the B cell. This molecule binds with the CD40 ligand on the surface of the T cell [68]. B cells then proceed through proliferation, differentiation, and internal isotype switching, inducing to production of specific antigen-stimulated antibodies, which leads to the formation of short-lived plasma cells that secrete antibody and memory B cells residing in the germinal lymph node centers, which will be available for future interactions with specific T cells. B lymphocytes can be characterized as either B1 or B2 cells, each having distinct markers and roles in facilitating immune reactions. B1 lymphocytes can be divided into B1a or B1b cells [68, 69]. These cells express IgM in greater quantities than IgG and are the primary source of natural antibodies produced in the absence of antigenic stimulation. These antibodies are polyreactive and cross-react with multiple antigens such as autoantigens, other immunoglobulins, and bacterial polysaccharides. Recently, Jensen et al. uncovered an important role for B1 lymphocytes in the progression of pre-eclampsia [70]. Preeclamptic placentas stained positive for markers of B1 B lymphocytes (CD19_CD5_). Furthermore, these authors demonstrated that B1 lymphocytes were stimulated to produce AT1-AA when co-cultured with sera from preeclamptic women but not from normal pregnant women. This study further illustrates the importance of B cells in the preeclamptic placenta and their stimulation by a soluble factor to produce AT1-AA and contribute to the progression of this disease. Furthermore, high levels of B1 cells is yet another important characteristic that preeclamptic women share with patients presenting with autoimmune diseases.

11.3.4 Activating Autoantibodies to the Angiotensin II Type I Receptor (AT1-AA)

Many studies in preeclamptic women have demonstrated increased circulating concentrations of an agonistic autoantibody to the angiotensin type 1 receptor (AT1-AA). AT1-AAs are implicated as a central mediator of several pathophysiological mechanisms in pre-eclampsia. During pre-eclampsia, AT1-AA induce NADPH oxidase and the MAPK/ERK pathway leading to NF-_B and tissue factor activation. AT1-AA stimulate sFlt-1 expression from trophoblast cells and IL-6 production from mesangial cells; they cause increased intracellular Ca^2_ signaling in platelets in women who went on to develop pre-eclampsia (Fig. 11.2) [65, 68, 71].

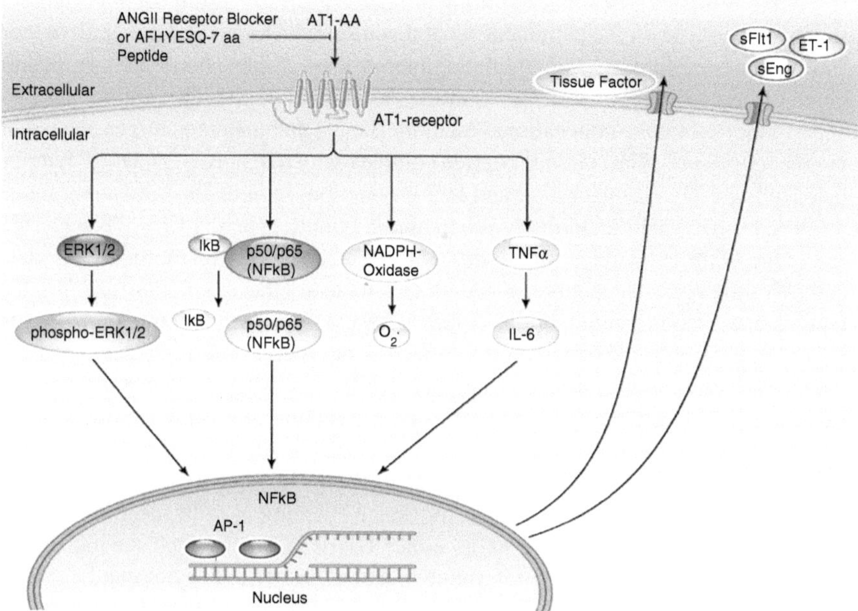

Fig. 11.2 Signal cascades of the angiotensin II type 1 receptor autoantibodies. AT1-AA induce signaling by the angiotensin II type 1 receptor (*AT1-receptor*), inhibited by AT1-receptor blocker (ARB) or the seven-amino acid peptide (*AFHYESQ*) mimicking the epitope of the AT1-AA in the second extracellular domain of the AT1-receptor. Intracellular cascades and promoter activations in the nucleus lead to an upregulation of endothelin-1 (*ET-1*), tissue factor, soluble fms-like tyrosine kinase-1 (*sFlt1*), soluble endoglin (*sEng*), and oxidative stress (Modified from La Marca et al. [75])

11.3.5 Inflammatory Cytokines

Several studies have shown an important role for inflammatory cytokines such as IL-6, IL-17 and TNF-α in the etiology of pre-eclampsia.

Studies in animal models have been important to show that moderate, long-term increases in cytokines during pregnancy raise blood pressure and compromise renal function. Mechanisms of hypertension during pregnancy in response to elevated cytokines appear to involve activation of ET-1, increased oxidative stress, and activation of AT1 receptors by AT1-AA. In addition, many laboratories have shown that TNF-α directly stimulates endothelial cells in culture to secrete ET-1 and sICAM, thus attracting leukocytes to adhere to vascular tissues determining edema, which could lead to temporary increases in blood pressure [67]. TNF-α mRNA is increased in preeclamptic placentas and thus could directly increase ET-1 in the placental unit.

IL-6 is important in both anti-inflammatory and pro-inflammatory processes and is a pivotal cytokine to influence activation of B cells as well as effector or regulatory T cells [68]. IL-6 is elevated in preeclamptic women, and AT1-AA-induced hypertensive pregnant mice.

IL-17 is a cytokine that has mostly been associated with autoimmune diseases but has recently gained attention in the aetiology of pre-eclampsia [67, 68]. Recent studies have shown that circulating IL-17 secreting TH17 cells are increased in preeclamptic patients compared with non pregnant patients [67]. Additionally, an important role for TH17 cells and IL-17 in the clearing of bacterial infections has been shown [68]. One important function of IL-17 producing TH17 cells is to recruit neutrophils and other phagocytic cells to a site of infection. IL-17 stimulates neutrophil activation, production of antimicrobial substances such as defensins and ROS, and phagocytosis of microbes or necrotic tissues [68]. Macrophages and neutrophils convert molecular oxygen into ROS by the phagocyte NADPH oxidase system. Activated neutrophils cause injury to normal host tissues, such as the placental unit, by the release of lysosomal enzymes, ROS, or nitric oxide. Preeclamptic women display oxidative stress, increased NADPH oxidase subunits within the placental unit, and elevated blood, urinary, and placental 8-isoprostanes, an indicator of whole body oxidative stress.

An additional cytokine gaining attention in the area of preeclamptic research is CD40/CD40 ligand. The CD40 antigen binds to the CD40 ligand on T cells and is important to stimulate B-lymphocyte proliferation, as previously mentioned [68]. A recent study compared the effect of maternal serum from preeclamptic patients and NP patients to induce apoptosis in cultured endothelial cells [72]. This study showed that endothelial dysfunction may be induced by this CD40/CD40 ligand. These authors found that altered morphology, decreased cell growth, and increased apoptosis were greater with CD40/CD40 ligand increased expression following exposure to preeclamptic sera versus sera from healthy normal pregnant women. However, in vivo studies revealing an important role for CD40/CD40 ligand during pregnancy are lacking. Furthermore, inhibition of this interaction would inhibit T cell-B cell communication and could clarify the role of either memory B cells vs. non memory B cells in the production of AT1-AA, as mentioned previously. Non memory B cells do not require this interaction with T cells for antibody secretion. Therefore, this could be a defining study revealing a role for the memory immune response as well as the route of production of AT1-AA during pre-eclampsia (Fig. 11.3).

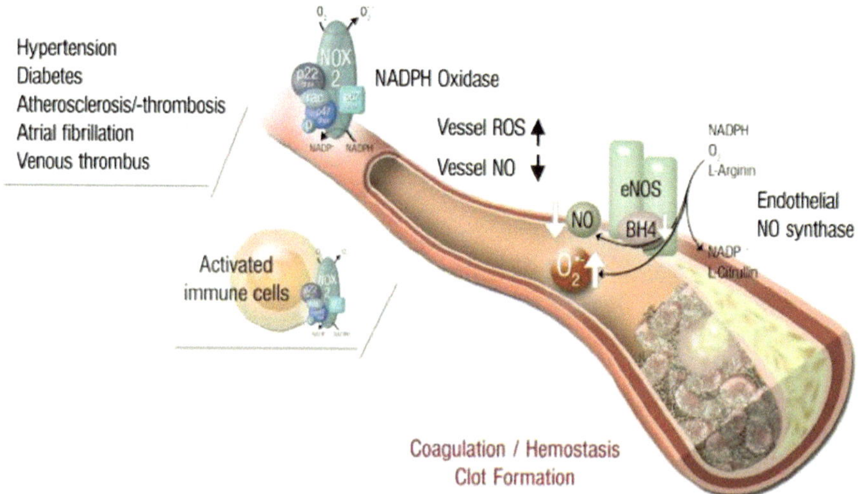

Fig. 11.3 Inflammatory cells, vascular dysfunction and atherothrombosis. The scheme illustrates the activation of immune cells and recruitment to vascular tissues leading to activation of secondary RONS sources such as NADPH oxidase and uncoupled eNOS, all of which contributes to vascular dysfunction. These processes lead to late-stage cardiovascular complication such as atherosclerosis with plaque formation and thrombosis. Vice versa, vascular RONS can activate immune cells and Trigger their Infiltration into the vascular wall (Modified from Karbach et al. *Curr Pharm Des* 2014)

References

1. Cunningham FG, Leveno KJ, Bloom SL, Hauth JC, Rouse DJ, Spong CY. Pregnancy hypertension. Williams obstetrics. 23rd ed. New York: McGraw Hill;2009.
2. Sibai B, Dekker G, Kupferminc M. Preeclampsia. Lancet. 2005;365:785–99.
3. Steegers EA, von Dadelszen P, Duvekot JJ, Pijnenborg R. Preeclampsia. Lancet. 2010;376: 631–44.
4. Redman CW, Sacks GP, Sargent IL. Preeclampsia: an excessive maternal inflammatory response to pregnancy. Am J Obstet Gynecol. 1999;180:499–506.
5. Rich-Edwards JW, Fraser A, Lawlor DA, Catov JM. Pregnancy characteristics and women's future cardiovascular health: an underused opportunity to improve women's health? Epidemiol Rev. 2014;36:57–70.
6. Feig DS, Shah BR, Lipscombe LL, Wu CF, Ray JG, Lowe J, Hwee J, Booth GL. Preeclampsia as a risk factor for diabetes: a population-based cohort study. PLoS Med. 2013;10:e1001425.
7. Gervasi MT, Chaiworapongsa T, Pacora P, Naccasha N, Yoon BH, Maymon E, Romero R. Phenotypic and metabolic characteristics of monocytes and granulocytes in preeclampsia. Am J Obstet Gynecol. 2001;185(4):792–7.
8. Martinez-Gonzalez MA, Bes-Rastrollo M. Dietary patterns, Mediterranean diet, and cardiovascular disease. Curr Opin Lipidol. 2014;25:20–6.
9. Xu H, Shatenstein B, Luo ZC, Wei S, Fraser W. Role of nutrition in the risk of preeclampsia. Nutr Rev. 2009;67:639–57.
10. Roberts JM, Balk JL, Bodnar LM, Belizán JM, Bergel E, Martinez A. Nutrient involvement in preeclampsia. J Nutr. 2003;133:1684S–92.
11. De-Regil LM, Palacios C, Ansary A, Kulier R, Pena-Rosas JP. Vitamin D supplementation for women during pregnancy. Cochrane Database Syst Rev 2012;(2):CD008873.

12. Imhoff-Kunsch B, Briggs V, Goldenberg T, Ramakrishnan U. Effect of n-3 long-chain polyunsaturated fatty acid intake during pregnancy on maternal, infant, and child health outcomes: a systematic review. Paediatr Perinat Epidemiol. 2012;26:91–107.
13. Conde-Agudelo A, Romero R, Kusanovic JP, Hassan SS. Supplementation with vitamins C and E during pregnancy for the prevention of preeclampsia and other adverse maternal and perinatal outcomes: a systematic review and metaanalysis. Am J Obstet Gynecol. 2011;204:503.e501–12.
14. Makrides M, Crowther CA. Magnesium supplementation in pregnancy. Cochrane Database Syst Rev 2001; (4):CD000937.
15. Duley L, Henderson-Smart D, Meher S. Altered dietary salt for preventing preeclampsia, and its complications. Cochrane Database Syst Rev 2005;(4):CD005548.
16. Patrelli TS, Dall'Asta A, Gizzo S, Pedrazzi G, Piantelli G, Jasonni VM, Modena AB. Calcium supplementation and prevention of preeclampsia: a meta-analysis. J Matern Fetal Neonatal Med. 2012;25:2570–4.
17. Lowe SA, Brown MA, Dekker G, Gatt S, McLintock C, McMahon L, Mangos G, Moore MP, Muller P, Paech M, Society of Obstetric Medicine of Australia and New Zealand, Walters B. Guidelines for the management of hypertensive disorders of pregnancy. 2008. [https://www.somanz.org/pdfs/somanz_guidelines_2008.pdf]
18. World Health Organization. WHO recommendations for prevention and treatment of preeclampsia and eclampsia. Geneva: WHO Press; 2011.
19. Brantsaeter AL, Myhre R, Haugen M, Myking S, Sengpiel V, Magnus P, Jacobsson B, Meltzer HM. Intake of probiotic food and risk of preeclampsia in primiparous women: the Norwegian Mother and Child Cohort Study. Am J Epidemiol. 2011;174:807–15.
20. Frederick IO, Williams MA, Dashow E, Kestin M, Zhang C, Leisenring WM. Dietary fiber, potassium, magnesium and calcium in relation to the risk of preeclampsia. J Reprod Med. 2005;50:332–44.
21. Goodarzi Khoigani M, Paknahad Z, Mardanian F. The relationship between nutrients intake and preeclampsia in pregnant women. J Res Med Sci. 2012;17:S210–7.
22. Gulsen S, Guner A. Nutrition habits and blood test results of preeclamptic and healthy pregnant women. J Res Med Sci. 2012;6:175–80.
23. Haugen M, Brantsaeter AL, Trogstad L, Alexander J, Roth C, Magnus P, Meltzer HM. Vitamin D supplementation and reduced risk of preeclampsia in nulliparous women. Epidemiology. 2009;20:720–6.
24. Kesmodel U, Olsen SF, Salvig JD. Marine n-3 fatty acid and calcium intake in relation to pregnancy induced hypertension, intrauterine growth retardation, and preterm delivery. Acta Obstet Gynecol Scand. 1997;76:38–44.
25. Klemmensen AK, Tabor A, Osterdal ML, Knudsen VK, Halldorsson TI, Mikkelsen TB, Olsen SF. Intake of vitamin C and E in pregnancy and risk of preeclampsia: prospective study among 57 346 women. BJOG. 2009;116:964–74.
26. Marcoux S, Brisson J, Fabia J. Calcium intake from dairy products and supplements and the risks of preeclampsia and gestational hypertension. Am J Epidemiol. 1991;133:1266–72.
27. Paknahad Z, Talebi N, Azadbakht L. Dietary determinants of pregnancy induced hypertension in Isfahan. J Res Med Sci. 2008;13:17–21.
28. Qiu C, Coughlin KB, Frederick IO, Sorensen TK, Williams MA. Dietary fiber intake in early pregnancy and risk of subsequent preeclampsia. Am J Hypertens. 2008;21:903–9.
29. Triche EW, Grosso LM, Belanger K, Darefsky AS, Benowitz NL, Bracken MB. Chocolate consumption in pregnancy and reduced likelihood of preeclampsia. Epidemiology. 2008;19:459–64.
30. Saftlas AF, Triche EW, Beydoun H, Bracken MB. Does chocolate intake during pregnancy reduce the risks of preeclampsia and gestational hypertension? Ann Epidemiol. 2010;20:584–91.
31. Wells GA SB, O'Connell D, Peterson J, Welch V, Losos M, Tugwell P. The Newcastle-Ottawa Scale (NOS) for assessing the quality of nonrandomised studies in meta-analyses. [http://www.ohri.ca/programs/clinical_epidemiology/oxford.asp]

32. Zhang J, Kai FY. What's the relative risk? A method of correcting the odds ratio in cohort studies of common outcomes. JAMA. 1998;280:1690–1.
33. Higgins JP, Thompson SG, Deeks JJ, Altman DG. Measuring inconsistency in meta-analyses. BMJ. 2003;327:557–60.
34. Geraldo Lopes Ramos J, Brietzke E, Martins-Costa SH, Vettorazzi-Stuczynski J, Barros E, Carvalho C. Reported calcium intake is reduced in women with preeclampsia. Hypertens Pregnancy. 2006;25:229–39.
35. Wei S-Q, Xu H, Xiong X, Luo Z-C, Audibert F, Fraser WD. Tea consumption during pregnancy and the risk of preeclampsia. Int J Gynaecol Obstet. 2009;105:123–6.
36. Borgen I, Aamodt G, Harsem N, Haugen M, Meltzer HM, Brantsaeter AL. Maternal sugar consumption and risk of preeclampsia in nulliparous Norwegian women. Eur J Clin Nutr. 2012;66:920–5.
37. Brantsaeter AL, Haugen M, Samuelsen SO, Torjusen H, Trogstad L, Alexander J, Magnus P, Meltzer HM. A dietary pattern characterized by high intake of vegetables, fruits, and vegetable oils is associated with reduced risk of preeclampsia in nulliparous pregnant Norwegian women. J Nutr. 2009;139:1162–8.
38. Chavarro JE, Halldorsson TI, Leth T, Bysted A, Olsen SF. A prospective study of trans fat intake and risk of preeclampsia in Denmark. Eur J Clin Nutr. 2011;65:944.
39. Clausen T, Slott M, Solvoll K, Drevon CA, Vollset SE, Henriksen T. High intake of energy, sucrose, and polyunsaturated fatty acids is associated with increased risk of preeclampsia. Am J Obstet Gynecol. 2001;185:451–8.
40. Longo-Mbenza B, Tshimanga BK, Buassa-bu-Tsumbu B, Kabangu J. Diets rich in vegetables and physical activity are associated with a decreased risk of pregnancy induced hypertension among rural women from Kimpese DR Congo. Niger J Med. 2008;17:265–9.
41. Morris CD, Jacobson SL, Anand R, Ewell MG, Hauth JC, Curet LB, Catalano PM, Sibai BM, Levine RJ. Nutrient intake and hypertensive disorders of pregnancy: evidence from a large prospective cohort. Am J Obstet Gynecol. 2001;184:643–51.
42. Oken E, Ning Y, Rifas-Shiman SL, Rich-Edwards JW, Olsen SF, Gillman MW. Diet during pregnancy and risk of preeclampsia or gestational hypertension. Ann Epidemiol. 2007;17:663–8.
43. Olafsdottir AS, Skuladottir GV, Thorsdottir I, Hauksson A, Thorgeirsdottir H, Steingrimsdottir l. Relationship between high consumption of marine fatty acids in early pregnancy and hypertensive disorders in pregnancy. BJOG. 2006;113:301–9.
44. Ortega RM, Martinez RM, Lopez-Sobaler AM, Andres P, Quintas ME. Influence of calcium intake on gestational hypertension. Ann Nutr Metab. 1999;43:37–46.
45. Richardson BE, Baird DD. A study of milk and calcium supplement intake and subsequent preeclampsia in a cohort of pregnant women. Am J Epidemiol. 1995;141:667–73.
46. Rifas-Shiman SL, Rich-Edwards JW, Kleinman KP, Oken E, Gillman MW. Dietary quality during pregnancy varies by maternal characteristics in Project Viva: a US cohort. J Am Diet Assoc. 2009;109:1004–11.
47. Rumbold AR, Maats FHE, Crowther CA. Dietary intake of vitamin C and vitamin E and the development of hypertensive disorders of pregnancy. Eur J Obstet Gynecol Reprod Biol. 2005;119:67–71.
48. Skajaa K, Dorup I, Sandstrom BM. Magnesium intake and status and pregnancy outcome in a Danish population. Br J Obstet Gynaecol. 1991;98:919–28.
49. Tande DL, Ralph JL, Johnson LK, Scheett AJ, Hoverson BS, Anderson CM. First trimester dietary intake, biochemical measures, and subsequent gestational hypertension among nulliparous women. J Midwifery Womens Health. 2013;58:423–30.
50. Timmermans S, Steegers-Theunissen RPM, Vujkovic M, Bakker R, den Breeijen H, Raat H, Russcher H, Lindemans J, Hofman A, Jaddoe VWV, Steegers EA. Major dietary patterns and blood pressure patterns during pregnancy: the Generation R Study. Am J Obstet Gynecol. 2011;205:337.e331–2.
51. Al MD, van Houwelingen AC, Badart-Smook A, Hasaart TH, Roumen FJ, Hornstra G. The essential fatty acid status of mother and child in pregnancy-induced hypertension: a prospective longitudinal study. Am J Obstet Gynecol. 1995;172:1605–14.

52. Atkinson J, Mahomed K, Williams M, Woelk G, Mudzamiri S, Weiss N. Dietary risk factors for preeclampsia among women attending Harare Maternity Hospital, Zimbabwe. Cent Afr J Med. 1998;44:86–92.
53. Duvekot EJ, de Groot CJ, Bloemenkamp KW, Oei SG. Pregnant women with a low milk intake have an increased risk of developing preeclampsia. Eur J Obstet Gynecol Reprod Biol. 2002;105:11–4.
54. Kazemian E, Dorosty-Motlagh AR, Sotoudeh G, Eshraghian MR, Ansary S, Omidian M. Nutritional status of women with gestational hypertension compared with normal pregnant women. Hypertens Pregnancy. 2013;32:146–56.
55. Reyes L, Garcia R, Ruiz S, Dehghan M, Lopez-Jaramillo P. Nutritional status among women with preeclampsia and healthy pregnant and non-pregnant women in a Latin American country. J Obstet Gynaecol Res. 2012;38:498–504.
56. Richards DG, Lindow SW, Carrara H, Knight R, Haswell SJ, Van der Spuy ZM. A comparison of maternal calcium and magnesium levels in pre-eclamptic and normotensive pregnancies: an observational case–control study. BJOG. 2014;121:327–36.
57. Schiff E, Friedman SA, Stampfer M, Kao L, Barrett PH, Sibai BM. Dietary consumption and plasma concentrations of vitamin E in pregnancies complicated by preeclampsia. Am J Obstet Gynecol. 1996;175:1024–8.
58. Sharbaf FR, Dehghanpour P, Shariat M, Dalili H. Caffeine consumption and incidence of hypertension in pregnancy. J Fam Reprod Health. 2013;7:127–30.
59. Zhang C, Williams MA, King IB, Dashow EE, Sorensen TK, Frederick IO, Thompson ML, Luthy DA. Vitamin C and the risk of preeclampsia—results from dietary questionnaire and plasma assay. Epidemiology. 2002;13:409–16.
60. Carlin Schooley M, Franz KB. Magnesium deficiency during pregnancy in rats increases systolic blood pressure and plasma nitrite. Am J Hypertens. 2002;15:1081–6.
61. Schoenaker DA, et al. The association between dietary factors and gestational hypertension and preeclampsia: a systematic review and meta-analysis of observational studies. BMC Med. 2014;12:157.
62. Torjusen H, et al. Reduced risk of preeclampsia with organic vegetable consumption: results from the prospective Norwegian Mother and Child Cohort Study. BMJ Open. 2014;4(9):e006143.
63. Lindsay KL. Probiotics in pregnancy and maternal outcomes: a systematic review. J Matern Fetal Neonatal Med. 2013;26(8):772–8.
64. Fukui A, Yokota M, Funamizu A, Nakamu R, Fukuhara R, Yamada K, Kimura H, Fukuyama A, Kamoi M, Tanaka K, Mizunuma H. Changes of NK cells in preeclampsia. Am J Reprod Immunol. 2012;67:278–86.
65. Wenzel K, Rajakumar A, et al. Angiotensin II type 1 receptor antibodies and increased angiotensin II sensitivity in pregnant rats. Hypertension. 2011;58:77–84.
66. Prins J, Boelens H, Heimweg J, Van der Heide S, Dubois A, Van Oosterhout A, Erwich J. Preeclampsia is associated with lower percentages of regulatory T cells in maternal blood. Hypertension Pregnancy. 2009;28:300–11.
67. Santner-Nanan B, Peek M, Khanam R, Richarts L, Zhu E, Fazekas de St Groth B, Nanan R. Systemic increase in the ration between FoxP3_ and IL-17producing CD4_ T cells in healthy pregnancy but not in preeclampsia. J Immunol. 2009;183:7023–30.
68. Abbus A, Lichtman A. Cellular and molecular immunology. In: General properties of the immune response, cells and tissue of the immune system. Philadelphia: Elsevier; 2005. p. 189–215.
69. Liao AH, Liu LP, Ding WP, Zhang L. Functional changes of human peripheral B lymphocytes in preeclampsia. Am J Reprod Immunol. 2009;61:313–21.
70. Jensen F, Wallukat G, Herse F, Budner O, El-Mousleh T, Costa SD, Dechend R, Zenclussen AC. CD19_CD5_ cells as indicators of preeclampsia. Hypertension. 2012;59:861–8.
71. Walther T, Wallukat G, Jank A, Bartel S, Schultheiss HP, Faber R, Stepan H. Angiotensin II type 1 receptor agonistic antibodies reflect fundamental alterations in the uteroplacental vasculature. Hypertension. 2005;46:1275–9.

72. Wu CF, Huang FD, Sui RF, Sun JX. Preeclampsia serum upregulates CD40/CD40L expression and induces apoptosis in human umbilical cord endothelial cells. Reprod Biol Endocrinol. 2012;10:28.
73. Chaiworapongsa T, Chaemsaithong P, Yeo L, Romero R. Preeclampsia part 1: current understanding of its pathophysiology. Nat Rev Nephrol. 2014;10(8):466–80.
74. European Society of Human Reproduction and Embryology. "Pregnancies following egg donation associated with more than 3-fold higher risk of hypertension." ScienceDaily. ScienceDaily, 2014. <www.sciencedaily.com/releases/2014/07/140701091446.htm>.
75. La Marca B et al. Elucidating immune mechanism causing hypertension during pregnancy. *Physiology* 2013;28:225–33

Lifestyle Intervention and Prevention of Spontaneous Preterm Delivery in Obese Pregnant Women 12

Christina Anne Vinter

Contents

12.1 Introduction

Obesity in pregnancy is a major source of preventable perinatal morbidity and one of the greatest challenges to practicing clinicians worldwide. Maternal obesity is associated to a number of complications during pregnancy and poor birth outcomes [1, 2] and represents an increasing public health burden [3, 4]. Maternal obesity during pregnancy also contributes to offspring obesity in early and later life.

During the last decades, we have seen a dramatic increase in the incidence of obesity. Among women aged 20–39 years of age in the USA, the prevalence of obesity (defined as body mass index (BMI) $\geq$ 30 kg/m^2) (Table 12.1) has reached

C.A. Vinter, MD, PhD
Department of Gynecology and Obstetrics, Odense University Hospital, Odense, Denmark
e-mail: christina.vinter@rsyd.dk

E. Ferrazzi, B. Sears (eds.), *Metabolic Syndrome and Complications of Pregnancy: The Potential Preventive Role of Nutrition*,
DOI 10.1007/978-3-319-16853-1_12

Table 12.1 The Institute of Medicine (IOM) recommendations for total weight gain during pregnancy

Prepregnancy BMI (WHO classification)	Recommended gestational weight gain (kg)
Underweight (BMI < 18.5 kg/m^2)	12.5–18
Normal weight (BMI 18.5–25 kg/m^2)	11.5–16
Overweight (BMI 25–30 kg/m^2)	7–11.5
Obese (BMI ≥ 30 kg/m^2)	5–9

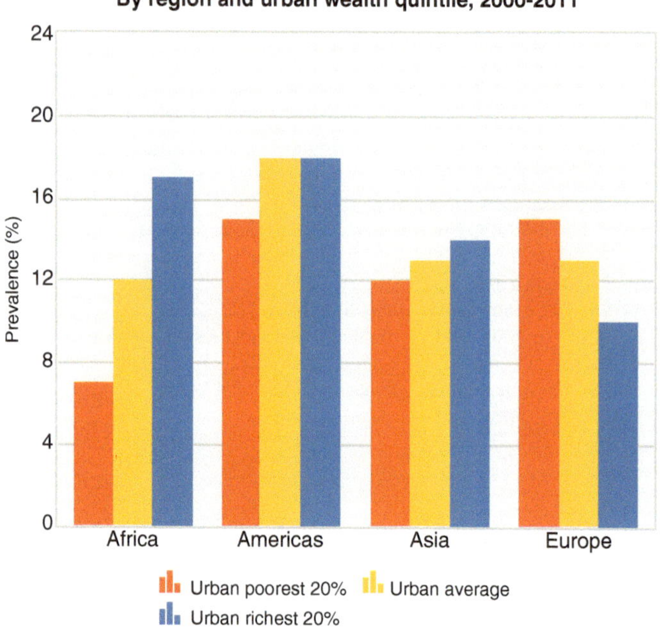

Fig. 12.1 WHO statistics on obesity worldwide stratified for income

36 % [7], and based on the latest WHO estimates, in European Union countries, overweight affects 30–70 % and obesity affects 10–30 % of adults. Unfortunately these epidemics encroached on urban rich people also in Africa and Asia mostly among those who adopted westernized lifestyles (Fig. 12.1). In England the prevalence of obesity is about 16 % [8]. Another major source of infant morbidity and mortality is preterm birth (PTB), defined as delivery before 37 weeks of gestation. Preterm birth affects 5–18 % of pregnancies in different settings [9].

There is evidence that obesity may be a risk factor for PTB, but the details of this relationship are not completely understood and often inconsistent [6, 10–12]. Results from new large population-based studies from Sweden [13] and California

[14] take into account a more complex interaction. In a review including results from both the Swedish and Californian studies, all together including almost 3.5 million deliveries, the phenotype of PTB is considered [5]. In the analysis the authors have in details looked at both spontaneous and medically induced deliveries, the impact of gestational age by dividing deliveries into extreme preterm (22–27 weeks), very preterm (28–31 weeks), and moderately preterm deliveries (32–36 weeks) as well as the dose-response relationship with increasing BMI and across ethnic backgrounds. They find that increasing levels of obesity leads to preterm delivery via two mechanisms: first of all by increasing the PTB-associated comorbidities of gestational diabetes (GDM) and hypertensive disorders in pregnancy. Preterm births secondary to these comorbidities occur in both spontaneous and medically induced deliveries and across all gestational ages. When removing women with the comorbidities, a second relationship reveals that appears to be due to obesity per se (Table 12.2). This relationship is mostly in the very preterm deliveries. Based on these studies, it is suggested that initiatives and intervention to reduce obesity are important strategies to reduce both spontaneous and medically induced PTB. Considering the high morbidity and mortality associated with extreme preterm-delivered infants, even small differences in risk may have consequences for future outcomes.

This chapter goes through a number of lifestyle intervention studies in obese pregnant women and the considerations about the difficulties in reducing clinical complications. Furthermore, the need for future clinical trials with focus on different aspects of PTB as a complex phenomenon is discussed.

12.2 Lifestyle Intervention in Obese Pregnant Women

Pregnancy offers the opportunity to manage or prevent obesity as many women are concerned with the health of their babies during pregnancy and are in frequent contact with their healthcare professionals. Excessive gestational weight gain (GWG) is associated with increased risk of maternal and fetal complications as well as postpartum weight retention. A recent meta-analysis found that excessive weight, also in the normal weight women, influences offspring obesity over the short and long term (Fig. 12.2) [15].

A number of clinical trials about lifestyle intervention in overweight and obese women have been published. The majority of these studies have focused on lifestyle changes including dietary or physical activity or a combination of both attempts. Several of the studies have used GWG as the primary outcome and/or whether women gained below, within, or above the American Institute of Medicine (IOM) recommendations on GWG. The IOM recommendations were revised in 2009 suggesting overweight women to gain 7–11.5 kg and obese women to gain 5–9 kg during pregnancy (Table 12.3) [16]. Most studies have not been powered to look at the clinical maternal and neonatal outcomes.

Table 12.2 Spontaneous preterm labor in women without hypertensive and diabetic disease [5]

	22–27 weeks[b]		28–31 weeks		32–36 weeks	
BMI[a]	*n* (%)	OR (95 % CI)	*n* (%)	OR (95 % CI)	*n* (%)	OR (95 % CI)
Normal (18.5 to <25)						
California	785 (0.15)	1 (ref)	1,164 (0.23)	1 (ref)	12 954 (2.56)	1 (ref)
Sweden[c]	679 (0.07)	1 (ref)	1,151 (0.12)	1 (ref)	19 855 (2.03)	1 (ref)
Overweight (25 to <30)						
California	481 (0.18)	**1.13 (1.01, 1.27)**	553 (0.21)	**0.85 (0.77, 0.94)**	6,166 (2.29)	**0.85 (0.82, 0.87)**
Sweden	319 (0.09)	**1.20 (1.04, 1.38)**	394 (0.11)	0.91 (0.81, 1.03)	6,813 (1.88)	**0.92 (0.89, 0.94)**
Obesity I (30 to <35)						
California	305 (0.25)	**1.58 (1.38, 1.80)**	253 (0.21)	**0.84 (0.73, 0.96)**	2,787 (2.27)	**0.82 (0.79, 0.86)**
Sweden	100 (0.10)	**1.25 (1.01, 1.56)**	142 (0.14)	1.07 (0.89, 1.29)	1,902 (1.85)	**0.86 (0.82, 0.90)**
Obesity II (35 to <40)						
California	128 (0.28)	**1.79 (1.48,2.16)**	103 (0.23)	0.92 (0.75, 1.13)	979 (2.17)	**0.78 (0.73, 0.84)**
Sweden	39 (0.14)	**1.62 (1.15, 2.26)**	42 (0.15)	1.09 (0.79, 1.50)	548 (1.96)	**0.86 (0.78, 0.94)**
Obesity III (40 +)						
California	84 (0.36)	**2.21 (1.76, 2.77)**	51 (032)	0.86 (0.65, 1.14)	515 (2.22)	**0.79 (0.72, 0.86)**
Sweden	19 (0.21)	**2.38 (1.48, 3.81)**	11 (0.12)	0.79 (0.42, 1.48)	167 (1.88)	**0.80 (0.69, 0.94)**

Bold numbers are significant at $p \leq 0.05$

[a]BMI in California based on measured height and reported prepregnancy weight; OR risk adjusted for maternal age, parity, education, maternal height, race/ethnicity, and prenatal care; BMI in Sweden based on measured weight and reported height at the initial first trimester visit; OR risk adjusted for maternal age, parity, education, maternal height, country of birth, smoking, and year of birth

[b]Weeks of gestation

[c]Swedish data from Cnattingius et al. [13], e-table 6, information on BMI from the first trimester

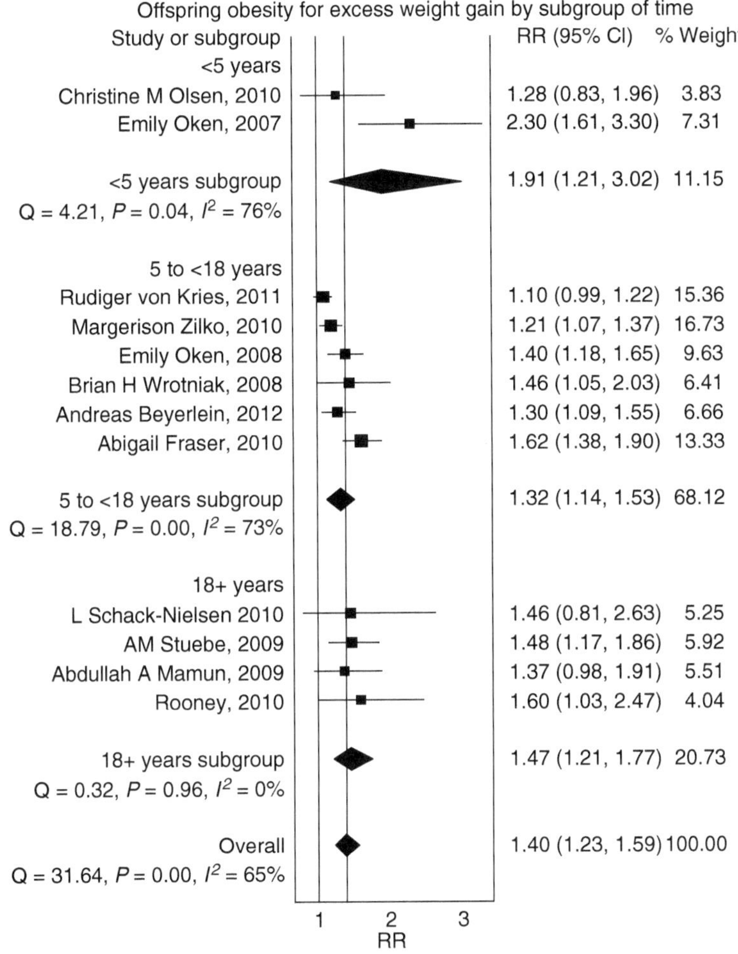

Fig. 12.2 Pooled estimates of offspring obesity due to maternal excess weight gain during pregnancy by quality effect model [15]

Table 12.3 WHO's BMI classification

BMI (kg/m^2)	Classification
<18.5	Underweight
18.5–24.9	Normal weight
25–29.9	Overweight
≥30	Obesity
30–34.9	Obesity class I
35–39.9	Obesity class II
≥40	Obesity class III

12.2.1 The Australian LIMIT Study

The Australian LIMIT study is the so far the largest published randomized controlled trial (RCT) with 2,212 overweight or obese pregnant women included [17]. Women randomized to lifestyle intervention were provided with dietary advices and individual diet plans and were encouraged to exercise. The behavioral strategies were provided during a face-to-face visit after inclusion and in gestational week 28 with a research dietician and followed up by three personal phone calls in between. The study did not succeed in reducing infants born large for gestational age (LGA) which was the primary outcome. Furthermore, there was no significant reduction in GWG between groups. But they found a significant reduction in the risk of birth weight above 4.5 kg, a reduction in respiratory distress in the neonates, as well as a shorter length of postnatal hospitalization. They also found a 26 % reduction in PTB and a 53 % reduction in preterm primary rupture of the membranes (PPROM), although these differences did not reach statistical significance [18].

12.2.2 The Irish ROLO Study

In the ROLO study (Randomized Control trial of low glycemic index diet to prevent macrosomia in euglycemic women) in Ireland, 800 euglycemic pregnant women in all BMI categories were randomized to receive low glycemic index and healthy eating diary advice in a group session before 22 weeks of gestation or to a standard control group [19]. Based on a 3-day food diary during each trimester, the intervention group had a significantly lower energy intake and reduced intake of food with high glycemic index. The intervention group had significantly lower GWG (kg) compared to the control group mean 11.5±4.2 vs. 12.6±4.4 kg, $p=0.003$ and a lower percentage of women in the intervention group exceeded the IOM recommendations on GWG. No difference in birth weight or neonatal abdominal circumference was seen. A lower neonatal waist circumference/length ratio was reported in the intervention, suggesting that a low glycemic index food intake limited central adiposity [20].

12.2.3 The Danish LiP Study

Among one of the most comprehensive randomized controlled trials on obese pregnant women is the Danish LiP (Lifestyle in Pregnancy) study [21]. In total, 360 obese pregnant women were included and randomized to intervention or control before 14 weeks of gestational age. Women randomized to intervention group received four individual diet counseling sessions during pregnancy and an exercise program consisting of aerobic classes (1 h weekly), free fitness membership during pregnancy, and exercise-motivating initiatives. The intervention group had significantly lower GWG (kg) compared to the control group (median [IQ-range]): 7.0 [4.7–10.6] vs. 8.6 [5.7–11.5]) ($p=0.01$). No significant differences in the clinical outcomes with respect to preeclampsia or pregnancy-induced hypertension, gestational diabetes, cesarean section, large for gestational age (LGA) infants, and admission to the neonatal intensive care unit were found. The study measured a number of metabolic outcomes throughout pregnancy and found that lifestyle intervention resulted in attenuation of the physiologic pregnancy-induced insulin resistance [22]. The intervention had no effect on duration of breastfeeding or postpartum weight retention [23]. The study is the first pregnancy intervention trial to publish detailed follow-up in the offspring, showing no anthropometric or metabolic effects at 2.5–3 years of age [24, 25].

12.2.4 The Danish TOP study

The TOP study (Treating Obesity in Pregnancy) is another Danish RCT with 425 obese pregnant women randomized into three intervention arms with physical activity (pedometer), physical activity and dietary counseling (dietician every second week), or control group [26]. Renault et al. found that physical activity intervention assessed by pedometer with or without dietary intervention reduced the GWG significantly compared to controls. They found no differences in any of the obstetric or neonatal outcomes. The study reported only a few cases of very preterm and preterm deliveries without any difference between groups.

12.2.5 Single-Center Interventional Studies

A number of other studies have focused on GWG and found different results. Wolff et al. [27], Claesson et al. [28], and Thornton et al. [29] reported significantly lower GWG in the intervention groups of obese women compared to controls, whereas Jeffries showed that overweight – but not obese women – gained significantly less weight after lifestyle intervention [30]. Quinlivan et al. [31] and Asbee et al. [32] succeeded in limiting GWG in women in the intervention group with mixed BMI categories. The "Fit for Delivery Study" by Phelan et al., a low-intensity behavioral RCT with 410 normal and overweight to obese women in the USA, found that the intervention significantly decreased the percentage of normal weight women who exceeded the 1990 Institute of Medicine (IOM) recommendations on GWG, but did not significantly affect GWG in overweight and obese women [33]. Olson's group reported significantly lower GWG in a subgroup of low-income women only [34]. Regarding obstetric outcomes, Quinlivan et al. found a significant reduction in GDM in the intervention group [31], Asbee reported a significant reduction in emergency cesarean delivery in the intervention group [32], and Luoto found a significant reduction in birth weight [35]. In a Belgian RCT from Guelinckx et al., a less intensive lifestyle education from nutritionists did not significantly affect GWG [6]. However, a later Belgian RCT found a significant reduction in GWG in the intervention group receiving antenatal lifestyle intervention focusing on mental and physical health [36].

Randomized controlled trials focusing on physical exercise only have evaluated on the effect of exercise intervention on GWG [37–40]. In these trials the group of exercising women had less GWG compared to control groups. However, these GWG differences were insignificant probably due to small sample sizes. A large Norwegian RCT with 855 healthy women reported results from a 12-week exercise program performed during the second trimester [41]. The primary aim of the study was to prevent GDM, but no effect was seen between intervention and control groups.

The use of online or electronic pregnancy interventions as a new and innovative initiative has not been much reported. To address this, the "e-Moms of Rochester" in the USA was developed and implemented in a RCT as an e-health intervention including a website and mobile phone applications [42]. Included in the intervention were a weight gain tracker and diet and physical activity goal-setting tools. The intervention had the highest engagement in high-income women in general but reached a relatively large group among minority and low-income women as well. A pilot study with SMS texts promoting appropriate GWG showed that this is a promising vehicle for behavior change among pregnant women [43].

12.2.6 Meta-Analysis and Systematic Reviews on Gestational Weight Gain Trials

Furthermore, a number of systematic reviews and meta-analysis have been performed recently. From these, we can conclude that despite the magnitude of the clinical problem with obesity in pregnancy and despite considerable efforts set in to prevent complications, we still do not have any specific evidence-based intervention to recommend. This knowledge gap is important to address in future studies. The latest systematic reviews consistently conclude that antenatal intervention is associated with restricted GWG [44–47], and it seems that dietary intervention was associated with the greatest reduction in GWG. Intervention might reduce the risk of preeclampsia and GDM, but this is not shown consistently. Furthermore, it is concluded that existing studies are of low to moderate quality, and therefore results should be interpreted with caution. Ongoing individual patient data (IPD) meta-analysis has provided data from 36 collaborators joining the network of international Weight Management in Pregnancy (iWIP) collaborative group [48]. Results from more than 9,000 women participating in RCTs about weight management in pregnancy will be included. The primary outcome of the study is GWG, but a number of secondary outcomes will be analyzed as well. Preterm delivery is one of the issues that will be addressed. The IPD meta-analysis will allow identifying and subsequently targeting the intervention to those groups that shows benefit with interventions in pregnancy with the so far best powered sample size.

Importantly, the beneficial effects as concluded from the mentioned studies need balancing against potential adverse outcomes as SGA, low birth weight, stillbirth, etc. From the performed studies, there has been no reporting of any adverse effects to the intervention programs.

12.2.7 Ongoing Interventional Trials on Gestational Weight Gain

Well-powered and comprehensive interventional trials are ongoing, and results are awaited. The UPBEAT study (UK Pregnancy Better Eating and Activity Trial) is a RCT designed to improve glycemic control and with the primary aim to reduce GDM and LGA [49]. The study randomizes more than 1,500 obese pregnant women into a behavioral intervention comprising dietary and physical activity changes. The DALI study (vitamin D and lifestyle intervention for gestational diabetes mellitus prevention) is a European multicenter trial with almost 900 obese pregnant women [50]. The intervention is based on coaching using the principles of motivational interviewing with focus on diet and physical activity and with an arm adding vitamin D or placebo. Primary outcome measures are GWG, fasting glucose, and insulin sensitivity. The Australian SPRING study (the Study of Probiotics IN the prevention of Gestational diabetes) is a RCT of probiotics in the prevention of GDM in 540 overweight and obese pregnant women [51]. Preterm birth is a secondary outcome in all these mentioned ongoing trials. However, the specific details of PTB are not predefined in the published protocols.

The RCTs listed above targeted and measured different lifestyle behaviors and interventions. Some studies included interventional force to behavioral changes, dietary habits, and physical activities, from the low-intensity behavioral studies to rather intense and repeated individual counseling and exercises. The inconsistency in setting, BMI, and intervention type and intensity makes comparison difficult. Furthermore, the low sample size in most of the performed studies makes it difficult to conclude on the clinical effects of intervention. Other reasons for lack of clinical effect may be the fact that intervention trials attract the healthiest women and not always representing the background population of overweight and obese pregnant women. Blinding of the intervention is not possible in most cases; thus, controls are motivated and aware of the ongoing intervention and may be influenced on lifestyle due to that. Another important issue is that interventions beginning in the second trimester, as most of the studies, may be all too late to overcome the early programming and preconceptional unfavorable metabolic state. The short period of pregnancy may be too short a window to change the implications of preexisting obesity. This fact may indeed be relevant for the risk of very preterm delivery.

A number of studies and clinical trials have been done toward the prediction and prevention of spontaneous PTB. Most clinical trials published have been on the administration of vaginal progesterone to women with a short cervix, the use of progesterone in women with a prior spontaneous preterm delivery, cervical cerclage to women with prior spontaneous delivery, and the use of antibiotics and tocolytics [9]. In a recent systematic review of interventions for PTB prevention, Meher and Alfiveric found that among 103 RCTs, no fewer than 72 different outcomes were reported [52], and this is a serious hindrance to progress in research and makes it difficult to draw useful conclusion about the clinical management and prevention of PTB. Based on that, the CROWN (CoRe Outcomes in WomeN's health) initiative has started [53]. In the CROWN collaboration, more than 50 editors and medical journals have come together to support researchers in the development of a set of core outcomes lists to be used in future studies when reporting on outcomes from RCTs (www.crowne-initiative.org). These outcomes are important to recognize and consider when planning future RCTs also on the managing of obesity in the prevention of PTB.

Conclusion

Lifestyle intervention in obese pregnant women may have the potential to limit the gestational weight gain which is important for reducing postpartum weight, limiting pregestational weight in the next pregnancy as well as the future weight trajectory. High-quality evidence proves the relationship between overweight, obesity, and preterm birth. However, interventional studies on diet and lifestyle have not been successful in reducing maternal and neonatal outcomes as PTB, GDM, preeclampsia, and macrosomia. Complications may all be associated with an unfavorable metabolic milieu in early gestation, and thus, interventions beginning in the second trimester might be too late and too short to overcome the negative impact of an early dysmetabolic condition. No lifestyle intervention studies in overweight and obese women have been designed with the specific primary aim to reduce the risk of spontaneous preterm delivery, and the existing intervention studies have not been powered to look into different outcomes about PTB. Results from the upcoming individual patient data meta-analysis on weight management in pregnancy (iWIP) will probably be able to shed light to some of the above-listed questions. Future intervention studies should carefully consider reporting and analyzing outcomes concerning PTB in a more detailed phenotypic way and not only reporting the simple dichotomy of birth before 37 completed weeks of gestation. Efforts should be considered to optimize pregestational bodyweight and the metabolic conditions before conception. Prevention of spontaneous PTB in obese women should be multidisciplinary and involve dieticians, physiotherapists, psychologists, endocrinologists, and obstetricians.

References

1. Ovesen P, Rasmussen S, Kesmodel U. Effect of prepregnancy maternal overweight and obesity on pregnancy outcome. Obstet Gynecol. 2011;118(2, Part 1):305–12.
2. Dodd JM, Grivell RM, Nguyen AM, Chan A, Robinson JS. Maternal and perinatal health outcomes by body mass index category. Aust N Z J Obstet Gynaecol. 2011;51(2):136–40.
3. Webber L, Divajeva D, Marsh T, McPherson K, Brown M, Galea G, et al. The future burden of obesity-related diseases in the 53 WHO European-Region countries and the impact of effective interventions: a modelling study. BMJ Open. 2014;4(7):e004787.
4. Wang YC, McPherson K, Marsh T, Gortmaker SL, Brown M. Health and economic burden of the projected obesity trends in the USA and the UK. Lancet. 2011;378(9793):815–25.
5. Gould JB, Mayo J, Shaw GM, Stevenson DK. Swedish and American studies show that initiatives to decrease maternal obesity could play a key role in reducing preterm birth. Acta Paediatr. 2014;103(6):586–91.
6. Smith GC, Shah I, Pell JP, Crossley JA, Dobbie R. Maternal obesity in early pregnancy and risk of spontaneous and elective preterm deliveries: a retrospective cohort study. Am J Public Health. 2007;97(1):157–62.

7. Flegal KM, Carroll MD, Kit BK, Ogden CL. Prevalence of obesity and trends in the distribution of body mass index among US adults, 1999–2010. JAMA. 2012;307(5):491–7.
8. Heslehurst N, Rankin J, Wilkinson JR, Summerbell CD. A nationally representative study of maternal obesity in England, UK: trends in incidence and demographic inequalities in 619 323 births, 1989–2007. Int J Obes (Lond). 2010;34(3):420–8.
9. Romero R, Dey SK, Fisher SJ. Preterm labor: one syndrome, many causes. Science. 2014;345(6198):760–5.
10. Torloni MR, Betran AP, Daher S, Widmer M, Dolan SM, Menon R, et al. Maternal BMI and preterm birth: a systematic review of the literature with meta-analysis. J Matern Fetal Neonatal Med. 2009;22(11):957–70.
11. McDonald SD, Han Z, Mulla S, Beyene J. Overweight and obesity in mothers and risk of preterm birth and low birth weight infants: systematic review and meta-analyses. BMJ. 2010;341:c3428.
12. Khatibi A, Brantsaeter AL, Sengpiel V, Kacerovsky M, Magnus P, Morken NH, et al. Prepregnancy maternal body mass index and preterm delivery. Am J Obstet Gynecol. 2012; 207(3):212.e1–7.
13. Cnattingius S, Villamor E, Johansson S, Edstedt Bonamy AK, Persson M, Wikstrom AK, et al. Maternal obesity and risk of preterm delivery. JAMA. 2013;309(22):2362–70.
14. Shaw GM, Wise PH, Mayo J, Carmichael SL, Ley C, Lyell DJ, et al. Maternal prepregnancy body mass index and risk of spontaneous preterm birth. Paediatr Perinat Epidemiol. 2014; 28(4):302–11.
15. Mamun AA, Mannan M, Doi SA. Gestational weight gain in relation to offspring obesity over the life course: a systematic review and bias-adjusted meta-analysis. Obes Rev. 2014;15(4):338–47.
16. Institute of Medicine. Weight gain during pregnancy: reexamining the guidelines. Washington, DC: The National Academy Press; 2009.
17. Dodd JM, Cramp C, Sui Z, Yelland LN, Deussen AR, Grivell RM, et al. The effects of antenatal dietary and lifestyle advice for women who are overweight or obese on maternal diet and physical activity: the LIMIT randomised trial. BMC Med. 2014;12(1):161.
18. Dodd JM, McPhee AJ, Turnbull D, Yelland LN, Deussen AR, Grivell RM, et al. The effects of antenatal dietary and lifestyle advice for women who are overweight or obese on neonatal health outcomes: the LIMIT randomised trial. BMC Med. 2014;12(1):163.
19. McGowan CA, Walsh JM, Byrne J, Curran S, McAuliffe FM. The influence of a low glycemic index dietary intervention on maternal dietary intake, glycemic index and gestational weight gain during pregnancy: a randomized controlled trial. Nutr J. 2013;12(1):140.
20. Horan MK, McGowan CA, Gibney ER, Donnelly JM, McAuliffe FM. Maternal low glycaemic index diet, fat intake and postprandial glucose influences neonatal adiposity–secondary analysis from the ROLO study. Nutr J. 2014;13:78.
21. Vinter CA, Jensen DM, Ovesen P, Beck-Nielsen H, Jorgensen JS. The LiP (Lifestyle in Pregnancy) study: a randomized controlled trial of lifestyle intervention in 360 obese pregnant women. Diabetes Care. 2011;34(12):2502–7.
22. Vinter CA, Jorgensen JS, Ovesen P, Beck-Nielsen H, Skytthe A, Jensen DM. Metabolic effects of lifestyle intervention in obese pregnant women. Results from the randomized controlled trial 'Lifestyle in Pregnancy' (LiP). Diabet Med. 2014;31(11):1323–30.
23. Vinter CA, Jensen DM, Ovesen P, Beck-Nielsen H, Tanvig M, Lamont RF, et al. Postpartum weight retention and breastfeeding among obese women from the randomized controlled Lifestyle in Pregnancy (LiP) trial. Acta Obstet Gynecol Scand. 2014;93(8):794–801.
24. Tanvig M, Vinter CA, Jorgensen JS, Wehberg S, Ovesen PG, Lamont RF, et al. Anthropometrics and body composition by dual energy X-ray in children of obese women: a follow-up of a randomized controlled trial (the Lifestyle in Pregnancy and Offspring [LiPO] study). PLoS One. 2014;9(2):e89590.
25. Tanvig M, Vinter CA, Jorgensen JS, Wehberg S, Ovesen PG, Beck-Nielsen H, et al. Effects of lifestyle intervention in pregnancy and anthropometrics at birth on offspring metabolic profile at 2.8 years – results from the Lifestyle in Pregnancy and Offspring (LiPO) study. J Clin Endocrinol Metab. 2015;100(1):175–83. doi:10.1210/jc.2014-2675.

26. Renault KM, Norgaard K, Nilas L, Carlsen EM, Cortes D, Pryds O, et al. The Treatment of Obese Pregnant Women (TOP) study: a randomized controlled trial of the effect of physical activity intervention assessed by pedometer with or without dietary intervention in obese pregnant women. Am J Obstet Gynecol. 2014;210(2):134.e1–9.
27. Wolff S, Legarth J, Vangsgaard K, Toubro S, Astrup A. A randomized trial of the effects of dietary counseling on gestational weight gain and glucose metabolism in obese pregnant women. Int J Obes (Lond). 2008;32(3):495–501.
28. Claesson IM, Sydsjo G, Brynhildsen J, Cedergren M, Jeppsson A, Nystrom F, et al. Weight gain restriction for obese pregnant women: a case-control intervention study. BJOG. 2008; 115(1):44–50.
29. Thornton YS, Smarkola C, Kopacz SM, Ishoof SB. Perinatal outcomes in nutritionally monitored obese pregnant women: a randomized clinical trial. J Natl Med Assoc. 2009;101(6): 569–77.
30. Jeffries K, Shub A, Walker SP, Hiscock R, Permezel M. Reducing excessive weight gain in pregnancy: a randomised controlled trial. Med J Aust. 2009;191(8):429–33.
31. Quinlivan JA, Lam LT, Fisher J. A randomised trial of a four-step multidisciplinary approach to the antenatal care of obese pregnant women. Aust N Z J Obstet Gynaecol. 2011;51(2):141–6.
32. Asbee SM, Jenkins TR, Butler JR, White J, Elliot M, Rutledge A. Preventing excessive weight gain during pregnancy through dietary and lifestyle counseling: a randomized controlled trial. Obstet Gynecol. 2009;113(2 Pt 1):305–12.
33. Phelan S, Phipps MG, Abrams B, Darroch F, Schaffner A, Wing RR. Randomized trial of a behavioral intervention to prevent excessive gestational weight gain: the Fit for Delivery Study. Am J Clin Nutr. 2011;93(4):772–9.
34. Olson CM, Strawderman MS, Reed RG. Efficacy of an intervention to prevent excessive gestational weight gain. Am J Obstet Gynecol. 2004;191(2):530–6.
35. Luoto R, Kinnunen TI, Aittasalo M, Kolu P, Raitanen J, Ojala K, et al. Primary prevention of gestational diabetes mellitus and large-for-gestational-age newborns by lifestyle counseling: a cluster-randomized controlled trial. PLoS Med. 2011;8(5):e1001036.
36. Bogaerts AF, Devlieger R, Nuyts E, Witters I, Gyselaers W, Van den Bergh BR. Effects of lifestyle intervention in obese pregnant women on gestational weight gain and mental health: a randomized controlled trial. Int J Obes (Lond). 2013;37(6):814–21.
37. Santos IA, Stein R, Fuchs SC, Duncan BB, Ribeiro JP, Kroeff LR, et al. Aerobic exercise and submaximal functional capacity in overweight pregnant women: a randomized trial. Obstet Gynecol. 2005;106(2):243–9.
38. Ong MJ, Guelfi KJ, Hunter T, Wallman KE, Fournier PA, Newnham JP. Supervised home-based exercise may attenuate the decline of glucose tolerance in obese pregnant women. Diabetes Metab. 2009;35(5):418–21.
39. Barakat R, Lucia A, Ruiz JR. Resistance exercise training during pregnancy and newborn's birth size: a randomised controlled trial. Int J Obes (Lond). 2009;33(9):1048–57.
40. Nascimento S, Surita F, Parpinelli M, Siani S, Pinto ES. The effect of an antenatal physical exercise programme on maternal/perinatal outcomes and quality of life in overweight and obese pregnant women: a randomised clinical trial. BJOG. 2011;118(12):1455–63.
41. Stafne SN, Salvesen KA, Romundstad PR, Eggebo TM, Carlsen SM, Morkved S. Regular exercise during pregnancy to prevent gestational diabetes: a randomized controlled trial. Obstet Gynecol. 2012;119(1):29–36.
42. Graham ML, Uesugi KH, Niederdeppe J, Gay GK, Olson CM. The theory, development, and implementation of an e-intervention to prevent excessive gestational weight gain: e-Moms Roc. Telemed J E Health. 2014;20(12):1135–42.
43. Pollak KI, Alexander SC, Bennett G, Lyna P, Coffman CJ, Bilheimer A, et al. Weight-related SMS texts promoting appropriate pregnancy weight gain: a pilot study. Patient Educ Couns. 2014;97(2):256–60.
44. Tanentsapf I, Heitmann BL, Adegboye AR. Systematic review of clinical trials on dietary interventions to prevent excessive weight gain during pregnancy among normal weight, overweight and obese women. BMC Pregnancy Childbirth. 2011;11(1):81.

45. Oteng-Ntim E, Varma R, Croker H, Poston L, Doyle P. Lifestyle interventions for overweight and obese pregnant women to improve pregnancy outcome: systematic review and meta-analysis. BMC Med. 2012;10:47. doi:10.1186/1741-7015-10-47.:47-10.
46. Thangaratinam S, Rogozinska E, Jolly K, Glinkowski S, Roseboom T, Tomlinson JW, et al. Effects of interventions in pregnancy on maternal weight and obstetric outcomes: meta-analysis of randomised evidence. BMJ. 2012;344:e2088. doi:10.1136/bmj.e2088.:e2088.
47. Agha M, Agha RA, Sandell J. Interventions to reduce and prevent obesity in pre-conceptual and pregnant women: a systematic review and meta-analysis. PLoS One. 2014;9(5):e95132.
48. Ruifrok AE, Rogozinska E, van Poppel MN, Rayanagoudar G, Kerry S, de Groot CJ, et al. Study protocol: differential effects of diet and physical activity based interventions in pregnancy on maternal and fetal outcomes-individual patient data (IPD) meta-analysis and health economic evaluation. Syst Rev. 2014;3(1):131.
49. Poston L, Briley AL, Barr S, Bell R, Croker H, Coxon K, et al. Developing a complex intervention for diet and activity behaviour change in obese pregnant women (the UPBEAT trial); assessment of behavioural change and process evaluation in a pilot randomised controlled trial. BMC Pregnancy Childbirth. 2013;13(1):148.
50. Jelsma JG, van Poppel MN, Galjaard S, Desoye G, Corcoy R, Devlieger R, et al. DALI: Vitamin D and lifestyle intervention for gestational diabetes mellitus (GDM) prevention: an European multicentre, randomised trial – study protocol. BMC Pregnancy Childbirth. 2013;13:142. doi:10.1186/1471-2393-13-142.:142-13.
51. Nitert MD, Barrett HL, Foxcroft K, Tremellen A, Wilkinson S, Lingwood B, et al. SPRING: an RCT study of probiotics in the prevention of gestational diabetes mellitus in overweight and obese women. BMC Pregnancy Childbirth. 2013;13:50.
52. Meher S, Alfirevic Z. Choice of primary outcomes in randomised trials and systematic reviews evaluating interventions for preterm birth prevention: a systematic review. BJOG. 2014;121(10):1188–94; discussion 95–6.
53. Khan K, Belizan JM. The CROWN initiative: journal editors invite researchers to develop core outcomes in women's health. Reprod Health. 2014;11:42.

Part IV

Future Dietary Strategies to Reduce Inflammation and Metabolic Syndrome by an Healthy Eating Plate

Maternal Diet, Developmental Origins, and the Intergenerational Transmission of Cardiometabolic Traits: A Window of Opportunity for the Prevention of Metabolic Syndrome?

13

Daniel C. Benyshek

Contents

13.1 Introduction: Maternal Prenatal Diet and the Developmental Origins of Health and Disease

During the late 1980s, British researchers were developing a new hypothesis about the causes of cardiometabolic disease in adults. Their theory pointed to critical windows of growth and development in utero in the etiology of many cardiometabolic disorders. Eventually named the "thrifty phenotype" hypothesis [1], it offered an alternative explanation to Neel's highly influential "thrifty genotype" hypothesis as

D.C. Benyshek, PhD
Department of Anthropology, University of Nevada, Las Vegas, NV, USA
e-mail: daniel.benyshek@unlv.edu

E. Ferrazzi, B. Sears (eds.), *Metabolic Syndrome and Complications of Pregnancy: The Potential Preventive Role of Nutrition*,
DOI 10.1007/978-3-319-16853-1_13

means of explaining obesity and cardiometabolic health problems—especially among the world's highest-risk populations. Hales and Barker's alternative hypothesis moved beyond simplistic (and inadequate) genetic or lifestyle explanations and eventually led to a new paradigm for understanding chronic disease risk. Their more integrated approach incorporates genetic heritability and lifestyle factors such as diet and activity levels into human health analysis but also recognizes the powerful role of *developmental plasticity*, the ability of a gene to generate a range of possible phenotypes depending on environmental experience. Indeed, life history theorists in evolutionary ecology and comparative biology were already familiar with these developmentally plastic biophysiological capacities, processes, and associated consequences [2, 3], but up until this time, they had largely been ignored in biomedicine. Now referred to as the Developmental Origins of Health and Disease (DOHaD), human developmental plasticity research within a biomedical context includes scientists from a broad range of disciplines. The paradigm has been especially useful in understanding the etiology of obesity and related cardiometabolic disorders such as metabolic syndrome.

A great deal of DOHaD research has focused on the investigation of the life course diet sequence associated with "nutrition transitions" in developing and developed countries around the world. Accordingly, there are two primary pathways associated with the developmental origins of cardiometabolic disease: the "famine" pathway and the "feast" pathway [4]. Much of the early DOHaD research investigated the famine developmental pathway to cardiometabolic disorders. The famine pathway is distinguished by a poor nutrition diet early in life (e.g., maternal undernutrition during pregnancy and while nursing), followed by energetically adequate diet in adulthood. Environments where this life course diet sequence has been most noted are in rapidly developing countries such as India where urbanization is spreading quickly [5] and among poor minority populations in developed countries [4]. The famine developmental pathway is further distinguished by an array of growth and adult phenotype characteristics, including low birth weight (especially < 2.5 kg), "catch-up" growth and an earlier adiposity rebound in childhood, abdominal obesity, dyslipidemia, hypertension, insulin resistance, and glucose intolerance in adulthood [4, 6].

Spurred by a worsening global obesity epidemic in recent years, the alternative feast developmental pathway to cardiometabolic disorders is increasingly receiving more attention. This pathway is typified by nutritional excess in early life (e.g., maternal high fat/sugar/energy diets), followed by a "Western" high-energy/low-fiber diet in adulthood [4, 7, 8]. The critical "early" nutrition/metabolic environment factors underpinning this dysregulated cardiometabolic developmental pathway go well beyond a mother's nutrition during pregnancy and nursing or formula feeding [9–11]. Indeed, preconceptual obesity and excessive weight gain during pregnancy are now considered independent risk factors for overweight offspring and those who exhibit abdominal obesity [12–15]. The hallmarks of the feast developmental cardiometabolic pathway include both low and high birth weight (especially > 4.0 kg), adolescent and adult obesity, dyslipidemia, hypertension, insulin resistance, and glucose intolerance [4, 16–18]. In both the feast and famine developmental pathways, developmentally programmed adjustments to early nutritional conditions represent pathological cardiometabolic traits in the context of their adult nutritional environments. Furthermore, these adjustments signify important factors in recent global epidemiological shifts that are often not recognized in the "nutrition transition" model or in current conventional efforts to stop the worldwide obesity epidemic [19].

In the past, DOHaD research focused simply on the associations between maternal diet during pregnancy and while nursing (e.g., under-/overnutrition) and the subsequent risk of cardiometabolic dysfunction. Researchers today are looking beyond those well-established correlations to find more nuanced, causal processes at work. DOHaD research now includes how early developmental environments affect regulatory systems, organs, and tissues that play important roles in cardiometabolic functioning. Some of these studies include hormone regulatory systems (e.g., hormones such as insulin and leptin and their interaction with appetite regulation and energy metabolism) [20], the hypothalamic-pituitary-adrenal axis [21], adipose tissue signaling and metabolism [22], cellular mitochondria [23], the structure and function of the pancreas [24, 25], and vascular system [26, 27] and altered placental function [28].

Today, the forefront of research into the developmental origins of health and disease is epigenetics—the investigation of the primary mechanisms that drive developmental programming and its transmission from one generation to the next.

The fundamental principles of epigenetics are not new; in fact they were first theorized by Waddington in 1942 (he also coined the term) [29]. Yet, his ideas are only now being fully appreciated and applied. Modern epigenetics investigates the system that turns genes on and off in plants and animals. Indeed, the study of the developmental origins of health and disease owes much to epigenetics, as it provides the primary mechanism by which developmental programming works.

One of the many facets of epigenetics is chromatin modification (the complex of nucleic acids and histone proteins that make up chromosomes), including DNA methylation, histone, and protamine modification. Additionally, changes to noncoding RNAs have also recently been implicated in epigenetic effects (see [30]). Presently, DNA methylation is an aspect of epigenetics that is fairly well understood, although much still remains a mystery [31]. Methyl groups are organic compounds that attach to DNA and signal a cell to either use or ignore a particular gene. Methyl groups adhere to DNA or to histone or protamine proteins that form DNA structural units, and this process is called methylation. The process works by blocking the attachment of transcription factors and other signaling proteins, thereby insuring a gene stays turned off [32]. Conversely, the process of demethylation turns a gene on. The precise role of methylation, histone and protamine modifications, and other epigenetic mechanisms remain an important focus of much research, particularly in the developmental origins of health and disease and more generally in phenotypic plasticity (see [33, 34]). Given the focus of the present chapter, the discussion of epigenetics will be limited to the latest research involving the transmission of developmentally programmed traits to subsequent generations.

13.2 The Intergenerational Transmission of Developmentally Altered Cardiometabolic Traits: Epigenetics and Alternative Developmental Pathways

Both human and animal studies surmise that the effects of developmentally programmed traits may be transmitted to subsequent generations and are not solely limited to the generation that was initially involved in the study [35, 36]. In rodent subjects, developmentally programmed traits, such as insulin resistance, are initially produced by directly exposing the rodent to early environmental conditions (e.g., poor-quality maternal diet). Those traits are then found in subsequent generations of offspring that *have not* been exposed to the same environmental conditions (e.g., adequate maternal diet) although often the traits diminish with each successive new generation [37, 38]. This pattern points to a fairly stable and heritable phenotypically plastic response (i.e., epigenetic), instead of one mediated by changes in DNA sequence (i.e., genomic change). According to Drake and Lui [36], there are three possible mechanisms that bring about these multigenerational outcomes: those due to persistent early development environmental exposures generation after generation, a single exposure to a maternal environment that produces identical traits in successive generations, and epigenetic effects that are transmitted through the germline.

13.3 Exposure to Persistent Environmental Conditions

One scenario is that persistent environmental exposure during critical developmental stages over many generations results in the same developmentally programmed traits each time. For instance, some researchers have hypothesized that perpetual sociopolitical disruptions, prejudice, and economic disadvantages suffered by ethnic/racial minority populations represent repeated environmental exposures to multiple generations that result in developmentally programmed traits. Those traits may play a role in the cardiometabolic health problems rampant in these populations [39]. Benyshek and colleagues have argued that the political/economic hardships and poor nutritional health suffered by many Native Americans during the reservation era are the very environmental conditions that bring about cardiometabolic disease via developmentally programmed pathways and suggest reassessing the type 2 diabetes epidemic among Native Americans in this light [40]. Similarly, Kuzawa and Sweet [41] make this same case for the disproportionate cardiovascular disease cases among African-Americans in the USA, suggesting it may be associated with the adverse social and economic conditions they have endured for so many generations (Fig. 13.1a represents this mechanism schematically). Thus, persistent, "external" (e.g., ecological, economic) environmental conditions "encode" the same developmentally formative traits generation after generation. This creates, the authors say, a trend that appears to be inherited and, therefore, genetically based. Such trends could be largely developmental, however, and thus conceivably preventable.

Experimental animal studies have produced similar generational effects when environmental stressors are placed upon successive generations of offspring. In a

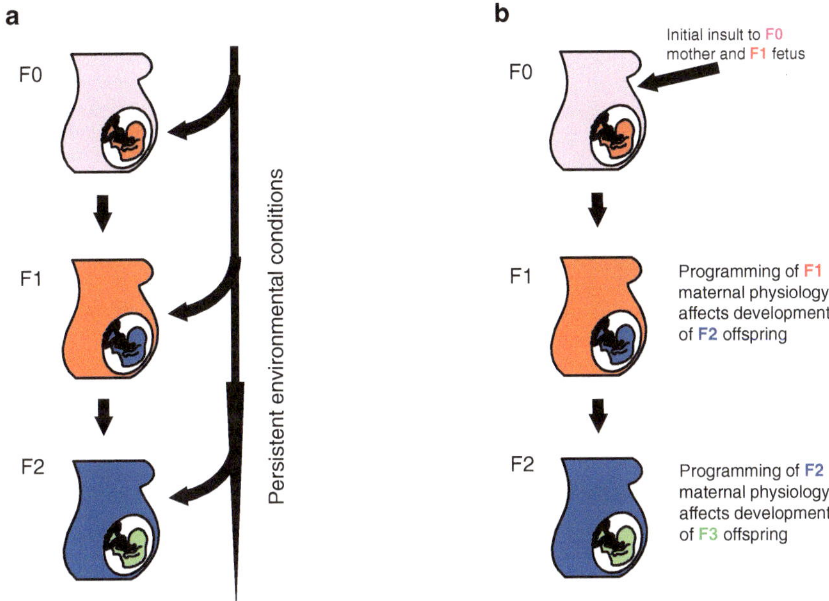

Fig. 13.1 Mechanisms for the intergenerational transmission of programming effects. (**a**) Persistence of an adverse external environment can result in the reproduction of the phenotype in multiple generations. (**b**) The induction of programmed effects in the F1 offspring following in utero exposure (e.g., programmed changes in maternal physiology or size) results in programmed effects on the developing F2 fetus and so on (Reproduced with permission Drake and Walker [35])

mouse study that used a persistent high-fat diet for each generation, F0 grandmothers and F1 mothers (all fed a high-fat diet during pregnancy and lactation) produced F2 male offspring that were also shown to be predisposed to obesity and hepatic steatosis [42]. In a study using rats that were overfed after birth, Plagemann and colleagues [43] purport an epigenetic model of obesity and the metabolic syndrome that is underpinned by the developmentally programmed dysregulation of hypothalamic body weight regulation. They conclude, based on their findings, that the "vicious intergenerative circle" of obesity and cardiometabolic disorders remains closed unless the maternal diet is modified during the nursing period ([43], p4974) (Fig. 13.1).

13.4 Maternal Environment Effects

Researchers have found that a single maternal (F0) environmental exposure can produce effects in F1 and F2 generation offspring via developmental programming. These observations are distinct from the developmentally programmed changes found only in the generations of offspring that are directly exposed to the stressed maternal environment (as discussed in the previous section). Thus, Skinner [44] has

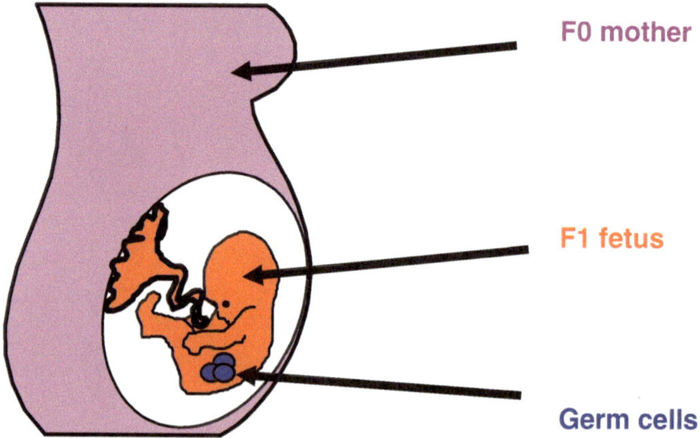

Fig. 13.2 Multigenerational exposure to an environmental effect. An environmental insult during pregnancy to a mother (F0 generation) might affect not only the developing fetus (F1 generation) but also the germ cells which will go on to form the F2 generation (Reproduced with permission Drake and Walker [35])

put forth that persistent exposure to environmental conditions should be referred to as a "multigenerational phenotype," distinguishable from "transgenerational inheritance" that is transmitted epigenetically via the germline (see below). In the case of the multigenerational phenotype, when a pregnant mother is consuming an inadequate, low-protein diet, three generations are effectively being exposed simultaneously to this dietary insult: the pregnant mother (F0), her fetal offspring (F1), and the primordial germ cells (PGCs)—the precursors of sperm and eggs—within the F1 fetus (Fig. 13.2).

As discussed previously, it has been well established in experimental animal studies and epidemiological literatures that a connection exists between low birth weight and subsequent adult risk for cardiometabolic syndrome [4, 45]. "Maternal constraint" was one of the first "maternal effects" studied by researchers. The maternal constraint of birth weight has been described in both maternal "supply" and "demand" terms [46]. Maternal constraint in terms of supply may be due to decreased uteroplacental blood flow, reduced blood volume, decreased oxygen-carrying capacity, prenatal nutrition, teratogens, and short birth intervals. Demand factors limiting fetal growth include such things as multiple gestations [47]. By using artificial insemination to cross small Shetland horses and large, draft, Shire horses, Walton and Hammond [48] demonstrated in their renowned crossbreeding study that offspring birth size was largely governed by the size of the gestating mother. In other words, smaller Shetland mothers gave birth to small foals regardless of parental genotype. A 37-year-long epidemiological study in Norway found concurring results. By analyzing birth weight, the researchers discovered that genetic factors accounted for only 31 % of birth weight variation [49]. Furthermore, several other population-based studies compared maternal birth weight and paternal birth weight with offspring birth weight and found the maternal effect to be considerably stronger [49–52], although there have been a few report findings to the contrary [53]. In the Cebu, Philippines, cohort study, however, maternal intergenerational birth weight correlations were not found to be stronger among taller women [50]. The authors surmised that reduced adult stature caused by a history of nutritional insufficiency did not lead to a further increased constraint of offspring birth weight. According to the authors, some of the mechanisms that might explain their findings include sex-linked genetic effects and indirect genetic, epigenetic, and shared environmental/cultural effects. It was noted that in every case the mechanism exerted its effect on birth weight for both the mother and child in utero [50]. In sum, maternal effects that disproportionately affect birth weight are complex and are probably influenced by a number of factors that reach well beyond adult maternal size and stature.

There is also corroborating evidence from human cohort studies concerning multigenerational maternal environment effects. In the Dutch "hunger winter" studies, it was found that mothers who were exposed to the famine during pregnancy (living on as little as 500 kcal/day) had female offspring (F1) with dysregulated lipid profiles (i.e., cholesterol and triglycerides) as opposed to offspring not exposed to famine conditions in utero [54]. They further found that the children of the exposed F1 females exhibited higher rates of neonatal obesity and were nearly twice as likely to develop cardiometabolic disease than the unexposed control group [55].

Multigenerational (i.e., F1, F2) effects have been documented through extensive experimental animal studies as well [36]. Using mostly rodent models, researchers have shown that a *single* (F0) maternal exposure generates cardiometabolic programming effects on F1 and F2 animals. A number of these studies restricted (F0) mothers to protein and/or energy diets during pregnancy and/or lactation and observed programmed effects in both F1 and F2 generation animals on insulin sensitivity and glucose tolerance [56–58], birth weight, blood pressure, kidney structure [59], and obesity [58]. Other studies exposed F0 mothers to excess glucocorticoids [60] or made surgical alterations to the placenta [61] and observed developmentally programmed effects on birth weight, glucose tolerance, and blood pressure.

Multigenerational effects linked to prenatal exposures to restrictive maternal diets are not the only models used in experiments of this kind. In feast pathway studies (as discussed above), researchers examined the cardiometabolic structure and function effects of maternal nutritional excess and/or obesity on offspring prior to conception, during pregnancy, and/or while nursing (see [8]). Studies have shown that *multigenerational* effects on obesity and other cardiometabolic traits can be tied to initial (F0) maternal nutritional excess. This environment during pregnancy influences body size and insulin sensitivity in both F1 and F2 offspring [62]. In an experiment utilizing mice, Gniuli et al. [63] report that a prenatal high-fat diet, especially if followed by a maternal high-fat diet while nursing, induces a "type 2 diabetes phenotype" in F1 offspring, which can then be transmitted to their F2 progeny, even if additional dietary insults are not provided. Indeed, the perinatal maternal nutritional environment alone has far-reaching implications. Srinivasan and colleagues [64] fed female rat pups a high-fat diet during the suckling period, resulting in obese adults. Their adult F2 offspring also became obese, even though their F1 mothers were fed a standard chow diet after weaning.

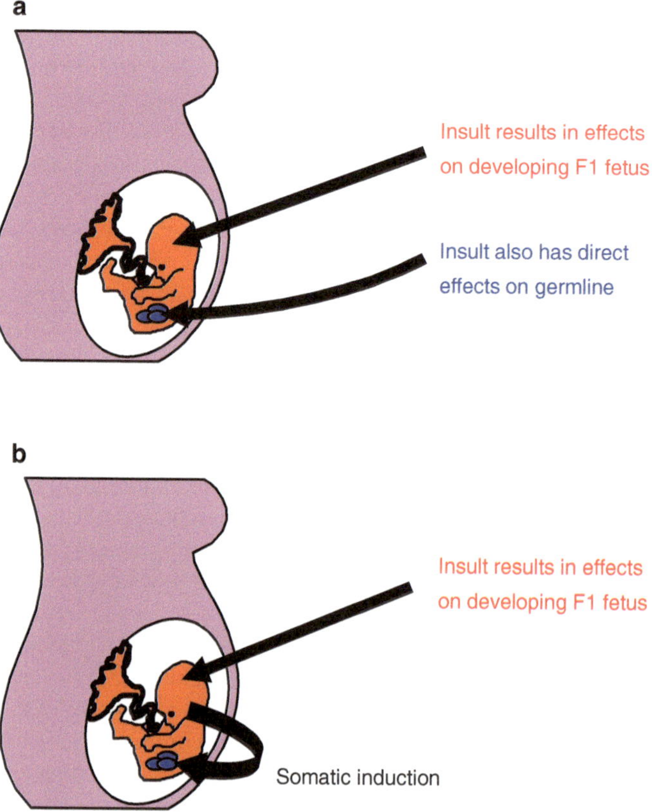

Fig. 13.3 Transmission of epigenetic effects through gametes. (**a**) An environmental exposure affects the developing F1 fetus but also has direct effects on the developing germ cells which form the F2 generation. (**b**) Alternatively, effects induced in the developing F1 fetus can be transmitted to the germ cells which will form the F2 generation (somatic induction) (Reproduced with permission Drake and Walker [35])

It remains unclear what mechanisms account for the intergenerational transmission of these developmentally programmed traits. Possible mechanisms include altered organ development, cellular signaling dysregulation, and epigenetic modifications. Perhaps, at least in some cases, the multigenerational programming effects of both the F1 and F2 generations are not due to the same, single maternal in utero exposure (e.g., F0 maternal low-protein diet) (Fig. 13.3). Alternatively, it could be that cardiometabolic dysfunction resulting from the early environment exposure of the F1 female gives rise to an altered intrauterine environment during her own pregnancy that is distinct from the one in which she was gestated (F0) but that also leads to the same developmentally programmed trait in her (F2) offspring. Indeed, some animal models of multigenerational transmission of glucose intolerance from F1 to F2 generations point to such a sequence. Several rodent studies have shown that glucose-intolerant, adult F1 animals whose mothers (F0) were fed a low-protein diet during pregnancy are insulin sensitive but have insufficient insulin secretory capacity as adults, which in turn results in glucose intolerance [65]. The glucose-intolerant adult (F2) offspring of these (F1) females, on the other hand (whose F1 mothers consumed a control diet during gestation/lactation), are insulin resistant (rather than insulin sensitive) and hyperinsulinemic (as opposed to insulin deficient) [56]. In this example, both F1 and F2 generation animals are glucose intolerant, apparently due to different developmental disruptions in glucose-insulin metabolism and due to distinct developmental programming pathways in the intrauterine environment. In this scenario, the intrauterine perturbation in one generation causes a metabolic cascade that leads to another (similar or dissimilar) cascade in the subsequent generation and so on (Fig. 13.1b).

Importantly, in most of the aforementioned multiple-generation animal studies, the research design did not include an F3 generation. Of the two studies that did include an F3 generation in their research design [59, 60], no evidence of transmission to F3 animals was found. The lack of F3 inheritance might suggest that the observed F1 and F2 effects were due to direct exposure (of the F1 fetus and F2 PGCs) in the (F0) intrauterine environment—lending some support to Skinner's notion of a "multigenerational phenotype" [44]. Both types of developmental programming inheritance may occur (Figs. 13.1b and 13.2).

13.5 Transgenerational Inheritance: Epigenetic Traits Transmissible Through the Germline

In order for developmentally programmed cardiometabolic traits to be transmitted to the F3 generation and subsequent generations after that (i.e., "transgenerational inheritance"), information about paternal and/or maternal exposure must be transmitted through the germline, since no direct exposure of the initial insult could exist for F3. Epigenetic inheritance research is now uncovering how this non-genomic inheritance may be possible in the germline when there are no changes in genetic structure (i.e., base pairs of DNA).

A relatively rare process of genomic imprinting was discovered in the 1980s [66], putting the epigenetic regulation of gene expression on the map. So although this mechanism has been recognized for some time, the possibility and importance of the transgenerational inheritance of epigenetic marks, and how it works, is only now beginning to be widely accepted and understood. Why did it take decades to come to light? The answer is that the traditional view in developmental biology and genetics held that epigenetic marks are erased and "reset" in the primordial germ cells (PGCs) in each generation. Since the epigenetic germline is reset, it allows the genetic regulatory system to be reestablished in each generation. This commonly known process has put the frequency and importance of epigenetic inheritance into doubt. However, new research discoveries have begun to alter that viewpoint [67, 68]. Through a process of chemical conversion and subsequent dilution during cell division, Hackett and colleagues [69] recently discovered how methylation marks are erased in mouse PGCs. They also determined how some (rare) methylation marks escape erasure, thereby providing a potential pathway for true transgenerational epigenetic inheritance. Researchers, in another breakthrough study, demonstrated that approximately 1 % of histone marks (located at key sequences with gene regulatory functions) remain in mouse sperm after cell differentiation, thereby furthering our nascent understanding of the inner workings of epigenetic inheritance [70].

These new findings may help us understand several epidemiological research discoveries that appear to reflect such processes at work in humans. In one such study, researchers analyzed three Swedish birth cohorts born in the late 1800s and early 1900s who experienced fluctuating food availability. The study's goal was to determine if food supply during the slow-growth phase (ages 8–2) of paternal grandfathers and grandmothers was linked to the risk of diabetes, cardiovascular disease, and longevity in their children and grandchildren. They discovered that low food intake by fathers during their slow-growth phase was associated with lower risk of diabetes and cardiovascular disease of sons. Conversely, an increased food intake during the paternal grandfather's slow-growth period was linked to increased risk for diabetes among grandsons [71, 72]. Food supply during the slow-growth phase of paternal grandfathers was associated with lifespan in grandsons, and likewise, food supply during fetal/infant life or the slow-growth period of paternal grandmothers was associated with lifespan in granddaughters [73].

The goal of Soubry and coworkers [74] was to determine if there is a relationship between parental obesity and DNA methylation at the insulin-like growth factor II (IGF-II) gene in their children (IFG-II is linked to a risk for obesity, gestational diabetes, and some forms of cancer). The researchers compared information about parental obesity to methylation patterns found in DNA from the umbilical cords of the fathers' newborn children. The results showed that the offspring of obese fathers had significantly lower DNA methylation at the IGF-II gene than did the children of nonobese fathers. The data augmented evidence for the transmission of epigenetic effects associated with obesity from males to their offspring.

Some animal studies have shown similar transgenerational effects. Throughout India, Southeast Asia, and Polynesia, chewing betel nuts is a popular practice. The betel nut contains the toxin nitrosamine and is known to increase risk for the cardiometabolic syndrome [75]. Three generations of experimental animals were used to model the effects of betel nut consumption on blood glucose. Boucher and colleagues [76] fed young mice betel nut in their standard chow for 4–6 days and then administered glucose tolerance tests to the F0 animals in adulthood. Consuming betel nut was found to significantly increase the risk of glucose intolerance in F0 animals. They also saw an increased risk in the F1 and F2 offspring of males that consumed betel nuts in their chow before mating.

Three consecutive generations were used in another rodent study to determine the effects of a (F0) maternal high-fat diet on offspring body size and glucose-insulin metabolism. Results revealed that, compared to control animals, both F1 and F2 generation animals were insulin resistant and had increased body length even though they were fed control diets. These effects were seen in both the paternal and maternal lineages. Animals were no longer insulin resistant in the F3 generation, but females inherited increased body length through the paternal line [77].

We [37] also experimented with three generations of rats. F0 female rats were fed a low-protein diet during pregnancy and lactation. The results showed reduced insulin secretory capacity in F1 rats and insulin resistance in their F2 offspring through the maternal line. F3 generation males also exhibited insulin resistance compared to controls, although it was less severe than in F2 animals. Changes in glucose-insulin metabolism in the F1, F2, and F3 generations can be traced to dietary alterations in F0 females, just as in the previous study. After weaning, all animals were fed control diets, as were pregnant and lactating F1 and F2 females. This means that at least some epigenetic effects connected with insulin-glucose metabolism survived germline epigenetic mark erasure by the F3 generation.

While evidence of inherited epigenetic alterations in the F2 generation has been confirmed in other animal studies, they found no evidence of transgenerational effects in F3 animals. Some of these experiments subjected pregnant F0 females to glucocorticoid overexposure [60] and low-protein diets during gestation [59].

The presence of F3 transgenerational epigenetic effects in some studies but not others requires explanation. A number of investigations modeled Skinner's "multi-generational phenotype" [44] that is due to direct exposure (Fig. 13.2) and therefore may lack F3 effects. In contrast, other studies were set up to allow the capture of "transgenerational inheritance" through the germline, via either direct effects on the developing germ cells in utero (Fig. 13.3a) or indirectly via "somatic induction" of the developing fetus [78] (Fig. 13.3b). Another possibility is that an epigenetic threshold was reached in some studies, but in others it was not. A threshold effect may calibrate to the type, intensity, duration, and/or timing of the initial F0 exposure and may determine the durability of epigenetic marks undergoing intergenerational epigenetic reprogramming. Or perhaps under some conditions, epigenetic marks that initially accumulate in the F1 generation and manage to avoid epigenetic erasure in F2 have become so "diluted" in subsequent generations that the phenotypic traits can no longer be identified. This might explain why some transgenerational studies found programmed effects diminished from F2 to F3 (e.g., 37). Since the reason(s) are still unclear, a comprehensive explanation of the mechanistic differences between multigenerational phenotypes and epigenetic transgenerational inheritance will have to wait for future studies of more than three generations, of which there are very few to date (Fig. 13.3).

13.6 The Intergenerational Transmission of Developmentally Programmed Cardiometabolic Traits: Implications for Prenatal Interventions

The existing worldwide obesity epidemic [79], in tandem with persistent undernutrition and poor food availability [80], emphasizes the importance of research involving the developmental origins and the intergenerational transmission of cardiometabolic dysregulation. The public health challenges associated with the scale of these disorders are staggering, and cost-effective and efficacious interventions are desperately needed. Is it possible that the principles of the developmental origins

Table 13.1 Metabolic syndrome prevention via prenatal maternal diet

Dietary factor	Findings	References
Genistein	Experimental animal studies suggest that early exposure to genistein may influence the adipogenesis processes and obesity-related diseases such as type 2 diabetes	[84]
EGCG	Experimental animal studies show maternal prenatal diet supplemented with green tea extract a rich source of (−)-epigallocatechin-3-gallate (EGCG) attenuates high-fat diet-induced insulin resistance in adult male offspring	[85]
Vitamin D	Several clinical trials have demonstrated improved insulin sensitivity and glucose tolerance among women with GDM when diets are supplemented with vitamin D and calcium	[86]
Omega-3 fatty acids	Experimental animal studies show improved insulin sensitivity among offspring whose mothers were fed omega-3 rich diets during pregnancy and pregnancy/lactation but were then fed either control or high-saturated-fat diets post-weaning; clinical trials suggest maternal prenatal omega-3 supplementation protects against low-birth-weight phenotype and is associated with improved body composition and insulin sensitivity in neonates	[87–90]

of cardiometabolic disease can also be leveraged to slow or reverse the current epidemiological trends? Based on the prevailing state of research, there is reason for both optimism and caution. Theoretically, the same physiological bases of developmental plasticity that lead to cardiometabolic dysregulation should be able to prevent, slow, or reverse the current trends. At the same time, developmental plasticity is itself shaped by evolutionary principles and processes that must be understood—and accounted for—if such interventions are to reach their full potential.

It has been over 20 years since the "thrifty phenotype" was first proposed, and today many researchers and public health officials continue to believe that the same developmentally plastic features of cardiometabolism that cause adult disease can be "reverse engineered" to improve health instead. Much of the research has targeted optimized fetal growth, with the goal of improved health later in life. To be sure, the possibilities surrounding the promise of such approaches during pregnancy and early postnatal are well represented in the DOHaD literature [40, 81, 82]. And indeed, a steadily increasing number of clinical trials and pharmacological and, especially, experimental animal studies continue to suggest the potential of interventions targeting the prenatal period to significantly improve cardiometabolic health outcomes later in life [83]. Some of the most promising metabolic syndrome-preventative strategies targeting early growth and development include maternal prenatal dietary supplementation with genistein, (−)-epigallocatechin-3-gallate (EGCG), vitamin D, and omega-3 fatty acids (see Table 13.1). Of these, maternal prenatal supplementation with omega-3 long-chain polyunsaturated fatty acids has been the most thoroughly studied, via experimental animal studies, human observational studies, and clinical trials.

Several experimental animal studies have investigated the effects of maternal prenatal/lactation diets rich in omega-3 LCPUFAs on systolic blood pressure, as well as levels of serum leptin and insulin in neonatal offspring [91]. Researchers have also investigated adult offspring weaned onto control [87] and "Western" diets high in saturated fat [88]. These studies all found that maternal diets rich in omega-3 LCPUFAs lead to improved cardiometabolic function (e.g., insulin resistance) in adult offspring consuming adequate or more than adequate diets. Observational and prospective studies have also associated higher intakes of omega-3 LCPUFAs during pregnancy with increased gestation duration and birth size (see [92] references) and reduction in deep placentation disorders. These associations, thereby, provide a possible mechanism for improved fetal growth and its associated improved cardiometabolic health outcomes [93]. Zhao and colleagues [94] recently assessed maternal and cord plasma fatty acids in relation to indicators of fetal insulin sensitivity in 108 mother-newborn pairs. Their findings showed that lower circulating levels of docosahexaenoic acid (DHA)—an important omega-3 LCPUFA—were associated with lower fetal insulin sensitivity. Several recent randomized clinical trials have confirmed and extended these findings by demonstrating that maternal prenatal omega-3 supplementation protects against the metabolic syndrome-inducing low-birth-weight phenotype [92] and is associated with improved body composition and insulin sensitivity in neonates [90]. It should be noted, however, that a study of the 19-year-old offspring of mothers supplemented with LCPUFA-rich fish oil during the third trimester of pregnancy failed to show enduring improvements in plasma lipids, blood pressure, or heart rate [95, 96].

13.7 Accounting for Evolution in Future Metabolic Syndrome Prevention Strategies

While the studies referred to above do offer hope that the current metabolic syndrome global pandemic might be slowed or reversed, to date, evidence from dozens of observational studies and controlled trials has tempered some of the more unbridled early optimism regarding the potential effectiveness of such interventions. In efforts to improve fetal growth as well as maternal and child health outcomes, researchers in many early studies supplemented maternal diet during pregnancy with targeted macro- and micronutrients. These studies have reported mixed results, however, and even when supplementation interventions were successful, often only small improvements were observed (see [97–99]). Although some of these approaches do appear to have potential [100], it is the species-specific timescales on which the developmental pathways are calibrated that may be to blame for their less than remarkable successes. As Kuzawa and Thayer point out, the "principles of evolutionary biology and adaptation lead us to hypothesize that many short term interventions that trigger large biological changes in short lived species, will have comparably small effects in humans" ([101], p229). In other words, differences in body size, lifespan, variability in the physical environment, and reproductive strategy of various mammalian species (e.g., rodents, guinea pigs, sheep, and humans) exert significant influence on the magnitude of developmentally programmed effects due to early life environments. Because of this, phenotypic plasticity operates under

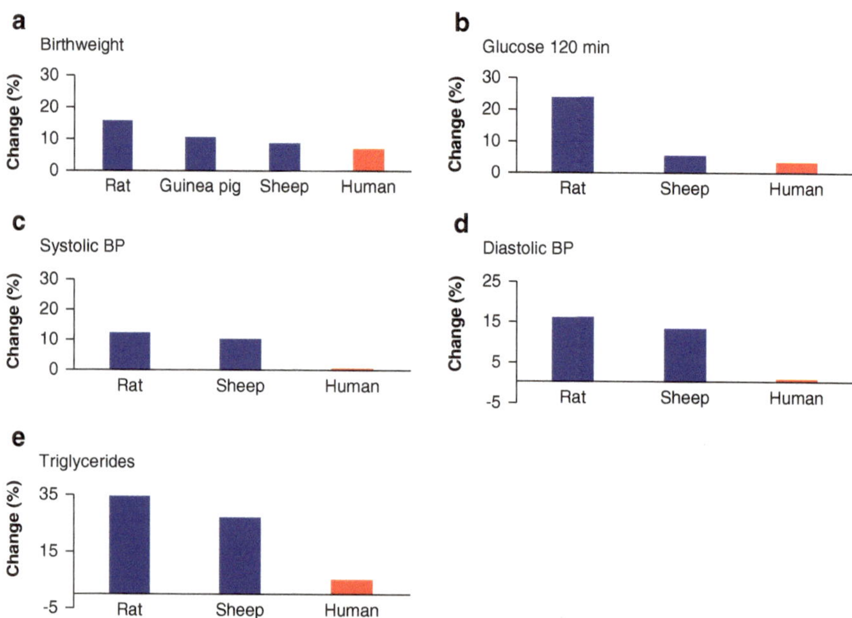

Fig. 13.4 Magnitude of change in offspring outcomes induced by maternal diet restriction during pregnancy, ordered by species. All animals born to mothers who experienced caloric restriction during early gestation (30–50 % caloric restriction). All values are calculated as the percentage difference between the control group and the case group and represent averaged male and female values. (**a**) Birth weight. Rat [102], guinea pig [103], sheep [104], human [105]: value represents conceived after famine control group versus conceived in middle or late gestation. (**b**) Glucose. Rat [106], values represent difference at 14 weeks of age; sheep [104], value represents difference at 3 years of age; human [105], value represents conceived after famine control versus early gestation exposure, measured in adulthood. (**c**, **d**) Systolic and diastolic blood pressure. Rat [102], value represents difference at 200 days postnatal; sheep [104], value represents difference at 3 years of age; human [105], value represents conceived after famine control versus early exposure, measured in adulthood. (**e**) Triglycerides. Rat [102], value represents difference at 200 days postnatal; sheep [107], value represents difference at 1 year of age; human [105], value represents conceived after famine control versus early exposure, measured in adulthood. *BP* Blood pressure

very different constraints for small-bodied, short-lived species that are subject to relatively little physical environmental variation over multiple generations (e.g., rodents) versus large-bodied, long-lived species that often occupy highly variable physical environmental conditions—often over just one reproductive life history stage (e.g., humans). Data from experimental animal studies, for example, assessing the effects—and effect sizes—of perturbations during gestation (e.g., maternal dietary restrictions during pregnancy), provide clear evidence of the consequence of these species-specific evolutionary processes (Fig. 13.4).

Recognizing these differences calls into question the "predictive adaptive response" (PAR) concept, which is one of the main tenets of a core concept in developmental origins research. PAR asserts that poor health results when there is a "mismatch" between early life environments and adult environments (e.g., poor maternal nutrition during pregnancy followed by overnutrition in adulthood) [108]. The epidemiological and experimental animal evidence consistent with the PAR theory is extensive; yet, several authors remain dubious of the concept. These authors are skeptical that environmental cues during early life (e.g., maternal nutrition during gestation) are reliable predictors of future adult environments in long-lived species like humans [109, 110]. These authors argue, alternatively, that the entire maternal phenotype—expressed as nutrients, hormones, metabolites, and growth and immune factors—transmits to the developing offspring (through the placenta and lactation) an integrated and averaged signal of multigenerational matrilineal experience. If it is true that maternal (and paternal) epigenomes do transmit multigenerational information that affects developmental programming, then this aspect of the evolution of phenotypic plasticity in humans must be accounted for in the structure and content of interventions to improve adult health.

To improve birth weight and other neonatal and maternal health outcomes that have proven resistant to short-term interventions in the past, one scenario might be to extend future interventions over longer periods of time and/or target multiple ages across reproductive life. If the hypothesis of a transmitted integrated signal that reflects longer-term nutritional conditions is correct [101, 109, 110], then possibly a more sustained intervention would be effectual, perhaps one that targets multiple generations in high-risk communities. There have been promising results from this kind of approach [100]. For example, nutritional supplement interventions for women could be used, not only throughout pregnancy but also immediately prior to conception and during lactation. Innovative interventions might even target boys' nutrition during the slow-growth phase of preadolescence and extend nutrition and body weight/composition interventions among fathers in the preconceptual period as well. Still others might analyze the crucial elements of metabolism by studying energy expenditure and physical activity during multiple sensitive periods of development [111, 112]. Finally, future efforts aimed at prevention might also seek to intervene with exogenous hormones and growth factor treatments, among others, postnatally, that might provide shortcuts to the type of long-term trend signals being transmitted to offspring during critical periods of early development [83, 101, 113].

At present, it remains uncertain whether or not the findings from these animal model treatment studies will ultimately provide the conceptual and empirical basis from which analogous interventions might be developed for humans. The results of the aforementioned studies do provide some reason for considerable optimism, however. Indeed, if such programs can be calibrated to account for humans' unique life history parameters, these interventions likely hold great promise in preventing metabolic syndrome in future generations.

References

1. Hales CN, Barker DJP. Type 2 (non-insulin-dependent) diabetes mellitus: The thrifty phenotype hypothesis. Diabetologia. 1992;35:595–601.
2. Stearns SC. The evolution of life histories. Oxford: Oxford University Press; 1992.

3. West-Eberhard MJ. Developmental plasticity and evolution. New York: Oxford University Press; 2003.
4. Benyshek DC. The developmental origins of obesity and related health disorders–prenatal and perinatal factors. Coll Antropol. 2007;31:11–7.
5. Popkin BM. Global nutrition dynamics: The world is shifting rapidly toward a diet linked with noncommunicable diseases. Am J Clin Nutr. 2006;84:289–98.
6. Eriksson JG. Patterns of growth: relevance to developmental origins of health and disease. In: Gluckman PD, Hanson MA, editors. Developmental origins of health and disease. Cambridge: Cambridge University Press; 2006. p. 223–32.
7. Alfaradhi M, Ozanne S. Developmental programming in response to maternal overnutrition. Front Genet. 2011;2:1–27.
8. Rkhzay-Jaf J, O'dowd JF, Stocker CJ. Maternal obesity and the fetal origins of the metabolic syndrome. Curr Cardiovasc Risk Rep. 2012;6:487–95.
9. Stettler N, Stallings VA, Troxel AB, Zhao J, Schinnar R, Nelson SE, Ziegler EE, Strom BL. Weight gain in the first week of life and overweight in adulthood a cohort study of European American subjects fed infant formula. Circulation. 2005;111:1897–903.
10. Singhal A, Cole TJ, Fewtrell M, Lucas A. Breastmilk feeding and lipoprotein profile in adolescents born preterm: follow-up of a prospective randomised study. Lancet. 2004;363: 1571–8.
11. Dewey KG, Heinig M, Nommsen L, Peerson J, Lönnerdal B. Breast-fed infants are leaner than formula-fed infants at 1 y of age: the darling study. Am J Clin Nutr. 1993;57:140–5.
12. Pirkola J, Pouta A, Bloigu A, Hartikainen A-L, Laitinen J, Järvelin M-R, Vääräsmäki M. Risks of overweight and abdominal obesity at age 16 years associated with prenatal exposures to maternal prepregnancy overweight and gestational diabetes mellitus. Diabetes Care. 2010; 33:1115–21.
13. Guénard F, Deshaies Y, Cianflone K, Kral J, Marceau P, Vohl M. Differential methylation in glucoregulatory genes of offspring born before vs after maternal gastrointestinal bypass surgery. Proc Natl Acad Sci U S A. 2013;110(28):11439–44.
14. Reynolds R, Osmond C, Phillips D, Godfrey K. Maternal BMI, parity, and pregnancy weight gain: Influences on offspring adiposity in young adulthood. J Clin Endocrinol Metab. 2010;95:5365–9.
15. Dabelea D. The predisposition to obesity and diabetes in offspring of diabetic mothers. Diabetes Care. 2007;30:S169–74.
16. Boney CM, Verma A, Tucker R, Vohr BR. Metabolic syndrome in childhood: association with birth weight, maternal obesity, and gestational diabetes mellitus. Pediatrics. 2005;115: e290–6.
17. Yu Z, Han S, Zhu J, Sun X, Ji C, Guo X. Pre-pregnancy body mass index in relation to infant birth weight and offspring overweight/obesity: a systematic review and meta-analysis. PLoS One. 2013;8:e61627.
18. Cnattingius S, Villamor E, Lagerros YT, Wikström AK, Granath F. High birth weight and obesity: a vicious circle across generations. Int J Obes (Lond). 2012;36:1320–4.
19. Gluckman PD, Hanson M, Zimmet P, Forrester T. Losing the war against obesity: the need for a developmental perspective. Sci Transl Med. 2011;3(93):93cm19.
20. Breton C. The hypothalamus-adipose axis is a key target of developmental programming by maternal nutritional manipulation. J Endocrinol. 2013;216:R19–31.
21. Sloboda DM, Newnham JP, Moss TJM, Challis JRG. The fetal hypothalamic-pituitary-adrenal axis: relevance to developmental origins of health and disease. In: Gluckman PD, Hanson MA, editors. Developmental origins of health and disease. Cambridge: Cambridge University Press; 2006. p. 191–205.
22. Feng B, Zhang T, Xu H. Human adipose dynamics and metabolic health. Ann N Y Acad Sci. 2013;1281:160–77.
23. McConnell JML. A mitochondrial component of developmental programming. In: Gluckman PD, Hanson MA, editors. Developmental origins of health and disease. Cambridge: Cambridge University Press; 2006. p. 75–81.

24. Portha B, Chavey A, Movassat J. Early-life origins of type 2 diabetes: fetal programming of the beta-cell mass. Exp Diabetes Res. 2011;2011:1–16.
25. Reusens B, Kalbe L, Remacle C. The developmental environment and the endocrine pancreas. In: Gluckman PD, Hanson MA, editors. Developmental origins of health and disease. Cambridge: Cambridge University Press; 2006. p. 233–43.
26. Thompson JA, Regnault TRH. In utero origins of adult insulin resistance and vascular dysfunction. Semin Reprod Med. 2011;29:211–24.
27. Napoli C, Pignalosa O, Rossi L, Botti C, Guarino C, Sica V, de Nigris F. The developmental environment and atherogenesis. In: Gluckman PD, Hanson MA, editors. Developmental origins of health and disease. Cambridge: Cambridge University Press; 2006. p. 300–9.
28. Myatt L, Roberts V. Placental mechanisms and developmental origins of health and disease. In: Gluckman PD, Hanson MA, editors. Developmental origins of health and disease. Cambridge: Cambridge University Press; 2006. p. 130–42.
29. Waddington CH. The epigenotype. Endeavour. 1942;1:18–20.
30. Lim JP, Brunet A. Bridging the transgenerational gap with epigenetic memory. Trends Genet. 2013;29:176–86.
31. Suzuki MM, Bird A. DNA methylation landscapes: provocative insights from epigenomics. Nat Rev Genet. 2008;9:465–76.
32. Bannister AJ, Kouzarides T. Regulation of chromatin by histone modifications. Cell Res. 2011;21:381–95.
33. Thayer ZM, Kuzawa CW. Biological memories of past environments: epigenetic pathways to health disparities. Epigenetics. 2011;6:798–803.
34. Burdge GC, Lillycrop KA. Nutrition, epigenetics, and developmental plasticity: Implications for understanding human disease. Annu Rev Nutr. 2010;30:315–39.
35. Drake AJ, Walker BR. The intergenerational effects of fetal programming: non-genomic mechanisms for the inheritance of low birth weight and cardiovascular risk. J Endocrinol. 2004;180:1–16.
36. Drake AJ, Liu L. Intergenerational transmission of programmed effects: public health consequences. Trends Endocrinol Metab. 2010;21:206–13.
37. Benyshek D, Johnston C, Martin J. Glucose metabolism is altered in the adequately-nourished grand-offspring (f 3 generation) of rats malnourished during gestation and perinatal life. Diabetologia. 2006;49:1117–9.
38. Benyshek DC, Johnston CS, Martin JF, Ross WD. Insulin sensitivity is normalized in the third generation (F3) offspring of developmentally programmed insulin resistant (F2) rats fed an energy-restricted diet. Nutr Metab (Lond). 2008;5:26.
39. Wells JCK. Maternal capital and the metabolic ghetto: An evolutionary perspective on the transgenerational basis of health inequalities. Am J Hum Biol. 2010;22(1):1–17.
40. Benyshek DC, Martin JF, Johnston CS. A reconsideration of the origins of the type 2 diabetes epidemic among Native Americans and the implications for intervention policy. Med Anthropol. 2001;20(1):25–64.
41. Kuzawa CW, Sweet E. Epigenetics and the embodiment of race: developmental origins of US racial disparities in cardiovascular health. Am J Hum Biol. 2009;21:2–15.
42. Li J, Huang J, Li J-S, Chen H, Huang K, Zheng L. Accumulation of endoplasmic reticulum stress and lipogenesis in the liver through generational effects of high fat diets. J Hepatol. 2012;56:900–7.
43. Plagemann A, Harder T, Brunn M, Harder A, Roepke K, Wittrock-Staar M, Ziska T, Schellong K, Rodekamp E, Melchior K. Hypothalamic proopiomelanocortin promoter methylation becomes altered by early overfeeding: an epigenetic model of obesity and the metabolic syndrome. J Physiol. 2009;587:4963–76.
44. Skinner MK. What is an epigenetic transgenerational phenotype?: F3 or F2. Reprod Toxicol. 2008;25:2–6.
45. Gluckman PD, Hanson MA. Developmental origins of health and disease. Cambridge: Cambridge University Press; 2006.
46. Gluckman PD, Hanson MA. Maternal constraint of fetal growth and its consequences. Semin Fetal Neonatal Med. 2004;9:419–25.

47. Hendrix N, Berghella V. Non-placental causes of intrauterine growth restriction. Semin Perinatol. 2008;32:161–5.
48. Walton A, Hammond J. The maternal effects on growth and conformation in Shire horse-Shetland pony crosses. Proc R Soc Lond B. 1938;125:311–35. Available from: http://rspb.royalsocietypublishing.org/content/125/840/311.
49. Lunde A, Melve KK, Gjessing HK, Skjærven R, Irgens LM. Genetic and environmental influences on birth weight, birth length, head circumference, and gestational age by use of population-based parent-offspring data. Am J Epidemiol. 2007;165:734–41.
50. Kuzawa CW, Eisenberg DT. Intergenerational predictors of birth weight in the Philippines: correlations with mother's and father's birth weight and test of maternal constraint. PLoS One. 2012;7(7):e40905.
51. Magnus P, Gjessing H, Skrondal A, Skjaerven R. Paternal contribution to birth weight. J Epidemiol Community Health. 2001;55:873–7.
52. Coutinho R, David RJ, Collins JW. Relation of parental birth weights to infant birth weight among African Americans and whites in Illinois: a transgenerational study. Am J Epidemiol. 1997;146:804–9.
53. Agnihotri B, Antonisamy B, Priya G, Fall CHD, Raghupathy P. Trends in human birth weight across two successive generations. Indian J Pediatr. 2008;75:111–7.
54. Lumey L, Stein AD, Kahn HS, Romijn J. Lipid profiles in middle-aged men and women after famine exposure during gestation: the Dutch hunger winter families study. Am J Clin Nutr. 2009;89:1737–43.
55. Painter R, Osmond C, Gluckman P, Hanson M, Phillips D, Roseboom T. Transgenerational effects of prenatal exposure to the Dutch famine on neonatal adiposity and health in later life. BJOG. 2008;115:1243–9.
56. Martin JF, Johnston CS, Han CT, Benyshek DC. Nutritional origins of insulin resistance: a rat model for diabetes-prone human populations. J Nutr. 2000;130:741–4.
57. Zambrano E, Martínez-Samayoa P, Bautista C, Deas M, Guillen L, Rodríguez-González G, Guzman C, Larrea F, Nathanielsz P. Sex differences in transgenerational alterations of growth and metabolism in progeny (f2) of female offspring (f1) of rats fed a low protein diet during pregnancy and lactation. J Physiol. 2005;566:225–36.
58. Jimenez-Chillaron JC, Isganaitis E, Charalambous M, Gesta S, Pentinat-Pelegrin T, Faucette RR, Otis JP, Chow A, Diaz R, Ferguson-Smith A. Intergenerational transmission of glucose intolerance and obesity by in utero undernutrition in mice. Diabetes. 2009;58:460–8.
59. Harrison M, Langley-Evans SC. Intergenerational programming of impaired nephrogenesis and hypertension in rats following maternal protein restriction during pregnancy. Br J Nutr. 2009;101:1020–30.
60. Drake AJ, Walker BR, Seckl JR. Intergenerational consequences of fetal programming by in utero exposure to glucocorticoids in rats. Am J Physiol Regul Integr Comp Physiol. 2005;288:R34–8.
61. Anderson CM, Lopez F, Zimmer A, Benoit JN. Placental insufficiency leads to developmental hypertension and mesenteric artery dysfunction in two generations of Sprague-Dawley rat offspring. Biol Reprod. 2006;74:538–44.
62. Dunn GA, Bale TL. Maternal high-fat diet promotes body length increases and insulin insensitivity in second-generation mice. Endocrinology. 2009;150:4999–5009.
63. Gniuli D, Calcagno A, Caristo ME, Mancuso A, Macchi V, Mingrone G, Vettor R. Effects of high-fat diet exposure during fetal life on type 2 diabetes development in the progeny. J Lipid Res. 2008;49:1936–45.
64. Srinivasan M, Mitrani P, Sadhanandan G, Dodds C, Shbeir-Eldika S, Thamotharan S, Ghanim H, Dandona P, Devaskar SU, Patel MS. A high-carbohydrate diet in the immediate postnatal life of rats induces adaptations predisposing to adult-onset obesity. J Endocrinol. 2008;197:565–74.
65. Dahri S, Snoeck A, Reusens-Billen B, Remacle C, Hote JJ. Islet function in offspring of mothers on low-protein diet during gestation. Diabetes. 1991;40:115–20.
66. Reik W, Collick A, Norris ML, Barton SC, Surani MA. Genomic imprinting determines methylation of parental alleles in transgenic mice. Nature. 1987;328(6127):248–51.

67. Brunner AM, Nanni P, Mansuy M. Epigenetic marking of sperm by post-translational modification of histones and protamines. Epigenetics Chromatin. 2014;7:2.
68. O'Doherty AM, McGettigan PA. Epigenetic processes in the male germline. Reprod Fertil Dev. 2014. doi:10.1071/RD14167.
69. Hackett JA, Sengupta R, Zylicz JJ, Murakami K, Lee C, Down TA, Surani MA. Germline DNA demethylation dynamics and imprint erasure through 5-hydroxymethylcytosine. Science. 2013;339:448–52.
70. Erkek S, Hisano M, Liang CY, Gill M, Murr R, Dieker J, Schübeler D, van der Vlag J, Stadler MB, Peters AH. Molecular determinants of nucleosome retention at CpG-rich sequences in mouse spermatozoa. Nat Struct Mol Biol. 2013;20(7):868–75.
71. Kaati G, Bygren LO, Edvinsson S. Cardiovascular and diabetes mortality determined by nutrition during parents' and grandparents' slow growth period. Eur J Hum Genet. 2002;10: 682–8.
72. Kaati G, Bygren LO, Pembrey M, Sjöström M. Transgenerational response to nutrition, early life circumstances and longevity. Eur J Hum Genet. 2007;15:784–90.
73. Pembrey ME, Bygren LO, Kaati G, Edvinsson S, Northstone K, Sjöström M, Golding J. Sex-specific, male-line transgenerational responses in humans. Eur J Hum Genet. 2006;14: 159–66.
74. Soubry A, Schildkraut JM, Murtha A, Wang F, Huang Z, Bernal A, Kurtzberg J, Jirtle RL, Murphy SK, Hoyo C. Paternal obesity is associated with igf2 hypomethylation in newborns: results from a newborn epigenetics study (NEST) cohort. BMC Med. 2013;11:29.
75. Lin WY, Chiu TY, Lee LT, Lin CC, Huang CY, Huang KC. Betel nut chewing is associated with increased risk of cardiovascular disease and all-cause mortality in Taiwanese men. Am J Clin Nutr. 2008;87:1204–11.
76. Boucher B, Ewen S, Stowers J. Betel nut (areca catechu) consumption and the induction of glucose intolerance in adult cd1 mice and in their f1 and f2 offspring. Diabetologia. 1994;37: 49–55.
77. Dunn GA, Bale TL. Maternal high-fat diet effects on third-generation female body size via the paternal lineage. Endocrinology. 2011;152:2228–36.
78. Jablonka E, Raz G. Transgenerational epigenetic inheritance: prevalence, mechanisms, and implications for the study of heredity and evolution. Q Rev Biol. 2009;84:131–76.
79. WHO [Internet]. Controlling the global obesity epidemic; 2013 [cited 2013 Mar 12]. Available from: http://www.who.int/nutrition/topics/obesity/en/.
80. FAO. The state of food insecurity in the world 2012: economic growth is necessary but not sufficient to accelerate reduction of hunger and malnutrition. Rome: Food and Agricultural Organization of the United Nations; 2012.
81. Gluckman PD, Hanson MA. The fetal matrix: evolution, development and disease. Cambridge: Cambridge University Press; 2004.
82. Forrester T. Developmental origins of health and disease: implications for primary intervention for cardiovascular and metabolic disease. In: Gluckman PD, Hanson MA, editors. Developmental origins of health and disease. Cambridge: Cambridge University Press; 2006. p. 436–45.
83. Ma N, Hardy DB. The fetal origins of the metabolic syndrome: can we intervene? J Pregnancy. 2012;2012:1–11.
84. Dolinoy DC, Weidman JR, Waterland RA, Jirtle RL. Maternal genistein alters coat color and protects Avy mouse offspring from obesity by modifying the fetal epigenome. Environ Health Perspect. 2006;114(4):567–72.
85. Li S, Tse IM, Li ET. Maternal green tea extract supplementation to rats fed a high-fat diet ameliorates insulin resistance in adult male offspring. J Nutr Biochem. 2012;23(12):1655–60.
86. Azemi M, Berisha M, Ismaili-Jaha V, Kolgeci S, Hoxha R, Grajçevci-Uka V, Hoxha- Kamberi T. Vitamin D - dependent rickets, type II case report. Mater Sociomed. 2014;26(1):68–70.
87. Sardinha FL, Fernandes FS, Tavares do Carmo MG, Herrera E. Sex-dependent nutritional programming: fish oil intake during early pregnancy in rats reduces age-dependent insulin resistance in male, but not female, offspring. Am J Physiol Regul Integr Comp Physiol. 2013;304(4):R313–20.

88. Benyshek DC, Kachinski JJ, Jin HB. F0 prenatal/lactation diets varying in saturated fat and long-chain polyunsaturated fatty acids alters the insulin sensitivity of F1 rats fed a high fat western diet postweaning. Open J Endocr Metab Dis. 2014;4:245–52.
89. Imhoff-Kunsch B, Briggs V, Goldenberg T, Ramakrishnan U. Effect of n-3 long-chain polyunsaturated fatty acid intake during pregnancy on maternal, infant, and child health outcomes: a systematic review. Paediatr Perinat Epidemiol. 2012;26(s1):91–107.
90. Courville AB, Harel O, Lammi-Keefe CJ. Consumption of a DHA-containing functional food during pregnancy is associated with lower infant ponderal index and cord plasma insulin concentration. Br J Nutr. 2011;106(2):208–12.
91. Korotkova TM, Eriksson KS, Haas HL, Brown RE. Selective excitation of GABAergic neurons in the substantia nigra of the rat by orexin/hypocretin in vitro. Regul Pept. 2002;104: 83–9.
92. Carlson SE, Colombo J, Gajewski BJ, Gustafson KM, Mundy D, Yeast J, Georgieff MK, Markley LA, Kerling EH, Shaddy DJ. DHA supplementation and pregnancy outcomes. Am J Clin Nutr. 2013;97(4):808–15.
93. Carvajal JA. Docosahexaenoic acid supplementation early in pregnancy may prevent deep placentation disorders. BioMed Res Int. 2014;2014:1–10.
94. Zhao JP, Levy E, Fraser WD, Julien P, Delvin E, Montoudis A, Spahis S, Garofalo C, Nuyy AM, Luo ZC. Circulating docosahexaenoic acid levels are associated with fetal insulin sensitivity. PLoS One. 2014;9(1):e85054.
95. Rytter D, Bech BH, Christensen JH, Schmidt EB, Henriksen TB, Olsen SF. Intake of fish oil during pregnancy and adiposity in 19-y-old offspring: follow-up on a randomized controlled trial. Am J Clin Nutr. 2011;94(3):701–8.
96. Rytter D, Christensen JH, Bech BH, Schmidt EB, Henriksen TB, Olsen SF. The effect of maternal fish oil supplementation during the last trimester of pregnancy on blood pressure, heart rate and heart rate variability in the 19-year-old offspring. Br J Nutr. 2012;108(8): 1475–83.
97. Merialdi M, Carroli G, Villar J, Abalos E, Gülmezoglu AM, Kulier R, Onis M. Nutritional interventions during pregnancy for the prevention or treatment of impaired fetal growth: an overview of randomized controlled trials. J Nutr. 2003;133:1626S–31.
98. Morton SMB. Maternal nutrition and fetal growth and development. In: Gluckman PD, Hanson MA, editors. Developmental origins of health and disease. Cambridge: Cambridge University Press; 2006. p. 98–129.
99. Kramer MS, Kakuma R. Energy and protein intake in pregnancy. Cochrane Database Syst Rev. 2010;3:1–74.
100. Behrman J, Calderon M, Preston S, Hoddinott J, Martorell R, Stein A. Nutritional supplementation in girls influences the growth of their children: prospective study in Guatemala. Am J Clin Nutr. 2009;90:1372–9.
101. Kuzawa CW, Thayer ZM. Timescales of human adaptation: the role of epigenetic processes. Epigenomics. 2011;3:221–34.
102. Ozaki T, Nishina H, Hanson MA, Poston L. Dietary restriction in pregnant rats causes gender-related hypertension and vascular dysfunction in offspring. J Physiol. 2001;530(1):141–52.
103. Kind KL, Simonetta G, Clifton PM, Robinson JS, Owens JA. Effect of maternal feed restriction on blood pressure in the adult guinea pig. Exp Physiol. 2002;87(4):469–77.
104. Gopalakrishnan GS, Gardner DS, Rhind SM. Programming of adult cardiovascular function after early maternal undernutrition in sheep. Am J Physiol. 2004;287(1):R12–20.
105. Roseboom TJ, Van Der Meulen JHP, Ravelli ACJ, Osmond C, Barker DJP, Bleker OP. Effects of prenatal exposure to the Dutch famine on adult disease in later life: an overview. Mol Cell Endocrinol. 2001;185(1–2):93–8.
106. Franco MC, Arruda RM, Dantas AP. Intrauterine undernutrition: expression and activity of the endothelial nitric oxide synthase in male and female adult offspring. Cardiovasc Res. 2002;56(1):145–53.
107. Gardner DS, Tingey K, Van Bon BWM. Programming of glucose-insulin metabolism in adult sheep after maternal undernutrition. Am J Physiol. 2005;289(4):R947–54.

108. Gluckman PD, Hanson MA. Living with the past: evolution, development, and patterns of disease. Science. 2004;305:1733–6.
109. Wells JCK. The thrifty phenotype as an adaptive maternal effect. Biol Rev. 2007;82: 143–72.
110. Kuzawa CW. Fetal origins of developmental plasticity: are fetal cues reliable predictors of future nutritional environments? Am J Hum Biol. 2005;17(1):5–21.
111. Huber K, Miles J, Norman A, Thompson N, Davison M, Breier B. Prenatally induced changes in muscle structure and metabolic function facilitate exercise-induced obesity prevention. Endocrinology. 2009;150:4135–44.
112. Miles J, Huber K, Thompson N, Davison M, Breier B. Moderate daily exercise activates metabolic flexibility to prevent prenatally induced obesity. Endocrinology. 2009;150: 179–86.
113. Vickers MH, Sloboda DM. Strategies for reversing the effects of metabolic disorders induced as a consequence of developmental programming. Front Physiol. 2012;3:242.

Anti-inflammatory Diets to Reduce Gestational Problems Caused by Obesity, Metabolic Syndrome, and Diabetes

14

Barry Sears

Contents

B. Sears, PhD
Inflammation Research Foundation, Marblehead, MA, USA
e-mail: bsears@drsears.com

E. Ferrazzi, B. Sears (eds.), *Metabolic Syndrome and Complications of Pregnancy: The Potential Preventive Role of Nutrition*,
DOI 10.1007/978-3-319-16853-1_14

14.1 Introduction

This entire book is dedicated to addressing the impact of obesity, metabolic syndrome, and diabetes on gestational problems. All of these clinical conditions are related to diet-induced inflammation. As a result, the use of anti-inflammatory diets in high-risk populations may be the most cost-effective way to engender improved pregnancy outcomes for both the mother and child.

Inflammation is a two-edged sword. It allows us to defend ourselves against microbial invasion and allows our injuries to heal. Yet on the other hand, if the inflammatory response is not sufficiency attenuated, inflammation can attack our own organs leading to earlier development of chronic diseases [1]. Maintaining inflammation in a zone that is not too low, but not high, is one of the key factors not only for a successful pregnancy but also a successful aging by the reduction of the earlier onset of chronic disease. However, in addition to microbial invasion or physical injuries that can activate our inflammatory responses, so can the diet.

Diets can be either pro-inflammatory or anti-inflammatory depending on the hormonal responses they generate. This is because these hormonal responses as well as specific nutrients in the diet are intimately connected with the most primitive part of our inflammatory responses: the innate immune system. This part of our immune system has been evolutionarily conserved for hundreds of millions of years and can be considered our first line of defense in the generation of inflammation. What is important is that the innate immune system is under considerable dietary control.

14.2 Inflammation at the Molecular Level

The central hub of the innate immune system is the gene transcription factor, nuclear factor kappaB (NF-κB). This is the master switch that turns on the expression of inflammatory gene products (COX-2, TNFα, IL-1β, IL-6, etc.) that amplify the initial inflammatory signals to nearby cells [2].

There are a number of dietary factors that can activate NF-κB. These factors include oxidative stress from excess calories and hormones derived from arachidonic acid [3, 4]. Additional dietary factors include saturated fatty acids, advanced glycosylated end products (AGE), and inflammatory cytokines from nearby cells all acting through specific receptors at the cell surface that can also activate NF-κB [5].

However, inflammation is not like a burning log whose fire eventually dies out. The inflammatory response consists of two distinct phases [5]. The first phase is the initiation of the inflammatory response. The second phase is the resolution of the inflammatory response. The resolution phase is controlled by a unique group of hormones (resolvins, protectins, and maresins) derived from omega-3 fatty acids [6]. As long as the initiation and resolution phases of inflammation are balanced, then you have homeostasis. On the other hand, if the initiation phase is too strong or the resolution phase is too weak, the end result is chronic low-level cellular inflammation. It is this chronic cellular inflammation below the perception of pain that is the driving force in the development of obesity, metabolic syndrome, and diabetes [7].

14.3 Measuring Cellular Inflammation

Since cellular inflammation is below the perception of pain, measuring it has posed a challenge. The earliest marker of cellular inflammation was high sensitivity C-reactive protein (hs-CRP) [8]. This protein is synthesized in the liver in response to elevated levels of IL-6 in the blood [9]. Unlike inflammatory cytokines that either have short half-lives or only enter the blood in very low concentrations [10], hs-CRP is relatively long-lived protein in the blood and therefore is more easily measured [11]. The major clinical drawback of hs-CRP is that even slight bacterial infections can rapidly elevate its levels, and as consequence it is not a very reliable marker [12]. Furthermore, it is a downstream marker of cellular inflammation as opposed to an early warning of the buildup of chronic cellular inflammation.

Inflammatory cytokines expressed by the activation of NF-κB (such as TNF, IL-1β, and IL-6) are better potential markers of cellular inflammation, yet there levels in the blood are very low and they are have very short half-lives making their use as analytical markers of cellular inflammation less feasible [9, 10].

Perhaps, the best upstream marker of cellular inflammation is the ratio of two fatty acids in the blood, the omega-6 fatty acid arachidonic acid (AA) and the omega-3 fatty acid eicosapentaenoic acid (EPA). AA is the building block of pro-inflammatory eicosanoids that stimulate inflammation. On the other hand, EPA is not only the competitive inhibitor of AA for the enzymes necessary for the production of inflammatory eicosanoids but also the building block for very powerful pro-resolution mediators such as resolvin E1 (RvE1) and resolvin E2 (RvE2). Thus, the AA/EPA ratio in the blood provides a detailed insight into the balance of inflammation and resolution in every cell in the body. Furthermore, unlike hs-CRP, the AA/EPA ratio is stable and reliable and often becomes elevated years ahead of the elevation of hs-CRP [13].

14.4 Definitions of Chronic Conditions That Can Be Treated by Anti-inflammatory Nutrition

Although virtually every chronic disease can be connected with increasing cellular inflammation, the three that are most germane to pregnancy are obesity, metabolic syndrome, and diabetes.

14.4.1 Obesity

Obesity can be defined as excess fat accumulation. Obesity presents little obstacle in becoming pregnant. However, it is when that excess fat becomes inflamed that obesity presents the problem during pregnancy [14]. Under normal conditions, the adipose tissue operates like a bank, taking in energy from the diet and storing them in the fat cells and then releasing that energy through the day. Normally, this process works very well unless disrupted by increased cellular inflammation [5, 13]. As the result, the subject is constantly fatigued. At the same time, cellular inflammation disturbs the intricate satiety mechanisms in the hypothalamus leading to increased hunger.

14.4.2 Metabolic Syndrome

Metabolic syndrome can be considered the first stage of the metastasis of cellular inflammation from the adipose tissue to other organs, in particular the liver and the muscles. Metabolic syndrome is not a defined condition but a cluster of associated clinical markers such as elevated waist measurement, high triglycerides, low HDL cholesterol, and hyperinsulinemia. All of these symptoms can be linked to insulin resistance [15]. Metabolic syndrome can be considered to be "prediabetes" as if left untreated the conversion rate to type 2 diabetes is 5–10 % per year [16].

14.4.3 Diabetes

Type 2 diabetes occurs with two different conjuring mechanisms: insulin resistance, due to lipid and cytokine damage to insulin receptors, occurring primarily within the muscles, liver, and fat tissue, and the destruction of beta cells in the pancreas leading to the inability to secrete sufficient amounts of insulin to control blood sugar levels. The proportion of insulin resistance versus beta cell dysfunction differs among individuals.

With this comes a rapid increase in blood glucose levels with a potential corresponding in increase advanced glycosylated end products (AGE) that can bind to receptors known as RAGE that also activates NF-κB [17].

The hydroxylated fatty acid (12-HETE), which is derived from arachidonic acid, appears to be a major player in the destruction of beta cells in the pancreas [18].

14.4.4 Hypertension and Cardiovascular Disease

Oxidative stress, due to caloric overload, chronic low-grade inflammation induced by adipose tissue dysfunction, represents a vicious cycle favoring the progression of endothelial dysfunction atherothrombosis, cardiac overload, and dysfunction. Increased food intake and insulin resistance have been shown also to rapidly enhance plasma leptin levels and subsequently tissue leptin resistance. The higher heart rate in the hyperleptinemic individuals will impose a greater myocardial workload and eventually predispose the heart to pathophysiological changes that encroach on the other adverse condition established by the "partners" of metabolic syndrome.

14.5 Building an Anti-inflammatory Diet

Since obesity, metabolic syndrome, and diabetes all ultimately rise from diet-induced inflammation, the logical approach to minimize their impact of these inflammation-related conditions on both the mother and fetus during pregnancy is to have the mother follow an anti-inflammatory diet. Before I describe the practical aspects of such an anti-inflammatory diet, let us first describe how various macronutrients in any diet can either be pro-inflammatory or anti-inflammatory [19].

14.5.1 Macronutrients and Inflammation

Omega-6 fatty acids are the basic building blocks for making a wide variety of pro-inflammatory eicosanoids. However, the real molecular foundation for pro-inflammatory eicosanoids is arachidonic acid, whereas the vast bulk of dietary omega-6 fatty consists of linoleic acid. The metabolic conversion of linoleic acid into arachidonic acid goes through several steps: the enzymes delta-6 and delta-5 desaturase are rate-limiting enzymes that normally control the flux of linoleic acid into arachidonic acid. Both of these enzymes are under hormonal and dietary control [20]. The hormone insulin (controlled by the amount of carbohydrate at a meal) activates these enzymes, whereas the hormone glucagon (controlled by the amount of protein at meal) inhibits their activity. The amount of insulin released in a meal depends on the glycemic load of the carbohydrates consumed. Refined carbohydrates such as found in bread, pasta, and processed foods are rapidly broken down to glucose. The more rapidly the glucose enters the bloodstream, the more rapidly insulin is released from the pancreas to remove excess glucose from the bloodstream. On the other hand, carbohydrates such as fruits and vegetables have a much lower glycemic load in a meal, meaning that they have a more limited impact (especially non-starchy vegetables) in the rise of blood glucose levels. As a result, insulin secretion is significantly reduced, and this reduces the potential activation of delta-6 and delta-5 desaturases.

Long-chain omega-3 fatty acids such eicosapentaenoic acid (EPA) and docosahexaenoic acid (DHA) are weak feedback inhibitors of these rate-limiting delta-6 and delta-5 desaturase enzymes necessary for the production of arachidonic acid. So as the levels of linoleic acid increase without a corresponding rise in omega-3 fatty acids, there is constant pressure to generate more arachidonic acid. When high levels of insulin (generated by a high-glycemic load diet) are coupled with high levels of linoleic acid from the diet, then the conversion of excess linoleic acid into arachidonic acid considerably increased. This is especially true if the levels of EPA and DHA are low. With the increased levels of arachidonic acid in cells, the likelihood of producing more pro-inflammatory eicosanoids is significantly enhanced.

The role of saturated fats in the generation of inflammation is more indirect compared to omega-6 fatty acids. Toll-like receptor 4 (TLR-4) interacts with the saturated fatty acid component of lipopolysaccharide (LPS). Saturated fats can also activate TLR-4, thus activating NF-κB although at a lower intensity than LPS itself [21, 22].

Whereas omega-6 and saturated fats are pro-inflammatory, omega-3 have anti-inflammatory effects. As mentioned above, omega-3 fatty acids are weak inhibitors of the rate-limiting enzymes required for the generation of arachidonic acid (AA). They also compete with AA for the enzymes required to generate eicosanoids. However, the different three-dimensional structures of EPA and DHA are quite different therefore imparting different effects. In particular, EPA and AA are very similar in three-dimensional structure, thus making EPA a better competitive inhibitor than DHA of the cyclooxygenase (COX) enzyme required to convert AA into eicosanoids, especially into prostaglandins and thromboxanes. As a result, the higher the level of EPA in the cell membrane relative to AA, the less likely that pro-inflammatory eicosanoids can be synthesized.

However, the real anti-inflammatory power of omega-3 fatty acids lies in their ability to function as substrates, a wide range of pro-resolution mediators that include resolvins, protectins, and maresins [5, 6]. These pro-resolution mediators are the key to reducing the levels of chronic cellular inflammation to bring any initial pro-inflammatory response back to homeostasis.

Monounsaturated fats such as oleic acid are virtually neutral in terms of eicosanoid actions. As a result, monounsaturated fats should be considered to be noninflammatory.

Finally, there is the role of polyphenols in inflammation [23, 24]. Polyphenols are the chemicals that give fruits and vegetables their color. At high enough levels, they have anti-inflammatory actions by activating the gene transcription factor PPAR-γ that inhibits the activation of NF-κB [23].

14.6 Putting It All Together

With the above short background on the hormonal effects of nutrients, it is now possible to put together the outlines of an anti-inflammatory diet.

A major problem in nutrition is that if one macronutrient nutrient goes up, then another must come down. That also means that the hormonal responses caused by a particular macronutrient nutrient will also rise and fall accordingly. The challenge is to find the right macronutrient combination to maintain the appropriate synergy of hormonal responses consistent with the continuous control of cellular inflammation.

In trying to find the appropriate balance of macronutrients, it follows a bell-shaped curve based on the protein-to-glycemic load ration as shown in Fig. 14.1.

If dietary carbohydrate content in the diet is too high, this will generate excess in insulin production. If this is coupled with high levels of omega-6 fatty acids, this can lead to increased cellular inflammation. At the other extreme when the carbohydrate content is too low, this can generate ketosis with corresponding rise in cortisol [25]. Between these two hormonal extremes lies a zone in which insulin levels and blood sugar levels are stabilized resulting in greater satiety and less fatigue.

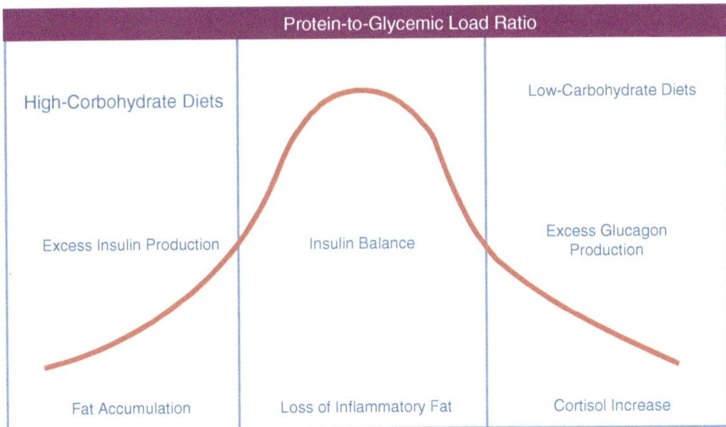

Fig. 14.1 Hormonal changes as a consequence of changing macronutrient composition

Another important question that has to be addressed is the level of calories required for an anti-inflammatory diet to be successful. This is important since it has been shown that the consumption of excess calories also creates inflammation in the hypothalamus leading to increased appetite [26].

14.7 History of Anti-inflammatory Diets

The first anti-inflammatory diet was proposed in the book, *The Zone*, published 20 years ago [19]. The central focus of this anti-inflammatory diet was one that was based on a bell-shaped curve of the protein-to-glycemic load described in Fig. 14.1. In addition there was a strong emphasis to reduce the levels of omega-6 and saturated fats with most of the fats in the diet coming from noninflammatory monounsaturated fats.

The midpoint of the protein-to-glycemic load for this anti-inflammatory diet had a slight excess of carbohydrates to low-fat protein. When the overall fat content was factored in the overall composition of the anti-inflammatory diet, it would be approximately 40 % low-glycemic-load carbohydrates, 30 % low-fat protein, and 30 % fat high in monounsaturated fats and low in omega-6 and saturated fatty acids. However, this proposed anti-inflammatory diet was also a calorie-restricted one to prevent the inflammatory effect of excess calories. Thus, the absolute levels of the various macronutrients of the proposed anti-inflammatory diet are shown in Table 14.1 at various total caloric intakes. The usual recommendation for females would be 1,200 cal per day and 1,500 cal per day for males.

It can be seen from Table 14.1 that at these caloric levels, the absolute levels of protein are adequate, the absolute levels of low-glycemic-load carbohydrates are moderate (although the volume on the plate would be significant), and the absolute levels of fats would be considered low. The macronutrient composition on a

Table 14.1 Macronutrient amounts of an anti-inflammatory diet at various caloric levels

Macronutrient	1,200 cal/day	1,500 cal/day
Carbohydrate	120 g/day	150 g/day
Protein	90 g/day	112 g/day
Fat	40 g/day	50 g/day

gram basis is 1 g of fat (primarily monounsaturated fats) for every 2 g of low-fat protein and 3 g of low-glycemic-load carbohydrates (primarily non-starchy vegetables and fruits).

14.8 Clinical Support for an Anti-inflammatory Diet

The first clinical trial to support such a macronutrient ratio in treating diabetics was reported in 1998 [27]. In this study, it was demonstrated that insulin resistance was significantly reduced within 4 days and before any weight loss. Carefully controlled clinical trials at Harvard Medical School in 1999 gave further support to the rapid hormonal changes and improvement in satiety using such the same macronutrient ratio in overweight children [28]. Researchers at Harvard Medical School confirmed these findings in satiety in 2000 in overweight adults [29]. More recent studies at Harvard Medical School have demonstrated that this macronutrient ratio is superior in reducing inflammation compared to isocaloric high-carbohydrate diets, even though the weight loss is identical [30].

In 2007, the Joslin Diabetes Center at Harvard Medical School announced their new dietary guidelines for treating obesity, metabolic syndrome, and diabetes [31]. These guidelines in terms of macronutrient composition and calorie content were virtually identical to those proposed more than a decade earlier [19]. Subsequent studies and other publications from the Joslin Diabetes Research Foundation have supported this anti-inflammatory diet concept [32, 33].

Numerous other clinical studies of this anti-inflammatory diet having 40 % of calories as carbohydrates, 30 % the calories as protein, and 30 % of calories as fat have demonstrated superior weight loss, fat loss, improved insulin levels, increased fat loss, increased satiety, and most importantly reduction of cellular inflammation [34–39].

From a visual standpoint, the composition of the plate for each meal is shown in Fig. 14.2.

At every meal, the plate should be divided into three equal sections. On one section should contain low-fat protein approximately the size and thickness of the palm of the hand. Appropriate protein choices would be chicken, fish, or protein-rich vegetarian sources. The other two-thirds of the plate should be filled with colorful carbohydrates (primarily non-starchy vegetables and limited amounts of fruits). This will simultaneously maintain a low glycemic load as well as provide adequate levels of polyphenols. Finally, the ideal added fat would be a dash of extra virgin olive oil (approximately 5 ml). The hormonal success of this dietary balance will be indicated by the lack of hunger and maintenance of mental acuity for the next 5 h.

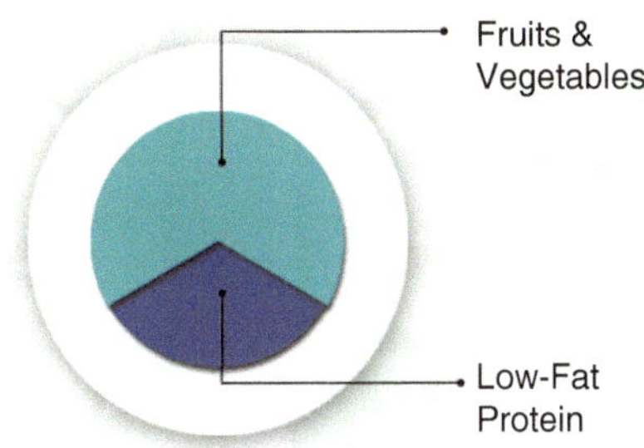

Fig. 14.2 Visual composition of typical anti-inflammatory meal

14.9 Clinical Markers of Inflammatory Risk and Their Ideal Ranges

There are three clinical markers that are important to achieve for an anti-inflammatory diet to be considered successful. Each of these markers relates to a different component of the inflammatory response, and all three markers should be within appropriate ranges to truly ensure that cellular inflammation is being managed.

14.9.1 AA/EPA Ratio

The first of these markers is the AA/EPA ratio. As discussed earlier, this is the first clinical marker that cellular inflammation is beginning to increase. The ideal ratio should be between 1.5 and 3. The average AA/EPA ratio in the Japanese population is 1.5 [40], whereas it is 18 in the average American population [41]. If the AA/EPA is less than 1, then the potential for bleeding increases, although there is significant reduction of cardiovascular events compared to the use of statins [42]. As long as the AA/EPA ratio remains above 1.2, there is no indication of any increased bleeding [43].

14.9.2 TG/HDL Ratio

This is a surrogate marker for insulin resistance in the liver and the beginning of the development of metabolic syndrome [44, 45]. The ideal ratio should be less than 1 (using mg/dl) or less than 0.4 (using mmoles/ml).

14.9.3 HbA1c

Glycosylated hemoglobin is a marker of long-term blood glucose control and is an indicator that type 2 diabetes is developing. It is generally accepted that HbA1c levels of greater 6.5 % is indicative of diabetes and increasing mortality [46].

Table 14.2 Clinical markers of an anti-inflammatory diet

Clinical maker	Optimal range
AA/EPA ratio	1.5–3
TG/HDL ratio	<1 (mg/dl) or <0.4 (mmoles/ml)
HbA1c	5 %

However, the optimal level of HbA1c should be 5 % as lower levels are also associated with increased mortality [47].

These optimal ranges are shown in Table 14.2.

All three clinical parameters must be within their optimal ranges to ensure the cellular inflammation is being controlled. If not, either a more strict anti-inflammatory diet should be employed, or the addition of anti-inflammatory supplements should be considered.

14.10 Potential Use for Anti-inflammatory Supplements

Often even a strict anti-inflammatory diet sometimes will not be sufficient to reach the desired ranges of the clinical markers described above. Under these circumstances, there are two additional anti-inflammatory supplements to consider.

14.10.1 Omega-3 Fatty Acids

The most important of these anti-inflammatory supplements would be highly refined omega-3 fatty acids that will help reduce the AA/EPA ratio and thus increase pro-resolution potential of the diet. The definition of a highly refined omega-3 fatty acid product would be one that has very low in PCB levels (5 ppb or lower). This is because all fish and the fish oils derived from them contain PCBs, which are known endocrine disruptors [48, 49].

A suggested serving would be about 2.5 g of supplemental EPA and DHA per day. However, the ideal dosage will be determined by titrating the blood levels of the mother to an appropriate AA/EPA ratio between 1.5 and 3. Adequate levels of these omega-3 fatty acids are critical not only for the proper neurological development of the fetus but also in reducing existing cellular inflammation in mother.

14.10.2 Polyphenol Extracts

As mentioned earlier, fruits and vegetables contain polyphenols. At high enough concentrations, polyphenol extracts can activate AMP kinase via interaction with the SIRT-1 gene [5, 23]. AMP kinase can be considered the central molecular switch that controls metabolism including blood glucose control. The supplementation with purified polyphenol extracts can further increase AMP kinase activity. An appropriate dose would be 500–1,000 mg of polyphenols per day.

14.11 Summary

Reducing the potential problems during pregnancy is best accomplished by first identifying high-risk populations with existing metabolic dysfunction caused by diet-induced inflammation and then working with such populations to reduce cellular inflammation by the use of an anti-inflammatory diet as described above. There are various time points at which such dietary interventions might be contemplated.

14.11.1 Peri-conception

The best time to prepare for the dramatic hormonal changes caused by pregnancy is lower cellular inflammation prior to conception. This is true for both parents. The rise in IVF treatments is an indication of the increasing difficulty of successful conception.

14.11.2 Pregnancy

It is known that the maternal diet can have significant effect on fetal programming with dramatic influence on the future health of the child [50–57]. The more closely a mother follows an anti-inflammatory diet, the better the future outcome for the child.

14.11.3 Postnatal

After birth, the brain is the most rapidly growing organ in the body of the child. Reducing cellular inflammation throughout the newborn's body with an anti-inflammatory diet is perhaps the best insurance policy for long-term metabolic health of the child. This is especially true as it is estimated that one-third of the children born in the United States after the year 2000 will develop diabetes [58].

Anti-inflammatory diets are ultimately based on new breakthroughs in molecular biology that support the ability of such a dietary strategy to reduce inflammation, increase resolution, and alter gene expression. The more quickly such diets are implemented in high-risk populations, the less the likelihood of long-term negative metabolic consequences for the offspring.

References

1. Serhan CN, Ward PA, Gilroy DW, Samir S. Fundamentals of inflammation. Cambridge, UK: Cambridge University Press; 2010.
2. Baker RG, Hayden MS, Ghosh S. NF-κB, inflammation, and metabolic disease. Cell Metab. 2011;13(1):11–22.
3. Mariotto S, Suzuki Y, Persichini T, Colasanti M, Suzuki H, Cantoni O. Cross-talk between NO and arachidonic acid in inflammation. Curr Med Chem. 2007;14(18):1940–4.

4. Calder PC. Dietary modification of inflammation with lipids. Proc Nutr Soc. 2002;61(3): 345–58.
5. Sears B. The mediterranean zone. New York: Random House; 2014.
6. Spite M, Claria J, Serhan CN. Resolvins, specialized proresolving lipid mediators, and their potential roles in metabolic diseases. Cell Metab. 2014;19(1):21–36.
7. Sears B. The anti-inflammation zone. New York: Regan Books; 2005.
8. Ndumele CE, Pradhan AD, Ridker PM. Interrelationships between inflammation, C-reactive protein, and insulin resistance. J Cardiometab Syndr. 2006;1(3):190–6.
9. Bastard JP, Maachi M, Lagathu C, Kim MJ, Caron M, Vidal H, et al. Recent advances in the relationship between obesity, inflammation, and insulin resistance. Eur Cytokine Netw. 2006; 17(1):4–12.
10. Mather SJ, Chianelli M. Radiolabelled cytokines. Q J Nucl Med. 1996;40(3):290–300.
11. Rifai N, Ridker PM. Inflammatory markers and coronary heart disease. Curr Opin Lipidol. 2002;13(4):383–9.
12. Tall AR. C-reactive protein reassessed. N Engl J Med. 2004;350:1450–2.
13. Sears B. Toxic fat. Knoxville: Thomas Nelson; 2008.
14. Lionetti L, Mollica MP, Lombardi A, Cavaliere G, Gifuni G, Barletta A. From chronic overnutrition to insulin resistance: the role of fat-storing capacity and inflammation. Nutr Metab Cardiovasc Dis. 2009;19(2):146–52.
15. Hotamisligil GS. Inflammation and metabolic disorders. Nature. 2006;444(7121):860–7.
16. De Fina LF, Vega GL, Leonard D, Grundy SM. Fasting glucose, obesity, and metabolic syndrome as predictors of type 2 diabetes: the Cooper Center Longitudinal Study. J Investig Med. 2012;60(8):1164–8.
17. Bierhaus A, Stern DM, Nawroth PP. RAGE in inflammation: a new therapeutic target? Curr Opin Investig Drugs. 2006;7(11):985–91.
18. Wei D, Li J, Shen M, Jia W, Chen N, Chen T, Su D, et al. Cellular production of n-3 PUFAs and reduction of n-6-to-n-3 ratios in the pancreatic beta-cells and islets enhance insulin secretion and confer protection against cytokine-induced cell death. Diabetes. 2010;59(2):471–8.
19. Sears B. The Zone. New York: Regan Books; 1995.
20. Brenner RR. Nutritional and hormonal factors influencing desaturation of essential fatty acids. Prog Lipid Res. 1981;20:41–7.
21. Huang S, Rutkowsky JM, Snodgrass RG, Ono-Moore KD, Schneider DA, Newman JW, et al. Saturated fatty acids activate TLR-mediated proinflammatory signaling pathways. J Lipid Res. 2012;53(9):2002–13.
22. Lee JY, Plakidas A, Lee WH, Heikkinen A, Chanmugam P, Bray G, et al. Differential modulation of Toll-like receptors by fatty acids: preferential inhibition by n-3 polyunsaturated fatty acids. J Lipid Res. 2003;44(3):479–86.
23. Scapagnini G, Vasto S, Sonya V, Abraham NG, Nader AG, Caruso C, et al. Modulation of Nrf2/ARE pathway by food polyphenols: a nutritional neuroprotective strategy for cognitive and neurodegenerative disorders. Mol Neurobiol. 2011;44(2):192–201.
24. Rahman I, Biswas SK, Kirkham PA. Regulation of inflammation and redox signaling by dietary polyphenols. Biochem Pharmacol. 2006;72(11):1439–52.
25. Ebbeling CB, Swain JF, Feldman HA, Wong WW, Hachey DL, Garcia-Lago E, et al. Effects of dietary composition on energy expenditure during weight-loss maintenance. JAMA. 2012;307(24):2627–34.
26. Zhang X, Zhang G, Zhang H, Karin M, Bai H, Cai D. Hypothalamic IKKbeta/NF-kappaB and ER stress link overnutrition to energy imbalance and obesity. Cell. 2008;135(1):61–73.
27. Markovic TP, Campbell LV, Balasubramanian S, Jenkins AB, Fleury AC, Simons LA, et al. Beneficial effect on average lipid levels from energy restriction and fat loss in obese individuals with or without type 2 diabetes. Diabetes Care. 1998;21:695–700.
28. Ludwig DS, Majzoub JA, Al-Zahrani A, Dallal GE, Blanco I, Roberts SB. High glycemic index foods, overeating, and obesity. Pediatrics. 1999;103(3):E26.
29. Agus MS, Swain JF, Larson CL, Eckert EA, Ludwig DS. Dietary composition and physiologic adaptations to energy restriction. Am J Clin Nutr. 2000;71(4):901–7.

30. Pereira MA, Swain J, Goldfine AB, Rifai N, Ludwig DS. Effects of a low-glycemic load diet on resting energy expenditure and heart disease risk factors during weight loss. JAMA. 2004;292(20):2482–90.
31. Joslin Diabetes Reseach Center. www.joslin.org/docs/Nutrition_Guideline_Graded.pdf. EPIC and Diabetes. 2007
32. Hamdy O, Carver C. The Why WAIT program: improving clinical outcomes through weight management in type 2 diabetes. Curr Diab Rep. 2008;8(5):413–20.
33. Hamdy O, Colberg SR. The diabetes breakthrough. Don Mills: Harlequin; 2014.
34. Layman DK, Boileau RA, Erickson DJ, Painter JE, Shiue H, Sather C, Christou DD. A reduced ratio of dietary carbohydrate to protein improves body composition and blood lipid profiles during weight loss in adult women. J Nutr. 2003;133:411–7.
35. Layman DK, Shiue H, Sather C, Erickson DJ, Baum J. Increased dietary protein modifies glucose and insulin homeostasis in adult women during weight loss. J Nutr. 2003;133(2):405–10.
36. Johnston CS, Tjonn SL, Swan PD, White A, Hutchins H, Sears B. Ketogenic low-carbohydrate diets have no metabolic advantage over nonketogenic low-carbohydrate diets. Am J Clin Nutr. 2006;83(5):1055–61.
37. Gannon MC, Nuttall FQ. Control of blood glucose in type 2 diabetes without weight loss by modification of diet composition. Nutr Metab. 2006;3:16.
38. Lasker DA, Evans EM, Layman DK. Moderate carbohydrate, moderate protein weight loss diet reduces cardiovascular disease risk compared to high carbohydrate, low protein diet in obese adults: a randomized clinical trial. Nutr Metab. 2008;5:30.
39. Layman DK, Evans EM, Erickson D, Seyler J, Weber J, Bagshaw D, et al. A moderate-protein diet produces sustained weight loss and long-term changes in body composition and blood lipids in obese adults. J Nutr. 2009;139(6):514–21.
40. Ohnishi H, Saito Y. Eicosapentaenoic acid (EPA) reduces cardiovascular events: relationship with the EPA/arachidonic acid ratio. J Atheroscler Thromb. 2013;20(12):861–77.
41. Harris WS, Pottala JV, Varvel SA, Borowski JJ, Ward JN, McConnell JP. Erythrocyte omega-3 fatty acids increase and linoleic acid decreases with age: observations from 160,000 patients. Prostaglandins Leukot Essent Fatty Acids. 2013;88(4):257–63.
42. Yokoyama M, Origasa H, Matsuzaki M, Matsuzawa Y, Saito Y, Ishikawa Y, et al. Effects of eicosapentaenoic acid on major coronary events in hypercholesterolaemic patients (JELIS): a randomised open-label, blinded endpoint analysis. Lancet. 2007;369(9567):1090–8.
43. Yee LD, Lester JL, Cole RM, Richardson JR, Hsu JC, Li Y, et al. Omega-3 fatty acid supplements in women at high risk of breast cancer have dose-dependent effects on breast adipose tissue fatty acid composition. Am J Clin Nutr. 2010;91(5):1185–94.
44. McLaughlin T, Reaven G, Abbasi F, Lamendola C, Saad M, Waters D, et al. Is there a simple way to identify insulin-resistant individuals at increased risk of cardiovascular disease? Am J Cardiol. 2005;96(3):399–404.
45. Salazar MR, Carbajal HA, Espeche WG, Leiva Sisnieguez CE, March CE, Balbin E, et al. Comparison of the abilities of the plasma triglyceride/high-density lipoprotein cholesterol ratio and the metabolic syndrome to identify insulin resistance. Diab Vasc Dis Res. 2013;10(4):346–52.
46. Levitan EB, Liu S, Stampfer MJ, Cook NR, Rexrode KM, Ridker PM, et al. HbA1c measured in stored erythrocytes and mortality rate among middle-aged and older women. Diabetologia. 2008;51(2):267–75.
47. Carson AP, Fox CS, McGuire DK, Levitan EB, Laclaustra M, Mann DM, et al. Low hemoglobin A1c and risk of all-cause mortality among US adults without diabetes. Circ Cardiovasc Qual Outcomes. 2010;3(6):661–7.
48. Ashley JT, Ward JS, Schafer MW, Stapleton HM, Velinsky DJ. Evaluating daily exposure to polychlorinated biphenyls and polybrominated diphenyl ethers in fish oil supplements. Food Addit Contam Part A Chem Anal Control Expo Risk Assess. 2010;27(8):1177–85.
49. Arsenescu V, Arsenescu RI, King V, Swanson H, Cassis LA. Polychlorinated biphenyl-77 induces adipocyte differentiation and proinflammatory adipokines and promotes obesity and atherosclerosis. Environ Health Perspect. 2008;116(6):761–8.

50. Yajnik CS. Fetal programming of diabetes: still so much to learn! Diabetes Care. 2010; 33(5):1146–8.
51. Ravelli AC, van Der Meulen JH, Osmond C, Barker DJ, Bleker OP. Obesity at the age of 50 y in men and women exposed to famine prenatally. Am J Clin Nutr. 1999;70(5):811–6.
52. Hanbauer I, Rivero-Covelo I, Maloku E, Baca A, Hu Q, Hibbeln JR, et al. The decrease of n-3 fatty acid energy percentage in an equicaloric diet fed to B6C3Fe mice for three generations elicits obesity. Cardiovasc Psychiatry Neurol. 2009;2009:867041.
53. Alvheim AR, Torstensen BE, Lin YH, Lillefosse HH, Lock EJ, Madsen L, et al. Dietary linoleic acid elevates the endocannabinoids 2-AG and anandamide and promotes weight gain in mice fed a low fat diet. Lipids. 2014;49(1):59–69.
54. Alvheim AR, Malde MK, Osei-Hyiaman D, Lin YH, Pawlosky RJ, et al. Dietary linoleic acid elevates endogenous 2-AG and anandamide and induces obesity. Obesity. 2012;20(10): 1984–94.
55. Muhlhausler BS, Ailhaud GP. Omega-6 polyunsaturated fatty acids and the early origins of obesity. Curr Opin Endocrinol Diabetes Obes. 2013;20(1):56–61.
56. Skinner MK. Endocrine disruptor induction of epigenetic transgenerational inheritance of disease. Mol Cell Endocrinol. 2014;398:1–3.
57. Schneider JE, Brozek JM, Keen-Rhinehart E. Our stolen figures: the interface of sexual differentiation, endocrine disruptors, maternal programming, and energy balance. Horm Behav. 2014;66(1):104–19.
58. Olshansky SJ, Passaro DJ, Hershow RC, Layden J, Carnes BA, Brody J, et al. A potential decline in life expectancy in the United States in the 21st century. N Engl J Med. 2005; 352(11):1138–45.

Let's Make It the Real Mediterranean Diet Not the "Supermarket Standard Feeding Plus a Leaf of Basil"

15

Angela Spadafranca and Lidia Lewandowski

Contents

15.1 Mediterranean Diet: Origins and Definition

The Mediterranean diet is born in the Mediterranean basin, a portion of land unique for its geography and considered by the historians "the cradle of society," because within its borders the whole history of the ancient world took place. The Mediterranean dietary pattern is the mirror of the history and the traditions of the people of Mediterranean basin. Besides foods as symbol of rural and agricultural culture such as bread, olive oil, and wine, triad of Greek and Roman tradition, other features of the Mediterranean diet are the results of the progress of the history; an example is the great historical impact of the discovery of America by Europeans. This discovery is also reflected in an importation of new foodstuffs such as potatoes, tomatoes, corn, peppers, and chili, as well as different varieties of beans. The tomato, "exotic curiosity," ornamental fruit only belatedly considered edible, was the first red vegetable that enriched our basket of plants and later became a symbol of the Mediterranean cuisine [1].

A. Spadafranca, PhD • L. Lewandowski (✉)
ICANS, International Centre for the Assessment of Nutritional Status,
University of Milan, Milan, Italy
e-mail: angela.spadafranca@unimi.it; lidia.lewandowski@tiscali.it

E. Ferrazzi, B. Sears (eds.), *Metabolic Syndrome and Complications of Pregnancy: The Potential Preventive Role of Nutrition*,
DOI 10.1007/978-3-319-16853-1_15

The definition of Mediterranean diet is not consensual, partly because this dietary pattern is fairly heterogeneous among Mediterranean countries and also within the countries themselves [2, 3]. However, many studies have defined the Mediterranean pattern identifying several typical foods, some of the common features of which are [4–7] a high consumption of plant foods such as legumes, cereals, fruits and vegetables, and nuts and seeds, low consumption of meat and dairy products and olive oil as main source of fat, and moderate consumption of wine.

15.2 Mediterranean Diet: A Choice of Good Health

Overall, the Mediterranean diet is considered a healthy prudent dietary pattern, and high adherence to it has been associated with a better health status, due to the protective effect against various chronic diseases such as coronary diseases and certain cancers [8–12].

The discovery of the health benefits of the Mediterranean diet is attributed to the American scientist Ancel Keys of the University of Minnesota School of Power, which pointed out the correlation between cardiovascular disease and diet for the first time [13]. Ancel Keys, in the 1950s, was struck by a phenomenon, which could not, at first, provide a full explanation. The poor population of small towns of southern Italy was, against all predictions, much healthier than the wealthy citizens of New York, either of their own relatives who emigrated in earlier decades in the United States. Keys suggested that this depended on food and tried to validate his original insight, focusing his attention on foods that made up the diet of these populations. Thus, he led the famous "Seven Countries Study" (conducted in Finland, Holland, Italy, United States, Greece, Japan, and Yugoslavia) in order to document the relationship between lifestyles, nutrition, and cardiovascular disease between different populations, including cross-sectional studies, being able to prove scientifically the nutritional value of the Mediterranean diet and its contribution to the health of the populations that adopted it [8]. From this study emerged clearly, as the populations that had adopted a diet based on the Mediterranean pattern presented a very low rate of cholesterol in the blood and, consequently, a minimum percentage of coronary heart disease. This was mainly due to the plentiful use of olive oil, bread, pasta, vegetables, herbs, garlic, red onions, and other foods of vegetable origin compared to a rather moderate use of meat [14].

Starting from Keys' studies, many other scientific researchers have analyzed the association between dietary habits and chronic diseases. It is now possible to say that there is a convergence of assessments agreed in the direction of full recognition of the beneficial qualities of the Mediterranean way of eating. Many studies and clinical trials have shown that the Mediterranean diet reduces the risk of cardiovascular disease and metabolic syndrome. A remarkable decrease of abdominal circumference, an increase in high-density lipoprotein (HDL), a decrease in triglycerides, a lowering of blood pressure, and a decrease in the concentration of glucose in the blood have been put into evidence [15, 16].

In a recent meta-analysis, the Mediterranean eating pattern turned out to be more effective than low-fat diets in inducing important long-term changes in cardiovascular risk factors and inflammatory markers [17]. Further evidence comes from the study conducted by the Epicor team in Italy which showed that women in the highest quartile of vegetables and olive oil consumption resulted to have lower incidence of coronary heart disease compared to those in the lowest quartile [18]. Good news came also for mental wellness. In addition to many studies supporting the beneficial effects of Mediterranean diet on the incidence of neurodegenerative disease as Parkinson's and Alzheimer's diseases [10, 19], a group of Spanish researchers found that higher adherence to Mediterranean diet is positively associated with better health-related quality of life [20].

15.3 Mediterranean Diet: In Pregnant Women

Recently, Mediterranean diet has been associated with the prevention of premature birth in pregnant women [21], lower incidence of gestational diabetes, and better degree of glucose tolerance [22].

The degree of adherence to the diet in 3,206 Caucasian pregnant mothers in Rotterdam was positively associated with plasma folate and serum vitamin B_{12} concentrations and showed an inverse relationship with homocysteine and high-sensitivity C-reactive protein plasma concentrations ($P < 0.05$). Important fetal size and placental parameters were associated with the degree of adherence to the diet, revealing a 72 g lower birth weight (95 % CI −110.8, −33.3) and a 15 g lower placental weight (95 % CI −29.8, −0.2) for women with low adherence to the diet. Therefore, low adherence to a Mediterranean diet in early pregnancy seems associated with decreased intrauterine size with a lower placental and a lower birth weight.

In the present study, women with low adherence to the Mediterranean diet did not only have smaller placentas but also tended toward higher uteroplacental vascular resistance [23].

This seems biologically plausible since early placentation is characterized by vascular remodeling, increased inflammation, oxidative stress, and rapid cell division.

The Mediterranean diet is an important source of methyl donors. Differences in quantitative methylation may affect genes implicated in placental and fetal size. These results might also suggest that fetal and placental programming can be affected by the use of the Mediterranean dietary pattern in early pregnancy. This is supported by recent findings that periconception folic acid use is associated with epigenetic changes in the insulin-like growth factor 2 gene in the child, thereby potentially affecting intrauterine programming [24]. This suggests that maternal diet may cause epigenetic modifications in the embryo, resulting in altered growth patterns. These results substantiate the importance of the Mediterranean diet and suggest the need for more attention and awareness in pregnancy.

15.4 Mediterranean Diet: Features and Practice

In January 1993, international experts on diet, nutrition, and health convened to review research on the composition and health implications of Mediterranean diets consumed during the past half century. In this conference called "Conference on The Diets of Mediterranean," the following Mediterranean patterns were defined:

- Abundant plant foods – fruits, vegetables, breads (whole grain), other forms of whole grain cereals, crucifers (broccoli and cauliflower), beans, nuts, and seeds)
- Minimally processed, seasonally fresh, and locally grown foods
- Fresh fruit as the typical daily dessert, with sweets based on nuts, olive oil, and concentrated sugars or honey consumed during feast days only
- Olive oil as the principal source of dietary fats
- Dairy products (mainly cheese and yogurt) consumed in low to moderate amounts
- Fewer than four eggs consumed per week
- Red meat consumed in low frequency and amounts, 1 per week
- Wine consumed in low to moderate amounts, generally with meals (red wine, only during meals and less than 125 ml, during pregnancy)

However, it must be said that this characteristic definition of the Mediterranean diet and its typical composition is not without ambiguities, which require certain considerations.

Due to multiple factors such as globalization and economic development, changes in food consumption have influenced and are still challenging traditional healthy food patterns in Mediterranean countries. Rui da Silva et al. [25] carried out a study aimed to analyze the worldwide trends of adherence to the Mediterranean diet, in 1961–1965 and 2000–2003. In order to have a sample from across the world, forty-one countries were selected, and data were obtained from the FAO food balance sheets in two periods: 1961–1965 and 2000–2003. The majority of the 41 countries in this study have tended to drift away from a Mediterranean-like dietary pattern. Mediterranean Europe and the other Mediterranean country groups suffered a significant decrease in their Mediterranean Index Adherence (MAI) values. The Mediterranean European group, especially Greece, experienced the greatest decrease in MAI value.

We cannot hide that Mediterranean societies are rapidly withdrawing from this eating pattern orienting their food choices toward products typical of the western diet pattern, which is rich in refined grains, animal fats, sugars, and processed meat but is quite poor in legumes, cereals, fruits, and vegetables. The reasons people keep on shifting from healthy to unhealthy dietary habits remain open to several interpretations. Social changes appear to have consistently contributed to radical reversal in dietary habits in European Mediterranean societies even though developing countries are somewhat turning into westernized diets as well. Among possible causes, increasing prices of some of the major food items of Mediterranean pyramid seem to have led people to give up this eating pattern in favor of less expensive products which allow to save money but are definitively unhealthy [26]. Nutrition policy actions to tackle dietary westernization and preserve the healthy prudent Mediterranean Diet are required.

15.5 Mediterranean Diet Pyramid: An Easy Model to Make the Real Mediterranean Diet

The "food pyramid" is an effective image designed for the first time in 1992 by the US Department of Agriculture which simply represents a fair and balanced way of eating, displaying the proportions and the frequencies with which foods should be consumed, a style that coincides with the Mediterranean model identified by the physiologist Ancel Keys.

The main concepts of the food pyramid are the "proportionality," that is, the right amount of foods to choose from each group; the "portion" standard quantity of food in grams, which is assumed as the unit of measurement to be a balanced feeding; the "variety," i.e., the importance of changing the choices within a food group; and "moderation" in the consumption of certain foods, such as fat or sweets.

In Fig. 15.1 there is a reproduction of Mediterranean pyramid: we can see that every day, we have to drink at least 8 glasses of water; to eat cereals (to avoid refined and to prefer wholemeal cereals), vegetables, and fruit; to dress with olive oil, herbs, and spices; to consume yogurt/milk/low-fat cheese, nuts, or dried fruit; and to drink a glass of red wine during the meal. This is an efficacy way to introduce energy, fibers, vitamins, antioxidants and anti-inflammatory compounds, minerals, and unsaturated fat (i.e., oleic acid from olive oil or balanced omega-3 and omega-6 from nut or dried fruit) with healthy effects. Interesting is to reflect upon the possible red wine consumption by pregnant women: until now generally gynecologists indicate to abstain from alcohol consumption in pregnancy for possible negative effects on fetal development; however, red wine is a rich source of polyphenol compounds with antioxidant effects that, if moderately consumed, could improve oxidative status of the women without damages for the baby. Few studies investigated this topic in pregnant women until now, controlling for smoking habits and binge drinking [27], and proved that when red wine is part of a healthy meal it improves placental weight and has no impact on fetus and newborn.

The food protein sources are important, and they must be in the diet every day, but it is mandatory to vary adequately the weekly frequency in order to modulate the impact of saturated fat associated to animal protein; for this reason, the consumption of vegetable proteins from legumes should be encouraged. We can find in Mediterranean diet a big variety of legumes: kidney beans, romano beans, fava beans, lima beans, chickpeas, peas, and lentils.

It is important to know that legumes associated with cereals improve their protein quality, because essential amino acid pool is completed. Legumes could be consumed with pasta, rice, spelt or couscous, and polenta in a plate but also as ingredient in a mixed salad or in a soup. The use of legumes as side dish is possible but only if associated with a moderate portion of other protein food such as fish, meat, or eggs; this is important to avoid an excess of protein intake.

Legumes, such as also whole grain, are a rich source of prebiotic fiber that stimulates in the colon the growth of *Bifidobacterium*, a beneficial bacterial genus. Moreover, many studies have shown the healthy effects of legumes on lipid and

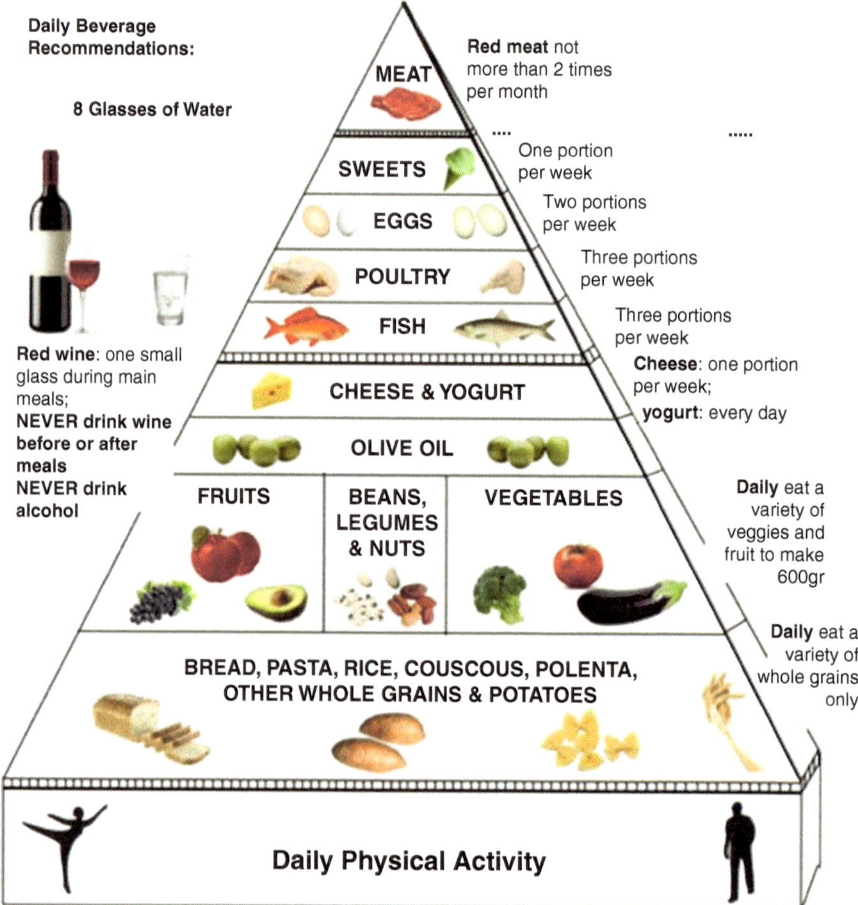

Fig. 15.1 Mediterranean diet pyramid: an easy model to make the real Mediterranean diet

glycemic serum human profile. Therefore, there are a lot of reasons to introduce the consumption of this typical Mediterranean food at least two to three times for week.

Besides legumes, fish consumption is advised at least twice a week. Health benefits (decreased risk of cardiovascular events and mortality) from fish consumption are ascribed to n-3 polyunsaturated fatty acids, eicosapentaenoic acid (EPA), and docosahexaenoic acid (DHA). DHA also appears important for neurodevelopment during gestation and infancy [28]. Women of childbearing age and nursing mothers should consume 2 seafood servings/week. Observational studies show positive associations between maternal DHA levels or fish intake during pregnancy and behavioral attention scores, visual recognition memory, and language comprehension in infancy. However, fish also contain contaminants such as mercury, dioxins, and polychlorinated biphenyls. The Environmental Protection Agency determined a reference dose, i.e., the allowable upper limit of daily intake, for methylmercury of

0.1 ug/kg per day (50 μg/week for a 70-kg woman, calculated from the lower 95 % confidence limit at which gestational exposure to mercury may produce abnormal neurologic test scores, multiplied by a tenfold uncertainty factor), and published a focused advisory for women of childbearing age, nursing mothers, and young children. The advisory specifically advises such individuals to avoid shark, swordfish, golden bass, and king mackerel (each containing 50 μg methylmercury per serving); sardines, salmon, crab, tuna, and trout are instead allowed [29].

The meat is a food with high protein content (from 15th to 25 %) and of high biological value, able to make all the amino acids necessary for protein synthesis (essential amino acids) in optimal amounts. It also provides B-complex vitamins, especially B12, and trace elements, particularly iron, zinc, and copper. However, among meat sources, it is better to prefer poultry and to limit red meat and white meat from small mammals – rabbit and hare – red meat is okay but only a few times per month since they are rich in cholesterol and saturated fat meat. A special characteristic of meat from mammalians is the different sialic acid of cell membrane, the difference between N-glycolylneuraminic acid (Neu5Gc) and *N*-acetylneuraminic acid (Neu5Ac) is tiny, but Neu5Gc is a weak immunogenic compound and its unbalanced and frequent consumption might be on the pro-inflammatory stimuli that play a negative role in long lifespan expected in modern humans [30].

Physical activity and other diet-related lifestyle factors contribute to wellness with Mediterranean patterns. Certain lifestyle factors are of particular interest: the social support and sense of community that accompanies sharing food with family and friends; lengthy meals that provide relaxation and relief from daily stress; and delicious meals, carefully prepared, that stimulate enjoyment of healthy diets.

"The Mediterranean diet is a set of traditional practices, knowledge and skills passed on from generation to generation and providing a sense of belonging and continuity to the concerned communities." This is the first reason cited by the UNESCO for recognizing the Mediterranean diet as an intangible cultural heritage. This international organization has officially ratified what science has been continuously demonstrating during the last decades. From what we read in the 5-point motivation, it appears quite clear that the UNESCO does not consider MD just as a mere collection of some selected foods but ascribes to the eating habits typical of the Mediterranean basin a cultural-promotion role deserving a special mention as plainly stated in the description of MD: "The Mediterranean diet encompasses more than just food. It promotes social interaction, since Mediterranean diet communal meals are the cornerstone of social customs and festive events. It has given rise to a considerable body of knowledge, songs, maxims, tales and legends. The system is rooted in respect for the territory and biodiversity, and ensures the conservation and development of traditional activities and crafts linked to fishing and farming in the Mediterranean communities of which Soria in Spain, Koroni in Greece, Cilento in Italy and Chefchaouen in Morocco are examples. Women play a particularly vital role in the transmission of expertise, as well as knowledge of rituals, traditional gestures and celebrations, and the safeguarding of techniques."

Mediterranean diet is a model culture of human health so let's make it the real Mediterranean diet not the "supermarket standard feeding plus a leaf of basil!"

To this purpose, don't forget the following *ten rules*:

1. Use olive oil as main dressing (40 ml/day).
2. Eat a portion of seasonal vegetables at every meal partly fresh or partly cooked (at least 200 g).
3. Eat a portion (150 g) of legumes at least twice a week.
4. Eat at least two portions of fish (200 g each) per week, including bluefish.
5. Limit meat once per week or one every fortnight, be it of good quality from extensive lawn breeding.
6. Eat fresh fruit every day and dry fruit as a snack (at least 200 g) (packaged juices do not belong to the healthy fruit category but rather to soft drinks or worse junk food if added with sugar and chemical colors).
7. Consume yogurt or milk every day, but use cheese in moderation (twice per week) (avoid milk and dairy products if you are lactose intolerant, as 25 % of Caucasians or 70 % of South Americans or 90 % of Chinese of Han ancestry).
8. Be sure to include whole grain bread or wholemeal cereals during your meals (consider to rotate among the variety of grains: wheat, rice, maize, spelt, buckwheat, barley; never use refined grains or refined flours, but as exceptions).
9. Drink wine (1–2 small glasses per day) always during meals (red wine is richer in polyphenols than white wine).
10. Leave sweets and soft drinks for special occasions.
11. Remember: Spices (ground black pepper, curcuma, chili pepper, oregano, basil, etc.) are good and great antioxidants; use them in abundance to make tasty plates and limit salt!

Tables 15.1 and 15.2 reported suggestions to easy practice Mediterranean diet.

Table 15.1 One day of Mediterranean diet: an example of 2,000 kcal

Breakfast	250 g of yogurt 40 g (4 spoons) of breakfast cereals or muesli 1 portion of fresh season fruit
Morning snack	30 g of whole crackers
Lunch	80 g of pasta with tomato sauce at pleasure, basil and/or vegetables 80 g of legumes (fresh, frozen, or tinned) 1 portion of cooked or uncooked seasonal vegetables (at least 200 g)
Afternoon snack	1 portion (20 g) of dry fruit (e.g., nuts, almonds)
Dinner	80 g of whole wheat bread 200 g of low-fat fish (codfish, place, or trout) 1 portion of cooked or uncooked seasonal vegetables (at least 200 g, except 50 g for salad) 1 portion of fresh season fruit
Throughout the day	40 g of virgin olive oil (4 spoons) to be added preferably after cooking (just before serving) 125 ml (1 glass) of red wine
Vinegar, lemon juice, aromatic herbs, and spices to taste	

Table 15.2 The variety is important: some useful suggestion to reach it

Breakfast	1 cup of milk (250 ml) (cow or goat) or 250 g of yogurt 40 g of wholemeal cereals, muesli, or 60 g of wheat bread 1 portion of fresh season fruit
Snack examples	30 g of crackers or 1 cereal bar or 60 g of bread or 20 g of dry fruit or seeds
Meal proposals	80 g of pasta with tomato sauce at pleasure, basil and/or vegetables or 80 g of rice, oat, spelt, or other cereals or 250 g of potato dumplings or 100 g of whole wheat bread or 300 g of potatoes or 80 g of maize flour or 150 g cooked maize porridge
	3 times a week: 200 g of low-fat fish or (max once a week tinned) 2 times a week: 150 g of white meat 1–2 times a month: 150 g of red meat 4 times a week: 150 g of legumes (fresh, frozen, or max once a week tinned) 1–2 times a week: 100 g of low-fat cheese 1 time a week: 100 g of bresaola or Prosciutto di Parma or ham, lean meat 1–2 times a week: 2 eggs
	1 portion of cooked or uncooked seasonal vegetables (at least 200 g, except 50 g for salad)
	1 portion of fresh season fruit
During the day	Virgin olive oil, vinegar, lemon juice, aromatic herbs, and spices 1 glass (125 ml) of red wine

References

1. Altomare R, Cacciabaudo F, Damiano G, Palumbo VD, Gioviali MC, Bellavia M, Tomasello G, Lo Monte AI. The Mediterranean diet: a history of health. Iranian J Publ Health. 2013;42:449–57.
2. Noah A, Truswell AS. There are many Mediterranean diets. Asia Pac J Clin Nutr. 2001; 10:2–9.
3. Karamanos B, Thanopoulou A, Angelico F, et al. Nutritional habits in the Mediterranean basin. The macronutrient composition of diet and its relation with the traditional Mediterranean diet. Multi-centre study of the Mediterranean Group for the Study of Diabetes (MGSD). Eur J Clin Nutr. 2002;56:983–91.
4. Willett WC, Sacks F, Trichopoulou A, Drescher G, Ferro-Luzzi A, Helsing E, Trichopoulos D. Mediterranean diet pyramid: a cultural model for healthy eating. Am J Clin Nutr. 1995; 61:1402S–6.
5. Trichopoulou A. Traditional Mediterranean diet and longevity in the elderly: a review. Public Health Nutr. 2004;7:943–7.
6. Serra-Majem L, Trichopoulou A, Ngo de la Cruz J, Cervera P, Garcia Alvarez A, La Vecchia C, Lemtouni A, Trichopoulos D. Does the definition of the Mediterranean diet need to be updated? Public Health Nutr. 2004;7:927–9.
7. Bach-Faig A, Geleva D, Carrasco JL, Ribas-Barba L, Serra- Majem L. Evaluating associations between Mediterranean diet adherence indexes and biomarkers of diet and disease. Public Health Nutr. 2006;9:1110–7.

8. Keys A, editor. Seven countries: a multivariate analysis of death and coronary heart disease. 1st ed. Cambridge: Harvard University Press; 1980.
9. Serra-Majem L, Roman B, Estruch R. Scientific evidence of interventions using the Mediterranean diet: a systematic review. Nutr Rev. 2006;64:S27–47.
10. Sofi F, Cesari F, Abbate R, Gensini GF, Casini A. Adherence to Mediterranean diet and health status: meta-analysis. BMJ. 2008;337:1344.
11. Helsing E, Trichopoulou A, editors. The Mediterranean diet and food culture – a symposium. Eur J Clin Nutr. 1989;43 Suppl 2:1–92.
12. Serra Majem L, Helsing E, editors. Changing patterns of fat intake in Mediterranean countries. Eur J Clin Nutr. 1993;47(Suppl 1):S1–100.
13. Keys AB, Keys M. How to eat well and stay well, the Mediterranean way. New York: Doubleday; 1975.
14. Menotti A, Keys A, Blackburn H, Kromhout D, Karvonen M, Nissinen A, et al. Comparison of multivariate predictive power of major risk factors for coronary heart diseases in different countries: results from eight nations of the seven countries study, 25-year follow-up. J Cardiov Risk. 1996;3:69–75.
15. Estruch R, Martínez-González MA, Corella D, et al. Effects of a Mediterranean-style diet on cardiovascular risk factors: a randomized trial. Ann Intern Med. 2006;145(1):1–11.
16. Fitó M, Guxens M, Corella D, Sáez G, Estruch R, de la Torre R, et al; PREDIMED Study Investigators. Effect of a traditional Mediterranean diet on lipoprotein oxidation: a randomized controlled trial. Arch Intern Med. 2007;167(11):1195–203.
17. Nordmann AJ, Suter-Zimmermann K, Bucher HC, Shai I, Tuttle KR, Estruch R, et al. Meta-analysis comparing Mediterranean to low-fat diets for modification of cardiovascular risk factors. Am J Med. 2011;124:841–51.
18. Bendinelli B, Masala G, Saieva C, Salvini S, Calonico C, Sacerdote C, et al. Fruit, vegetables, and olive oil and risk of coronary heart disease in Italian women: the EPICOR Study. Am J Clin Nutr. 2011;93:275–83.
19. Sofi F, Abbate R, Gensini GF, Casini A. Accruing evidence on benefits of adherence to the Mediterranean diet on health: an updated systematic review and meta-analysis. Am J Clin Nutr. 2010;92:1189–96.
20. Henríquez Sánchez P, Ruano C, de Irala J, Ruiz-Canela M, Martínez-González MA, Sánchez-Villegas A. Adherence to the Mediterranean diet and quality of life in the SUN Project. Eur J Clin Nutr. 2012;66(3):360–8.
21. Mikkelsen TB, Østerdal ML, Knudsen VK, Haugen M, Meltzer HM, Bakketeig L, Olsen SF. Association between a Mediterranean-type diet and risk of preterm birth among Danish women: a prospective cohort study. Acta Obstet Gynecol. 2008;87:325–30.
22. Karamanos B, Thanopoulou A, Anastasiou E, Assaad-Khalil S, Albache N, Bachaoui M, Slama CB, El Ghomari H, Jotic A, Lalic N, Lapolla A, Saab C, Marre M, Vassallo J, Savona-Ventura C, the MGSD-GDM Study Group. Relation of the Mediterranean diet with the incidence of gestational diabetes. Eur J Clin Nutr. 2014;68(1):8–13.
23. Timmermans S, Steegers-Theunissen RP, Vujkovic M, den Breeijen H, Russcher H, Lindemans J, Mackenbach J, Hofman A, Lesaffre EE, Jaddoe VV, Steegers EA. The Mediterranean diet and fetal size parameters: the Generation R Study. Br J Nutr. 2012;108(8):1399–409.
24. Steeegers-Theunissen RPM, Obermann-Borst SA, Kremer D, et al. Periconceptional maternal folic acid use of 400 micrograms per day is related to increased methylation of the IGF2 gene in the very young child. PLoS One. 2009;4:7845.
25. da Silva R, Bach-Faig A, Raido´Quintana B, Genevieve B, Vaz de Almeida MD, Serra-Majem L. Worldwide variation of adherence to the Mediterranean diet, in 1961–1965 and 2000–2003. Public Health Nutr. 2009;12(9A):1676–84.
26. Bonaccio M, Iacoviello L, De Gaetano G, on behalf of the Moli-sani investigators. The Mediterranean diet: the reasons for a success. Thromb Res. 2012;29:401–4.
27. Lundsberg LS, Illuzzi JL, Belanger K, Triche EW, Bracken MB Low-to-moderate prenatal alcohol consumption and the risk of selected birth outcomes: a prospective cohort study. Ann Epidemiol. 2015;25(1):46–54.e3.

28. Wang C, Harris WS, Chung M, et al. n-3 Fatty acids from fish or fish-oil supplements, but not {alpha}- linolenic acid, benefit cardiovascular disease outcomes in primary- and secondary-prevention studies: a systematic review. Am J Clin Nutr. 2006;84:5–17.
29. Mozaffarian D, Rimm EB. Evaluating the risks and the benefits fish intake, contaminants, and human health. JAMA. 2006;296(15):1885–99.
30. Hedlund M, Tangvoranuntakul P, Takematsu H, et al. *N*-Glycolylneuraminic acid deficiency in mice: implications for human biology and evolution. Mol Cell Biol. 2007;27(12):4340–6.

Nutrition Around the Clock and Inflammation: The Right Food at the Right Time Makes the Difference

16

Attilio Speciani

Contents

16.1 Introduction

The metabolic effects of circadian desynchronization, and their apparent promotion of an obese phenotype, often in the absence of increased energy intake, are intriguing findings that underscore the significance of the endogenous timing system in the regulation of metabolism.

This might have even a greater impact in pregnancy, when hormonal and metabolic factors change the metabolic plasticity to adapt to changes in circadian rhythms. The perception of circadian rhythms depends on internal and environmental signaling: light or darkness, available energy from meals or from tissue storage,

A. Speciani, MD
Nutrition Department, SMA Srl – Associated Medical Services, Milan, Lombardia, Italy
e-mail: attilio.speciani@me.com

E. Ferrazzi, B. Sears (eds.), *Metabolic Syndrome and Complications of Pregnancy: The Potential Preventive Role of Nutrition*,
DOI 10.1007/978-3-319-16853-1_16

daily physical activity and adequate night rest, psychological and metabolic stressors such as caffeine, etc. In order to achieve a correct circadian rhythm, both the excess of sleep and its deprivation should be prevented to avoid adverse affect on weight gain during pregnancy. The proper distribution of meals during the day, with a hearty breakfast and a light dinner; a good balance in all meals of complex carbohydrates from veggies, fruit, and cereals and healthy proteins; a proper overnight fasting; all of them are key issues to meet the requirements of circadian rhythms both in terms of metabolism and of interaction of nutrients with intestinal microbiota.

16.2 Pregnancy: A Unique Opportunity to Focus on Healthy Diet for the Whole Family

The Institute of Medicine guidelines for weight gain in pregnancy were initially developed in 1990 to promote adequate gestational weight gain with the goal of preventing premature births and small-for-gestational-age infants [1]. However, with an increasing number of women entering pregnancy who are overweight and obese, the Institute of Medicine guidelines for weight gain in pregnancy were recently updated in 2009 with a shift of focus toward maternal health outcomes and the reduction of postpartum weight retention and childhood adiposity [2].

Pregnancy for a woman, but more generally for the entire family, represents a unique moment in which there is greater attention to the recommendations to improve health through nutrition. This should prompt physicians, gynecologists, and researchers to understand which aspects of everyday life most influence the metabolic response of the organism and to correct them.

The metabolic effects of circadian desynchronization, and their apparent promotion of an obese phenotype, often in the absence of increased energy intake, are intriguing findings that underscore the significance of the endogenous timing system in the

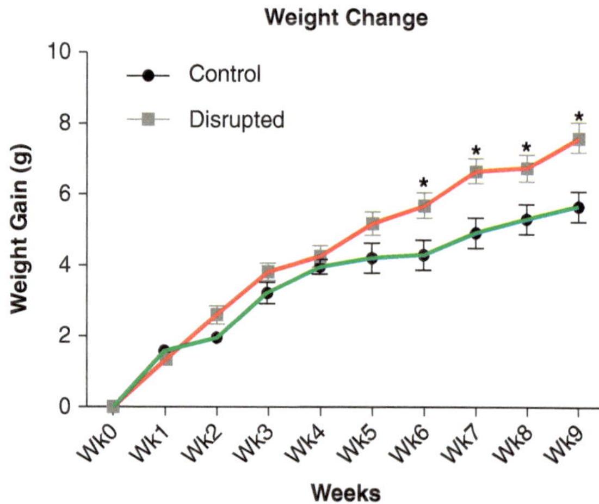

Fig. 16.1 Mice subjected to circadian disruption (CD) show statistically significant weight gain starting at 6 weeks. By the 10th week, CD mice weigh significantly more than mice without circadian disruption (t test, $P = 0.0037$; D), and at the end of the experiment, they show significantly higher plasma leptin and plasma insulin [3]

regulation of metabolism (Fig. 16.1) [3]. It can be hypothesized that the circadian system could be implicated in the effectiveness of weight loss intervention. Indeed, the most important factors of energy homeostasis, including the sleep–wake cycle, thermogenesis, feeding, and glucose, protein, and lipid metabolism, are subjected to time regulation. This circadian rhythm synchronizes energy intake and expenditure with changes in the external environment. Interestingly the reduced response to circadian synchronizing found in low responders to diet intervention is one of the hallmarks of aging. An attenuated amplitude of this response has been observed in elderly subjects as well as in obese and in Alzheimer's patients [4]. This evidence has fostered increasing interest in the notion that metabolic syndrome and obesity are associated with chronodisruption. This is also supported by the fact that obese individuals appear to be less responsive to environmental cues, and diurnal variations in body temperature are diminished in obese humans. Bandin et al. [4] investigated the possible relationship between total weight loss and circadian rhythmicity in order to assess whether it could be a marker of weight loss effectiveness. He found that low diet-responder women had significant alterations of circadian wrist temperature usually measured to monitor physiologic temperature changes during the day.

16.3 Day and Night: Different Signals for Losing Weight

Circadian rhythmicity influences the central regulation of behavior, reproduction, metabolism, and virtually every other physiological parameter. The disruption of the key signal of the circadian pacemaker, environmental light, might explain part of the many of the chronic diseases associated with western lifestyle and social organization. The highly inheritable functional properties of the circadian pacemaker could be at the root of genetic vulnerability to obesity. Epidemiological evidence links human obesity to exposure to electrical light [5] and to circadian desynchronization [6]. Furthermore, genetic evidence supports an association between obesity and variations in the expression of genes induced by time in humans [7]. Taken together, this data supports the concept that human phenotype is driven toward obesity and metabolic dysfunction also through an interaction of circadian desynchronization induced by artificial light and the individual inheritable properties of the circadian pacemaker.

In 2012, Wise and coworkers [8] explained why light is so important in the regulation of circadian rhythm of the human body. He found that latitude lines are significantly related to the properties of circadian pacemaker and can affect individual susceptibility to circadian desynchronization and its metabolic consequences. For example, humans recently migrating north from equatorial zones seem to be more vulnerable to the metabolic effects of circadian desynchronization and susceptibility to obesity when they are exposed to the variable day length of northern latitudes [9]. Furthermore, these migrants are generally considered to be at increased risk of obesity, with individuals of African ancestry particularly susceptible to obesity and metabolic dysfunction as they migrate to the north. An interesting corollary to this argument is the question of whether humans native in northern zones are more compliant to circadian rhythms that make them less vulnerable to the effects of circadian desynchronization.

Additional epidemiological evidence is provided by the reduced susceptibility to metabolic syndrome of Yup'ik Eskimos in spite of westernization and a high prevalence of increased central adiposity [10]. Although these native North American people acquire a more modern American lifestyle, their circadian resilience might protect them against some of the effects of obesity. This data in humans are in agreement with findings in lower animals. As early humans migrated north of the Equator, they encountered photoperiods that were less predictable, with the timing of sunrise and sunset showing daily variation. It is likely that human fitness was optimized by the regular photoperiod at the Equator and that migration into the variability of northern places came at the expense of circadian resonance. But this was most likely a worthwhile trade-off for better climatic conditions, food, or extended territories.

Data on the relationship between sleep–wake cycle in pregnancy and weight gain are conflicting, and Restall et al. [11] find that more than 10 h of night sleep on weekdays are positively correlated with higher gestational weight gain than women who reported sleeping less than 8 h. These results are opposite to the findings by Althuizen, who correlated short nocturnal sleep with increased gestational weight gain [12]. Recently a larger study concluded that sleep deprivation is a risk factor for higher gestational weight gain [13].

16.4 Ruler of Circadian Hormones

One of the possible connections between alteration of the phases of light and metabolism is the production of melatonin. In humans, the melatonin is produced by the pineal gland, a small endocrine gland located in the center of the brain but outside the blood–brain barrier. Production of melatonin is inhibited by light hitting the retina and facilitated by darkness. The melatonin signal forms part of the system that regulates the sleep–wake cycle by chemically causing drowsiness and lowering the body temperature, although it is the central nervous system (specifically the suprachiasmatic nuclei) that controls the daily cycle in most components of the paracrine and endocrine systems rather than the melatonin signal alone. The anti-obesogenic and the weight-reducing effects of melatonin depend on several mechanisms and actions [14]. Experimental evidence demonstrates that melatonin is necessary for the proper synthesis, secretion, and action of insulin [15]. Melatonin is a powerful chronobiotic being partly responsible for the daily distribution of metabolic processes: daytime activity/feeding phase is associated with high insulin sensitivity; nighttime rest/fasting is associated with insulin-resistant metabolic phase of the day [16]. Furthermore, melatonin commands energy flow to and from the stores and energy expenditure through the activation of brown adipose tissue. Table 16.1 summarizes some of the major aspects of melatonin functions [18].

Finally, there is a large body of evidence that melatonin is one of the major scavengers of both oxygen- and nitrogen-based reactive species. The lipophilic nature of melatonin helps indolamine to cross cell membranes to easily reach subcellular compartments, including the mitochondria: melatonin interacts with lipid bilayers and stabilizes mitochondrial inner membranes, which may improve electron transport chain activity, and, consequently ATP production (Fig. 16.2) [19].

Table 16.1 Biochemical effects to explain the anti-obesogenic and the weight-reducing roles of melatonin [14–19]

Biochemical effects of melatonin
Experimental evidence demonstrates that melatonin is necessary for proper synthesis, secretion, and action of insulin. The reduction in melatonin production induces insulin resistance and glucose intolerance
Melatonin is responsible for the establishment of an adequate energy balance mainly by regulating energy flow to and from fat stores
Melatonin may improve electron transport chain activity and, consequently, ATP production
Melatonin is one of the major scavengers of both oxygen- and nitrogen-based reactive species
The complex actions of melatonin on both the metabolic side and the control of oxidative stress go in the direction of explaining how the respect of a proper circadian rhythm with appropriate sleep duration can help to prevent metabolic disorders

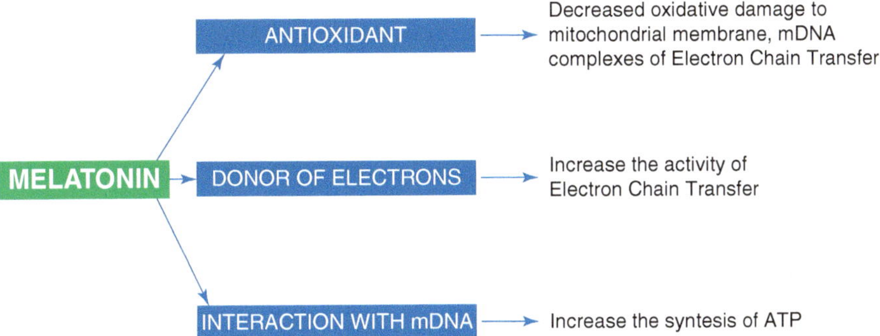

Fig. 16.2 A synoptic view of the roles of melatonin on energy metabolism via mitochondria [19]

The reduction in melatonin production, as during aging, night-working shifts, or illuminated environments, induces insulin resistance, glucose intolerance, sleep disturbance, and metabolic circadian disorganization characterizing a state of chronodisruption leading to obesity. It is evident that the complex actions of melatonin on both the metabolic side and the control of oxidative stress go in the direction of explaining how the respect of a proper circadian rhythm with an appropriate sleep can help prevent metabolic disorders of pregnant women and, consequently, even an excessive weight gain.

16.5 The Importance of a Correct Timing of the Three Daily Meals

Current evidence suggests that the timing of meals can influence metabolic syndrome by affecting circadian rhythms. In particular, there is huge scientific evidence that breakfast is one of the most important daily moments to give a strong signal of metabolic activation to the whole body, in order to stop obesity and ease weight loss. Odegaard et al. described the strategic importance of breakfast in the fight against at least four "wealth diseases" [20]: obesity, metabolic syndrome, hypertension, and diabetes. This study, like many others under different perspectives, found that those subjects having breakfast only occasionally had the tendency to put on weight, while those having breakfast regularly were significantly protected against the abovementioned disorders, showing a very significant loss of weight compared to the controls: almost 2 kg less in those regularly having breakfast compared to the subjects having it only occasionally or never. To comply with a proper circadian rhythm, breakfast should be the most rich meal of the day.

16.6 Breakfast: The Most Important Signal of Richness to Activate Metabolism

After breakfast, caloric intake should be reduced gradually until having a light dinner early in the evening. Also the composition of breakfast has great importance in the regulation of the mechanisms of satiety during the day. An interesting scientific work proposed by Fallaize et al. [21] compared three different types of breakfasts, with equal energy intake, to evaluate its effect on satiety, hunger, and subsequent calorie intake throughout the day. The first proposed breakfast consisted of eggs with toast, the second cereals, milk, and toast, while the third was a croissant and juice. The ones who had eaten eggs in the morning had significantly reduced their energy intake during lunch and dinner, despite having available unlimited amount of food. The first choice, which showed the highest effect on satiety, was characterized by having a higher protein intake and the lowest percentage in carbohydrates. The choices that are made in the morning affect diet throughout the day by modulating feeding behavior. These evidences are totally forgotten by the lifestyle counseling offered by the vast majority of doctors in southern European countries where breakfast is limited to refined carbohydrates, like biscuits, white bread, or sugar disguised in jam, coffee, or tea or even worse is totally skipped but for a cup of coffee.

16.7 Proteins in Every Meal to Stimulate Metabolism and Build Lean Mass

To lose weight properly, every meal has to be combined with the right amount of protein. Mamerow et al. [22] have in fact precisely defined that the amount of protein required during a day must be distributed in a balanced manner among all three meals. The authors of this study examined the effects of protein distribution on skeletal muscle protein synthesis in healthy adult men and women and measured changes in muscle protein synthesis in response to isoenergetic and isonitrogenous diets with protein at breakfast, lunch, and dinner evenly distributed or skewed. The authors of this study proved that the best balance occurs when the amount of protein of the day is distributed evenly within the three meals.

Table 16.2 Molecular and metabolic role of fat-specific protein 27 (FSP27) [23–26]

Molecular role	Metabolic role
FSP27 is a lipid-droplet-associated protein that is expressed in white adipose tissue or in the liver and is a direct mediator of PPAR-dependent hepatic steatosis, which suggests that expression of FSP27 may promote lipid-droplet formation in hepatocytes	Studies on lipid metabolism in the liver and in the white adipose tissue have given more importance to the mechanism of the metabolic adaptation to fasting overnight
FSP27 during adaptation to fasting is highly induced (about 800-fold), mainly in the early period (up to 15 h of fasting). Over longer periods of fasting (24 h), the expression of PPARα target genes remains high, but the expression of FSP27 decreases fourfold with respect to its levels after 15 h of fasting	In the first phase of fasting, the body mobilizes fat reserves to support the metabolic needs of the organism. This process of adaptation to fasting is effective only in the first 15 h. With more prolonged period of caloric restriction, the body changes its strategy, storing fats in liver and white adipose tissue
Another member of the family of proteins linked to FSP27 may be involved in the maturation of VLDL by interacting with apoB-100/-48 suggesting that FSP27 protein could play a role in the accumulation/export of newly synthesized triglyceride in the early steps of fasting adaptation process	The fatty acids from adipose tissue to the liver are reesterified and sent to various tissues through the formation of VLDL

16.8 Eating and Fasting at the Right Time to Activate Metabolism and Fat Consumption

Studies on lipid metabolism in the liver and in the white adipose tissue underline the importance given to fasting overnight. Vilà-Brau et al. [23] studied how the expression of certain molecules deposit of lipids is modified in response to fasting. One of these accumulated liver proteins is the fat-specific protein 27 (FSP27), which belongs to a family of proteins that play critical roles in controlling metabolic homeostasis (Table 16.2) [24, 25]. This data suggest that FSP27 protein could play a role in the accumulation/export of the newly synthesized triglyceride in the early steps of the fasting adaptation process. In the first phase of fasting, the body mobilizes fat reserves to support the metabolic needs of the organism. The fatty acids from adipose tissue to the liver are reesterified and sent to various tissues through the formation of VLDL. This process of adaptation to fasting is effective only in the first 12–15 h. With more prolonged period of caloric restriction, the body changes its strategy, preserving fat reserves in the liver and white adipose tissue. So, proper distribution of meals allows taking advantage of the period of physiological overnight fasting to induce better mobilization and use of fat reserves in excess [26].

16.9 Microbioma and Distribution of Meals During the Day

The distribution of meals during the day also influences the response of the intestinal bacterial flora. At every meal the intestinal flora is modified by the specific composition of the meal, timing of meals, the digestive capacity of the individual, and the bacterial flora already present in the gut. The framework is made extremely complicated by the fact that the gut itself follows an intrinsic homeostatic clock [27]. Alterations of symbiosis between microbiota and intestinal epithelial cells are associated with intestinal and systemic pathologies. Interactions between bacterial products and Toll-like receptors are known to be mandatory for intestinal epithelial cells homeostasis. Mukherji et al. [28] explain how the interactions between the intestinal bacterial flora and intestinal epithelial cells are essential to define a proper circadian rhythm in the intestine. To quote the authors own words “Alterations of symbiosis between microbiota and intestinal epithelial cells (IEC) are associated with intestinal and systemic pathologies. Interactions between bacterial products (MAMPs) and Toll-like receptors (TLRs) are known to be mandatory for IEC homeostasis, but how TLRs may time homeostatic functions with circadian changes is unknown. Interestingly, microbiota signaling deficiencies induce a prediabetic syndrome due to ileal corticosterone overproduction consequent to clock disruption.” According to this seminal paper, gut inflammation depends not only on the type of food usually eaten, but also on the circadian dietary habits chosen. These can definitely make the difference between those who gain weight without knowing why and those, instead, who can eat without getting fat. For a few years now, it has become clearer that a low-grade inflammatory state promoted by abnormal relationship between the intestinal microbiota and the gastroenteric immune cells may lead to insulin resistance. An interesting study analyzed the differences in gut microbioma sometimes found in identical twins, one of which is lean while the other one fat despite following the same diet. Ridaura et al. [29] showed that by transferring gut bacteria from a fat mouse into a germ-free mouse, the latter starts to put on weight; instead, if gut bacteria from a lean mouse are also transferred together with those from the fat one, the balancing effect given by the lean mouse microbes is sufficient to stop weight gain. Alterations in the gastrointestinal microbiota have been implicated in obesity in mice and humans, and the key microbial functions influencing host energy metabolism and adiposity is mediated by a microbe–host dialogue that functionally regulates host lipid metabolism and plays a profound role in cholesterol metabolism and weight gain in the host [30].

References

1. Institute of Medicine (US) Committee on Nutritional Status During Pregnancy and Lactation. Nutrition during pregnancy: part I weight gain: part II nutrient supplements. Washington DC: National Academies Press (US); 1990.
2. Institute of Medicine (US) and National Research Council (US) Committee to Reexamine IOM Pregnancy Weight Guidelines, Rasmussen KM, Yaktine AL. Weight gain during pregnancy: reexamining the guidelines. Washington DC: National Academies Press (US); 2009.
3. Karatsoreos IN, Bhagat S, Bloss EB, et al. Disruption of circadian clocks has ramifications for metabolism, brain, and behavior. Proc Natl Acad Sci U S A. 2011;108:1657–62. doi:10.1073/pnas.1018375108.
4. Bandín C, Martinez-Nicolas A, Ordovas JM, et al. Circadian rhythmicity as a predictor of weight-loss effectiveness. Int J Obes. 2014;38:1083–8. doi:10.1038/ijo.2013.211.
5. Wyse CA, Selman C, Page MM, et al. Circadian desynchrony and metabolic dysfunction; did light pollution make us fat? Med Hypotheses. 2011;77:1139–44. doi:10.1016/j.mehy.2011.09.023.

6. Suwazono Y, Dochi M, Sakata K, et al. A longitudinal study on the effect of shift work on weight gain in male Japanese workers. Obesity (Silver Spring). 2008;16:1887–93. doi:10.1038/oby.2008.298.
7. Garaulet M, Corbalán-Tutau MD, Madrid JA, et al. PERIOD2 variants are associated with abdominal obesity, psycho-behavioral factors, and attrition in the dietary treatment of obesity. J Am Diet Assoc. 2010;110:917–21. doi:10.1016/j.jada.2010.03.017.
8. Wyse CA. Does human evolution in different latitudes influence susceptibility to obesity via the circadian pacemaker?: migration and survival of the fittest in the modern age of lifestyle-induced circadian desynchrony. Bioessays. 2012;34:921–4. doi:10.1002/bies.201200067.
9. Luke A, Guo X, Adeyemo AA, et al. Heritability of obesity-related traits among Nigerians, Jamaicans and US black people. Int J Obes Relat Metab Disord. 2001;25:1034–41. doi:10.1038/sj.ijo.0801650.
10. Boyer BB, Mohatt GV, Plaetke R, et al. Metabolic syndrome in Yup'ik Eskimos: the Center for Alaska Native Health Research (CANHR) Study. Obesity (Silver Spring). 2007;15:2535–40. doi:10.1038/oby.2007.302.
11. Restall A, Taylor RS, Thompson JMD, et al. Risk factors for excessive gestational weight gain in a healthy, nulliparous cohort. J Obes. 2014;2014:148391. doi:10.1155/2014/148391.
12. Althuizen E, van Poppel MNM, Seidell JC, van Mechelen W. Correlates of absolute and excessive weight gain during pregnancy. J Womens Health (Larchmt). 2009;18:1559–66. doi:10.1089/jwh.2008.1275.
13. Abeysena C, Jayawardana P. Sleep deprivation, physical activity and low income are risk factors for inadequate weight gain during pregnancy: a cohort study. J Obstet Gynaecol Res. 2011;37:734–40. doi:10.1111/j.1447-0756.2010.01421.x.
14. Cipolla-Neto J, Amaral FG, Afeche SC, et al. Melatonin, energy metabolism, and obesity: a review. J Pineal Res. 2014;56:371–81. doi:10.1111/jpi.12137.
15. Shi S-Q, Ansari TS, McGuinness OP, et al. Circadian disruption leads to insulin resistance and obesity. Curr Biol. 2013;23:372–81. doi:10.1016/j.cub.2013.01.048.
16. Wolden-Hanson T, Mitton DR, McCants RL, et al. Daily melatonin administration to middle-aged male rats suppresses body weight, intra-abdominal adiposity, and plasma leptin and insulin independent of food intake and total body fat. Endocrinology. 2000;141:487–97. doi:10.1210/endo.141.2.7311.
17. Stanford KI, Middelbeek RJW, Townsend KL, et al. Brown adipose tissue regulates glucose homeostasis and insulin sensitivity. J Clin Invest. 2013;123:215–23. doi:10.1172/JCI62308.
18. Cazzola R, Rondanelli M, Faliva M, Cestaro B. Effects of DHA-phospholipids, melatonin and tryptophan supplementation on erythrocyte membrane physico-chemical properties in elderly patients suffering from mild cognitive impairment. Exp Gerontol. 2012;47:974–8. doi:10.1016/j.exger.2012.09.004.
19. Leon J, Acuña-Castroviejo D, Sainz RM, et al. Melatonin and mitochondrial function. Life Sci. 2004;75:765–90. doi:10.1016/j.lfs.2004.03.003.
20. Odegaard AO, Jacobs DR, Steffen LM, et al. Breakfast frequency and development of metabolic risk. Diabetes Care. 2013;36:3100–6. doi:10.2337/dc13-0316.
21. Fallaize R, Wilson L, Gray J, et al. Variation in the effects of three different breakfast meals on subjective satiety and subsequent intake of energy at lunch and evening meal. Eur J Nutr. 2013;52:1353–9. doi:10.1007/s00394-012-0444-z.
22. Mamerow MM, Mettler JA, English KL, et al. Dietary protein distribution positively influences 24-h muscle protein synthesis in healthy adults. J Nutr. 2014;144:876–80. doi:10.3945/jn.113.185280.
23. Vilà-Brau A, De Sousa-Coelho AL, Gonçalves JF, et al. Fsp27/CIDEC is a CREB target gene induced during early fasting in liver and regulated by FA oxidation rate. J Lipid Res. 2013;54:592–601. doi:10.1194/jlr.M028472.
24. Jensen MD, Ekberg K, Landau BR. Lipid metabolism during fasting. Am J Physiol Endocrinol Metab. 2001;281:E789–93.
25. Ye J, Li JZ, Liu Y, et al. Cideb, an ER- and lipid droplet-associated protein, mediates VLDL lipidation and maturation by interacting with apolipoprotein B. Cell Metab. 2009;9:177–90. doi:10.1016/j.cmet.2008.12.013.

26. Speciani AF, Necchi M, Speciani MC. Colazione e brunch per il benessere. Milan: LSWR; 2014.
27. Moore SR, Pruszka J, Vallance J, et al. Robust circadian rhythms in organoid cultures from PERIOD2: LUCIFERASE mouse small intestine. Dis Model Mech. 2014;7:1123–30. doi:10.1242/dmm.014399.
28. Mukherji A, Kobiita A, Ye T, Chambon P. Homeostasis in intestinal epithelium is orchestrated by the circadian clock and microbiota cues transduced by TLRs. Cell. 2013;153:812–27. doi:10.1016/j.cell.2013.04.020.
29. Ridaura VK, Faith JJ, Rey FE, et al. Gut microbiota from twins discordant for obesity modulate metabolism in mice. Science. 2013;341:1241214. doi:10.1126/science.1241214.
30. Joyce SA, MacSharry J, Casey PG, et al. Regulation of host weight gain and lipid metabolism by bacterial bile acid modification in the gut. Proc Natl Acad Sci USA. 2014;111:7421–6. doi:10.1073/pnas.1323599111.